Master

gy

Commissioning Editor: Timothy Horne
Development Editor: Barbara Simmons
Project Manager: Emma Riley
Designer: Stewart Larking
Illustration Manager: Bruce Hogarth

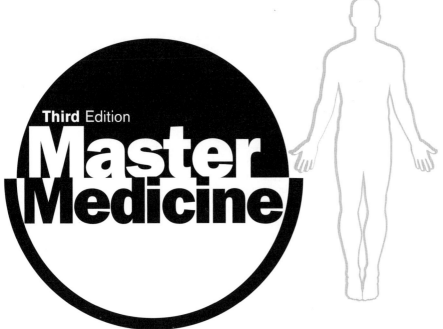

Third Edition

Master Medicine

Medical Pharmacology

A clinical core text for integrated curricula with self-assessment

SIMON CONSTABLE
BSc MRCP(UK) PGCert (LTHE)
Lecturer in Clinical Pharmacology
University of Liverpool;
Honorary Specialist Registrar
Royal Liverpool University Hospital

PETER WINSTANLEY
MD FRCP DTM&H
Professor of Clinical Pharmacology
University of Liverpool;
Honorary Consultant Physician
Royal Liverpool University Hospital

TOM WALLEY
MD FRCP FRCPI
Professor of Clinical Pharmacology
University of Liverpool;
Honorary Consultant Physician
Royal Liverpool University Hospital

CHURCHILL LIVINGSTONE

ELSEVIER

Edinburgh London New York Oxford Philadelphia St Louis Sydney Toronto 2007

CHURCHILL
LIVINGSTONE
ELSEVIER

An imprint of Elsevier Limited

© Pearson Professional Limited 1996
© 2002, Elsevier Limited. All rights reserved.
© 2007, Elsevier Limited. All rights reserved.

First edition 1996
Second edition 2002
Third edition 2007

ISBN: 978-0-443-10291-2

British Library Cataloguing in Publication Data
A catalogue record for this book is available from the British Library

Library of Congress Cataloging in Publication Data
A catalog record for this book is available from the Library of Congress

Note
Knowledge and best practice in this field are constantly changing. As new research and experience broaden our knowledge, changes in practice, treatment and drug therapy may become necessary or appropriate. Readers are advised to check the most current information provided (i) on procedures featured or (ii) by the manufacturer of each product to be administered, to verify the recommended dose or formula, the method and duration of administration, and contraindications. It is the responsibility of the practitioner, relying on their own experience and knowledge of the patient, to make diagnoses, to determine dosages and the best treatment for each individual patient, and to take all appropriate safety precautions. To the fullest extent of the law, neither the Publisher nor the Authors assumes any liability for any injury and/or damage to persons or property arising out of or related to any use of the material contained in this book.

The Publisher

ELSEVIER   your source for books,
journals and multimedia
in the health sciences

www.elsevierhealth.com

The
publisher's
policy is to use
paper manufactured
from sustainable forests

Working together to grow
libraries in developing countries

www.elsevier.com | www.bookaid.org | www.sabre.org

ELSEVIER   BOOK AID   Sabre Foundation
International

Printed in China

Contents

Using this book **1**

1   **Basic principles** **3**
2   **The autonomic nervous system** **21**
3   **Drugs in cardiovascular disease 1: prevention** **33**
4   **Drugs in cardiovascular disease 2: treatment** **51**
5   **Drugs and the blood** **71**
6   **Drugs used in CNS disease** **85**
7   **Analgesics** **107**
8   **Drugs used in anaesthesia** **115**
9   **Drugs for arthritis** **125**
10 **Respiratory disorders and hypersensitivity** **135**
11 **Drugs and the gastrointestinal system** **149**
12 **Drugs for endocrine and metabolic disorders** **165**
13 **Antibiotics (antimicrobials)** **191**
14 **Chemotherapy for fungi, viruses and protozoa** **211**
15 **Anticancer chemotherapy** **223**
16 **Drugs and the skin** **233**
17 **Drug overdose and poisoning** **241**
18 **Substance dependency and abuse** **251**
19 **Drugs in pregnancy, breastfeeding, children and the elderly** **263**
20 **Effects of disease state on drug response** **273**
21 **Adverse drug reactions and drug interactions** **283**
22 **New drugs and clinical trials** **293**

Index **303**

Using this book

Philosophy of the book

What drugs are used for hypertension? How do they work? What adverse effects do they have, and who should *not* receive them? This book will help you with these, and similar, questions with the general aims of both passing the examination and retaining an understanding of pharmacology for your future career.

Drugs have always been, and remain, one of the main ways of treating and preventing disease. Broadly, the discipline of *pharmacology* is concerned with how drugs work and how they reach their site of action, while *therapeutics* is concerned with their clinical use. Most doctors have expertise in therapeutics – they use it every day of practice. However, although detailed expertise in pharmacology is not needed by all doctors, most retain a degree of 'background knowledge' which renders their therapeutic use of drugs more rational.

Your aim should be to develop an understanding of the principles which govern the clinical use of drugs.

Layout of the book

This book is organised along clinical rather than strictly pharmacological lines to render it more accessible to medical students. Consequently the chapters focus on anatomical systems (e.g. the cardiovascular system) or the therapy of specific diseases (e.g. cancer chemotherapy) rather than on mechanisms of drug action. In each chapter we have tried to set out mechanisms and principles, rather than lists, and have tried to link together sections of the book where the same topic is dealt with from different angles.

The chapters are subdivided into sections, each dealing with a therapeutic area (the cardiovascular chapter, for example, includes sections on hypertension, angina and arrhythmias), and we have tried to construct these in a reasonably uniform way. Each section includes a brief description of the clinical context: there would be little point learning about antiepileptic drugs, for example, if you did not understand the nature of epilepsy. Many diverse drugs may be relevant to the therapy used to treat the same condition: we have grouped similar drugs under the same class heading (e.g. the benzodiazepines). For most drug classes we describe:

- mode of action: at the molecular, cellular, organ and whole-body levels where relevant
- examples and clinical pharmacokinetics: there are usually several drugs of each class in common use; we describe the commoner examples and contrast their pharmacokinetic properties
- therapeutic uses: a drug class can be used for several indications (e.g. although beta-blockers are described in the ischaemic heart disease section of Chapter 3, they are also used for hypertension, anxiety and migraine)
- adverse effects: are described in detail under subheadings and, because some subgroups of the population are at particular risk from certain drugs (e.g. beta-blockers precipitate asthma), these *contraindications* are listed
- interactions: patients often take more than one drug at a time: potential adverse interactions, and their clinical consequences, are described.

The final section of each chapter allows self-assessment; we have tried to set questions that require thought rather than recollection of facts. Self-assessment is in the form of case histories (which require short answers), traditional multiple choice questions, 'extended matching items' questions and some essays. The answers are given along with a detailed explanation in each case. Some aspects of a topic may be covered for the first time in this section of the book.

Approach to examinations

There is no correct way to revise for an examination and by this stage in your career you have already passed many, so your own system cannot be too bad. However, your performance may be improved by reading the brief notes below.

Before starting to prepare for the examination, you need to know:

- the scope of the syllabus in your medical school (these vary quite widely); consult the list of lectures/tutorials given, or the study guides presented at the start of the course
- the format of the examination (consult past papers if you can)
- how many examinations you will be sitting at once (your revision plan will need to divide time between subjects).

The *notes* you made during lectures, tutorials or group sessions are probably the ideal revision material; the subject was described by, or your reading was guided by, those who set the exam, and reading your notes should stimulate your memory. Large *textbooks of clinical pharmacology* are useful as a reference source during revision, as they were during the course, but you should not try to read them from cover to cover. Furthermore, it is probably unwise to buy more than one reference text; different books may cover the same topic in differing ways, causing confusion. Condensed 'crammers' which rely heavily on lists are probably best avoided: they encourage retention of facts rather than understanding and, on the whole, pharmacology does not lend itself to lists. The present book covers most, though not all, of the topics likely to crop up in undergraduate examinations, and can be used to complement your own notes.

Tips on methods of examination

Multiple choice questions (MCQs)

For the most part, these test your recall of facts. Read the stem of the question with care, paying attention to words such as *only, rarely, usually, never* and *always*.

The most common forms of MCQs involve *either* choosing the most appropriate answer from a list (usually one out of five) *or* answering true/false to each part of the question.

Remember to check the marking system – many MCQ exams employ negative marking.

Short notes

The examiners will have decided on a marking system for each important fact. You should set out your knowledge in a concise manner – no marks will be gained for superfluous information.

Case histories

This type of question may be designed to test both recall of factual knowledge and its application to a clinical therapeutic problem. Formats vary, but a common form is an evolving case history, with information being presented sequentially and responses to specific questions (e.g. on choice of drug or anticipated adverse effects). As with '*Short notes*' you should aim to be concise.

Extended matching items questions

In these questions you must choose the option from the list provided that best fits the given statement or question. This type of question, not normally associated with negative marking, is used in United States licensing examinations and similar examinations for other bodies, and is also used by several undergraduate schools. These questions can easily be adapted to fit multidisciplinary ('integrated') assessments.

Basic principles

1.1	**Pharmacokinetics**	**3**
1.2	**Pharmacokinetic parameters**	**8**
1.3	**Pharmacodynamics**	**10**
	Self-assessment on Chapter 1: questions	**15**
	Self-assessment on Chapter 1: answers	**18**

Overview

A drug can be taken to mean any molecule or compound used to alter body functions to prevent or treat disease. Although a drug generally produces the same *type* of effect in different people, there can be wide variation in the *degree* of that effect. The factors underlying such interindividual variation in drug response have obvious clinical importance and are the main theme of this chapter. *Pharmacokinetics* is the description of processes affecting the amount of a drug reaching its target location (e.g. rates of absorption and distribution) and its ultimate fate (e.g. metabolism and excretion) – the effect of the body on the drug. *Pharmacodynamics* describes the physiological and biochemical effects of drugs in the whole animal and at the tissue and molecular level – the effect of the drug on the body. Most drugs exert their effects by interacting with macromolecular 'targets', which may be receptors, enzymes or structural proteins.

- appreciate that most drugs are partially bound to plasma proteins but it is the unbound drug fraction that is active
- be aware of the influence of disease on plasma protein binding
- appreciate that biotransformation usually converts drugs into inactive water-soluble compounds for elimination in urine or bile
- be aware that biotransformation is very prone to interindividual variation (caused by genetic and environmental factors)
- know that drugs can be excreted in bile and by the kidneys.

Clinical response to a drug can sometimes be directly measured with accuracy, like the effect of insulin on blood sugar or warfarin on clotting, and this measurement alone can be enough to predict *how much* drug is needed and *how often*. More usually, however, such direct measurements are impossible and an indirect approach (using drug concentrations and their rates of change) can be used to predict the magnitude and duration of action of a drug. Variation in drug concentration and their rates of change (because of differences in *absorption*, *distribution*, *metabolism* or *excretion*) is the other major cause of interindividual variability in drug response: the underlying concepts are termed *pharmacokinetics*.

1.1 Pharmacokinetics

Learning objectives

At the end of this section you should:
- appreciate that most drugs act systemically and need to be absorbed; a proportion of a topical drug may also be absorbed
- be able to describe the Henderson–Hasselbach equation and follow its relevance to drug disposition

Clinical sketch

A man with angina pectoris has not understood instructions on the use of glyceryl trinitrate tablets. He swallows them instead of putting them under his tongue. There is no therapeutic benefit.

Comment: this drug is subject to extensive first-pass metabolism.

Absorption

Most drugs require absorption for activity. Topical drugs may also be absorbed, giving rise to unwanted effects.

Factors affecting the rate and degree of absorption

Lipid solubility

Drugs must cross lipid cell membranes in order to be absorbed. The lipid solubility of a drug is largely determined by factors such as molecular weight and structure. However, lipid solubility of an individual drug is variable: only the *unionised* fraction of the drug is lipid soluble. Most drugs are weak acids or bases, and their degree of ionisation is determined by the surrounding pH and their pK_a (the pK_a is the pH at which the drug is 50% ionised). The Henderson–Hasselbach equation allows the unionised fraction to be calculated:

for acids: $pH = pK_a + \log$ (ionised conc./ unionised conc.)

for bases: $pH = pK_a + \log$ (unionised conc./ ionised conc.)

Thus, weak bases are predictably better absorbed from the small bowel. Weak acids might be expected to be absorbed from the stomach, but factors such as surface area influence this.

Surface area

The greater the surface area, the faster absorption takes place. The surface area of the small bowel exceeds that of the stomach to such a degree that even acidic drugs will usually be more extensively absorbed from this site. So if given orally, the rate of absorption of most drugs is greatly influenced by the rate of gastric emptying. Small bowel surface area can be reduced by diseases.

Other factors

The drug must spend an adequate time at the absorption site. Short transit time (e.g. during gastroenteritis) may reduce the degree of absorption. Blood flow is another important factor. For example, in severe hypotension, blood flow to muscle may be low and intramuscular (i.m.) drugs may be absorbed slowly.

Bioavailability

Bioavailability refers to the fraction of the dose which proceeds *unaltered* from the site of administration to the systemic circulation. When a drug is given intravenously (i.v.), 100% of the dose enters the systemic circulation, and bioavailability is 1.0. While incomplete absorption often accounts for low bioavailability, there are other possible explanations (Fig. 1):

- it may be broken down by acid conditions in the gut, e.g. benzylpenicillin
- it may be metabolised by enzymes in the gut wall or liver before reaching the systemic venous blood (e.g. glyceryl trinitrate). This is termed the first pass effect.

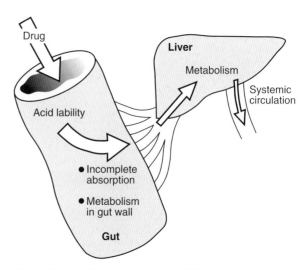

Fig. 1 Causes of incomplete bioavailability.

Distribution

Clinical sketch

A man takes phenytoin for his epilepsy. Unknown to him, his plasma albumin falls markedly over the next few weeks, without the dose of phenytoin being changed. He develops marked ataxia.

Comment: the clinical relevance of plasma protein binding is often much less clear cut than in this example. Here, the patient's ataxia has resulted from an increase in the free concentration of phenytoin.

Clinical sketch

A patient with meningitis is treated with gentamicin. The organism is very sensitive to the antibiotic in vitro, but the patient shows no improvement.

Comment: this would be very unacceptable clinical practice and the patient might well die. Gentamicin does not readily cross the blood–brain barrier.

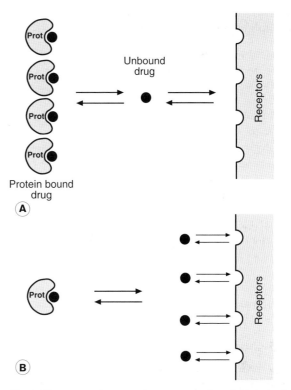

Fig. 2 Variation in plasma protein concentration. **A**. High levels of plasma proteins; **B**. reduced levels of plasma proteins.

Plasma protein binding

Most drugs travel in the plasma partly in solution in the plasma water and partly bound to plasma proteins – the ratio of one to the other varies between drugs. Binding is reversible and the bound and unbound drug fractions are always in a state of dynamic equilibrium. Only the *unbound* drug fraction is available to cross membranes and produce an effect. Acidic drugs mainly bind to albumin, while basic drugs bind more avidly to α_1-acid glycoprotein. Plasma protein binding can be clinically important when, because of a disease state (see Ch. 20), plasma protein concentrations fall (e.g. albumin concentrations in liver cirrhosis) or rise (e.g. α_1-acid glycoprotein in acute infection) (Fig. 2). Warfarin and diazepam are examples of drugs extensively bound to proteins (90% or more). Examples of drugs with less extensive protein binding include digoxin and gentamicin.

Tissue distribution

Most drugs have their effects in the tissues. The degree to which a given drug is likely to accumulate in a tissue can be predicted (without accuracy) from knowledge of its lipophilicity and the blood flow of the tissue. A highly lipophilic drug crosses membranes readily even in the presence of tight junctions between endothelial cells (e.g. into the central nervous system (CNS)); the principal determinant of tissue distribution is organ blood flow. For example, the anaesthetic thiopental is highly lipophilic and accumulates to a greater degree in brain than in muscle because of the much higher blood flow to the former. In contrast, a hydrophilic drug (such as gentamicin) crosses membranes poorly. The principal determinant of tissue distribution will, therefore, be the degree of 'leakiness' of the capillary endothelium. For example, gentamicin accumulates to a greater degree in muscle than in brain because of the leaky nature of muscle capillaries.

Metabolism

Clinical sketch

The risk of drug toxicity from isoniazid (used for tuberculosis) is higher in Egyptians than in Eskimo (Inuit and Yupik) populations.

Comment: there is a genetic polymorphism in the metabolism of isoniazid: Egyptians are likely to metabolise it slowly (and are called 'slow acetylators' or 'poor metabolisers'), while Eskimos usually metabolise it rapidly (and are called 'fast acetylators' or 'extensive metabolisers'). This is one of the first recognised examples of pharmacogenetics – the study of genetic variability in drug metabolism.

Most metabolism (biotransformation) takes place in the liver (other sites include the gut wall (e.g. contraceptive steroids) and plasma (succinylcholine)). The chemical processes involved are numerous and are broadly classified into phase I and phase II reactions, which (confusingly) does not mean that phase I necessarily precedes or is followed by phase II. Phase I processes include oxidation, reduction and hydrolysis. Of these, oxidation reactions are most common and are often catalysed by one of the family of cytochrome P450 enzymes (CYP450). Phase I usually results in:

- introduction or exposure of a polar group
- increased water solubility
- abolition of pharmacological activity.

However, this is not invariable: the phase I products of some drugs have pharmacological activity while the parent compound does not (the so-called prodrugs, e.g. enalapril, see Ch. 3) while in other cases the phase I products are highly toxic, for example in paracetamol poisoning (see Ch. 17). Phase II processes (often termed conjugation) involve the attachment to the drug of an endogenous substance, such as glucuronide, sulphate or acetyl groups. The result-ing conjugate is almost invariably polar, water soluble and without pharmacological activity (morphine is an exception, see Ch. 7).

Variation in biotransformation

Genetic factors (genetic polymorphisms)

Genetic differences have profound effects on the levels of certain drugs in the body. For instance, several drugs are eliminated by acetylation (e.g. isoniazid (Ch. 13), procainamide (Ch. 3) and hydralazine (Ch. 3)). 'Slow acetylators' are at risk of toxicity from these drugs. The proportions of fast and slow acetylators vary between ethnic groups. Other genetically determined variations include poor metabolisers of the muscle relaxant succinylcholine (Ch. 8). An increasing amount is being understood about the effect of polymorphisms in the genes encoding the drug-metabolising CYP450 isoenzymes.

Induction and inhibition of cytochrome P450 enzymes

Some drugs can increase the rate of synthesis of cytochrome P450 enzymes and this enzyme induction can enhance the clearance of other drugs. Usually such induction requires exposure to the inducing agent for over a week before effects are seen. Examples of inducing agents are:

- rifampicin
- carbamazepine
- phenobarbital
- phenytoin.

Other drugs can inhibit cytochrome P450 enzymes (usually by competing for the enzyme's active site). This is usually seen rapidly after drug exposure (within a couple of days). Examples of enzyme-inhibiting agents are:

- cimetidine
- erythromycin
- ciprofloxacin
- isoniazid.

Concentration-dependent biotransformation

Most drugs are metabolised by concentration-independent mechanisms: in other words there is always excess enzyme 'capacity' irrespective of drug concentration. Consequently, the proportion of drug metabolised in a set time is constant. However, some drugs can saturate a rate-limiting enzyme within the therapeutic range. Under these circumstances (sometimes called zero order processes) the proportion of drug metabolised in a set time diminishes as its concentration rises. A good clinical example of this is the antiepileptic drug phenytoin (Ch. 6).

Disease-induced factors

Diseases affecting the liver are particularly important in drug metabolism: for example, the metabolism of opiates is slower in patients with liver disease (see Ch. 20).

Excretion

Some drugs (e.g. aminoglycosides, atenolol, gliclazide and digoxin) are mainly excreted without metabolism; renal disease will cause such drugs to accumulate. Most drug metabolites are inactive; hence biotransformation is the vital step in terminating drug action. If, however, metabolites are active (e.g. the principal metabolite of diazepam), drug action may only be terminated by excretion.

Clinical sketch

A patient with congestive cardiac failure is being treated with loop diuretics. She has severely impaired renal function. The diuresis obtained by enormous doses of furosemide is modest.

Comment: we tend to think of renal excretion as a terminator of drug action. In the case of the loop diuretics, the drug works on ion transporters in the luminal membrane. Therefore, drug action correlates with glomerular filtration rate, and furosemide tends to work poorly in patients with renal failure.

Clinical sketch

A patient is given digoxin for atrial fibrillation. He has impaired renal function. No measurements of digoxin concentration are made, and the patient develops complete heart block.

Comment: digoxin is eliminated unchanged, and accumulates in renal impairment. Extreme caution under these circumstances is necessary including the use of therapeutic drug monitoring. This patient has developed a serious, potentially life-threatening toxicity – but this is predictable based on the known pharmacology of digoxin.

Renal excretion

Glomerular filtration

Renal blood flow is about 1.5 L/min, and about 10% of this, by volume, appears as glomerular filtrate. Only unbound drug may be filtered since protein molecules are too large.

Tubular secretion

Cells of the proximal convoluted tubule can actively secrete some compounds, mostly relatively strong acids and bases, into the lumen of the nephron (e.g. penicillin). Under these circumstances and assuming that no reabsorption occurs, the rate of excretion of a drug exceeds its rate of filtration.

Tubular reabsorption

Active reabsorption has evolved to help to conserve nutrients. Certain drugs too may be extensively reabsorbed: such compounds tend to be lipid soluble and unionised at urine pH (see the Henderson–Hasselbach equation on p. 4). This is of most importance in drug poisoning. For example, in aspirin overdose:

- aspirin is an acid with a pK_a of 3.5
- if the urinary pH is 2.5 then the ratio of ionised : unionised drug is 0.1 (antilog of −1), i.e. 90% of the drug is unionised, it crosses membranes readily and will be reabsorbed
- if the urine pH were 5.5 then the same ratio would be 100 (antilog of 2), i.e. only 1% of the drug is unionised and it crosses membranes poorly.

Other routes of excretion

Biliary

Parent drugs and metabolites with molecular weights greater than 350 may be actively excreted into the bile; examples include many drug conjugates (products of phase II metabolism). This process may be followed by loss of the drug in the faeces. However, drug conjugates may be broken down by gut bacteria, releasing the parent drug, which may be reabsorbed. The resulting enterohepatic circulation may have important clinical consequences, for example with oral contraceptive steroids.

One

Clinical sketch

A young female patient is taking the oral contraceptive pill. She is given a short-course of the broad spectrum antibiotic doxycycline for a sexually transmitted infection. She is advised by the doctor at the genitourinary clinic to use condoms as well as the pill for the duration of the antibiotic treatment as well as for 7 days after stopping.

Comment: broad spectrum antibiotics may reduce the efficacy of oestrogen-containing contraceptive pills because they may kill the normal gut bacterial flora responsible for the recycling of oestrogen from the large bowel. There will hence be reduced enterohepatic circulation, less systemic exposure to oestrogen, potentially leading to ovulation and a failure of contraception. This is only a short-term problem. The use of condoms would also seem sensible if the patient is to avoid transmission of this infection to her partner(s).

Minor routes

Drugs may be excreted in saliva, sweat, tears and expired air, but none of these is a major route. Lactating mothers excrete some drugs in breast milk, with potentially important consequences for the breast-fed infant.

1.2 Pharmacokinetic parameters

Learning objectives

At the end of this section you should:
- be able to describe the phases of the concentration versus time curves of a drug after oral administration
- appreciate that, to make useful clinical predictions, drug disposition must be 'reduced' to numerical parameters, such as half-life, clearance and apparent volume of distribution
- be aware that pharmacokinetic parameters allow predictions to be made regarding the duration of drug action and the effects of disease states, interindividual variation and other drugs on drug disposition.

Clinical sketch

A patient with moderately severe renal failure needs gentamicin for septicaemia. The clinical team consults Appendix 3 of the BNF and is advised to give the drug at reduced dose and longer dose interval.

Comment: gentamicin is eliminated by the kidney and its half-life is longer in patients with renal failure.

Clinical sketch

A patient is admitted after a large overdose of amitriptyline. The clinical team consults the local poisons unit and is told that haemodialysis would not contribute to management.

Comment: amitriptyline has a large volume of distribution (around 18 L/kg). This indicates that most of the drug is in the tissues. Therefore, only a small proportion of the drug in the body would pass through the haemodialysis machine.

Pharmacokinetics allows predictions to be made regarding the activity of a drug in the body; to be useful, these predictions must be reduced to numerical parameters such as half-life, clearance and volume of distribution (VD).

Half-life

Half-life is the easiest pharmacokinetic parameter to envisage and is the time taken for concentration to fall to half its original value; the unit of measurement is hours. Drug concentration data are usually plotted against time, as illustrated in Figure 3. When concentration data are plotted arithmetically (Fig. 3A), an exponential curve results, and the data are often easier to handle if the vertical scale is logarithmic (Fig. 3B). Half-life is the main determinant of dose frequency (Fig. 4). A drug achieves 50% of its steady-state concentration after one half-life, 75% after two half-lives, 88% after three, 94% after four and 97% after five half-lives. So, for example, for a drug with a half-life of 6 hours, with regular dosing, steady-state concentrations should be achieved after approximately 30 hours.

Area under the curve

The area under the curve (AUC) refers to the area under a concentration versus time curve for a drug and is used in the calculation of most other parameters. In Figure 5, which represents data obtained after an oral dose, AUC can be calculated from the time of dosing to the last data point by summation of the trapezoids. Extrapolation of the elimination phase (the dotted line in Fig. 5A) allows calculation of the AUC to infinity; the unit of measurement is of the form grams per litre per hour (g/L per h).

Clearance

For the majority of drugs the rate of elimination E is directly proportional to the drug concentration c. In other words: $E = kc$, where k is a constant. This constant is termed clearance (C) and can be envisaged

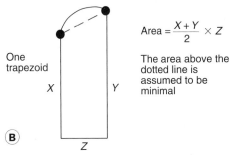

Fig. 5 Calculation of the area under the curve (AUC) from summation of trapezoids. **A**. Data from multiple oral doses. **B**. One trapezoid.

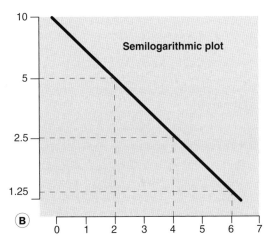

Fig. 3 The half-life of a drug. **A**. Arithmetic plot. **B**. Semilogarithmic plot.

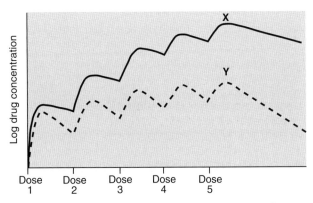

Fig. 4 Two drugs given at the same interval. The half-life of drug X is half that of drug Y. Drug X therefore accumulates to a greater degree.

as the *volume* of plasma that is 'cleared' completely of the drug per unit time; the unit of measurement is, therefore, of the form litres per hour (L/h).

Apparent volume of distribution

Once in the tissue, most drugs bind to macromolecules: some of this binding mediates drug action, while other binding is 'inert'. Some drugs, like aspirin, mainly stay in the circulation and undergo little tissue binding whereas others, like the tricyclic antidepressants, are so extensively bound in the tissues (mostly in an 'inert' manner) that plasma concentrations are small. Figure 6 shows the effect of tissue binding on the plasma concentration of the drug and on its VD. VD is calculated from the amount of drug in the body, divided by the plasma concentration. Where drugs have minimal tissue binding (Fig. 6A) the VD is close to the plasma volume. Where tissue binding is high, the apparent VD is high, 300 litres in Figure 6B. In the real world, we never know precisely how much drug is in the tissues of a living subject – it cannot be measured – but VD gives an *indirect* measure of the degree of tissue distribution. The units of measurement are those of volume (millilitre or litre) and are often adjusted for body weight. VD values range from

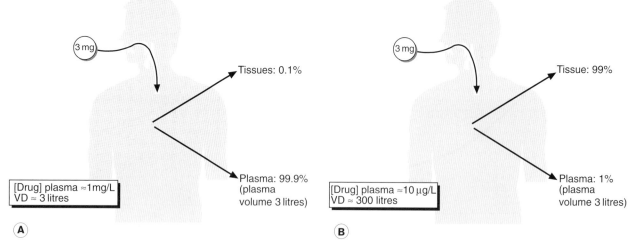

Fig. 6 Apparent volume of distribution (VD). **A**. A drug that is minimally tissue bound would have, for example, 0.1% in the tissues and 99.9% left in the plasma; for a 3 mg dose, this would leave 2.997 mg in the plasma. In a 70 kg adult with a plasma volume of 3 litres, the plasma concentration would be 0.999 mg/L. VD is the drug in the body divided by that in the plasma, i.e. 3 ÷ 0.999 = 3.003l. This is roughly equal to the plasma volume. **B**. An extremely tissue-bound drug might have 99% in the tissues and in this case a 3 mg dose would give a plasma concentration of 10 μg/L and VD of 300 litres.

about 0.1 L/kg body weight (e.g. for salicylate or warfarin), through 1–10 L/kg (e.g. digoxin or propranolol) to 20 L/kg (e.g. tricyclics).

1.3 Pharmacodynamics

Learning objectives

At the end of this section you should:
- be able to classify the ways in which drugs work at the molecular level
- be able to describe the main forms of regulatory *receptors*, the secondary processes that are usually initiated within the cell and the role of 'second messengers'
- be able to define the terms *agonist* and *antagonist*
- know the mechanisms underlying interindividual responses to drugs
- be able to describe the relationships between drug concentration and response or toxic effects
- be able to define the term therapeutic index and list some drugs with small and large indices.

Most drugs exert their effects on the body by interacting with macromolecules, which are usually on the surface of, or within, cells. Variation in these macromolecule targets (such as the number available and the concentration of other compounds competing for binding to the target) is one cause of interindividual variability in drug response. The processes underlying these concepts are termed pharmacodynamics.

Clinical sketch

A 70-year-old man has been taking beta-blockers for many years for his angina. He develops intermittent claudication, and his doctor stops the beta-blocker suddenly. His angina worsens within days, and he is admitted to hospital with a myocardial infarction.

Comment: it is likely that receptor numbers are increased ('upregulated') in the presence of prolonged 'blocking'. Sudden withdrawal of the drug can produce marked effects, as here.

Clinical sketch

A 45-year-old woman with asthma takes both salbutamol and aminophylline for her disease.

Comment: both these drugs act via the same 'second messenger', cyclic AMP. Salbutamol increases cyclic AMP production by interacting with a G-protein-linked receptor, while aminophylline 'blocks' the enzyme that metabolises cyclic AMP.

Drug action at the tissue and molecular level

The target macromolecules may be regulatory receptors, enzymes or structural proteins. A few drugs can interact directly with transport mechanisms and some can exert direct physical effects (e.g. the osmotic diuretic mannitol).

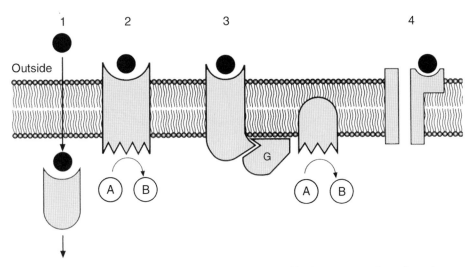

Fig. 7 Drug receptors. **1**. Membrane solubility allows lipid-soluble drugs to cross the cell membrane and bind to intracellular receptors. **2**. Transmembrane proteins bind the drug at the extracellular side of the cell membrane and binding activates an intracellular enzyme site. **3**. The transmembrane protein is linked to an enzyme via a G-protein. **4**. The receptor is a transmembrane ion channel.

Target macromolecules

Receptors

Regulatory molecules have evolved to allow endogenous chemical signals (including neuronal and hormonal activity) to affect the internal function of cells; these are termed receptors (Fig. 7). Some receptors are intracellular, for example those for glucocorticoids and thyroid hormone. Clearly, in these cases, the drug must be lipid soluble in order to cross the cell membrane. Where the drug–receptor complex influences DNA transcription, the resultant mRNA encodes for the synthesis of a new protein that alters cell function: such complicated processes are slow.

Many receptors are situated in the cell membrane and act in various ways to pass the message to the cell interior.

Transmembrane enzymes. These may have a drug (or hormone) binding site lying outside the cell membrane (e.g. the receptor for insulin) and an enzyme moiety at the intracellular end; insulin receptors work in this way. Binding of hormone (or drug) to the receptor causes the enzyme to become active, catalysing a reaction.

Other transmembrane receptors act via G-protein. Binding of hormone (or drug) to the extracellular receptor causes interaction with a G-protein on the inside aspect of the cell membrane. The G-protein may 'amplify' the initial signal (because the G-protein may remain 'active' long after the receptor has dissociated from the agonist molecule) and interacts with an intracellular enzyme, the product of which (a *second messenger*) changes cell function.

Such second messengers include cyclic AMP, inositol polyphosphates and cyclic GMP. Clinical examples of such receptors include β-adrenoceptors and angiotensin, histamine H_2, 5-hydroxytryptamine (5-HT, or serotonin) and muscarinic acetylcholine receptors.

Ion channels. These transmembrane proteins have a central channel down which selected ions may flow when the channel is open. They permit more rapid responses needed for neuronal function, and the cardiac conducting system. These receptors bridge the lipid bilayer and, when activated, open to allow the passive diffusion of specific ions. Diffusion of the ion along a concentration gradient changes the transmembrane potential, which elicits further intracellular responses. Clinical examples include sodium channels in heart muscle (see cardiac arrhythmia in Ch. 4).

Other target macromolecules

Enzymes. Lipid-soluble drugs often alter cell function by impairing enzyme activity. The drug may resemble the enzyme's natural substrate, with which it may compete for binding. Alternatively, the drug may bind irreversibly to the active site of the enzyme. Examples of enzymes that may be inhibited by drugs are numerous and include angiotensin converting enzyme (ramipril), dihydrofolate reductase (methotrexate), xanthine oxidase (allopurinol) and monoamine oxidase (selegiline).

Structural proteins. An example of a drug targeting structural proteins is the binding of colchicine (used for gout) to tubulin. Drug binding inhibits tubulin polymerisation and, therefore, interferes with the migration and mitosis of cells of the immune system.

Transport mechanisms. Living cells maintain internal concentrations of ions such as Na^+, K^+, Cl^- and Ca^{2+} that differ from external concentrations. Therefore, the passive entry of ions via specific channels must be opposed by active pumping in the reverse direction to maintain gradients. Such pumps are usually enzyme systems that consume energy in the form of ATP. Examples include Na^+/K^+-ATPase (which is inhibited by digoxin) and H^+/K^+-ATPase (which is inhibited by omeprazole).

Drugs with physicochemical effects

Some drugs have direct physicochemical effects, for example antacids (used for dyspepsia), resins (such as those used for hypercholesterolaemia) and osmotically active compounds (such as mannitol).

Relationship between dose and response

Agonists

Agonists are compounds that bind to receptors and stimulate them. In in vitro systems, the relationship between concentration and response resembles that in Figure 8. The maximum drug effect is often termed E_{max} and the concentration of drug required for half the maximum effect is termed EC_{50} ('effective concentration 50%'). Agonists can be subdivided into *full* agonists (Fig. 9, compound A), which induce a maximal response when all receptors are occupied, and *partial* agonists, which produce a submaximal response even when all receptors are occupied (Fig. 9, compound B). Compound A in Figure 9 has greater efficacy than compound B. The term potency

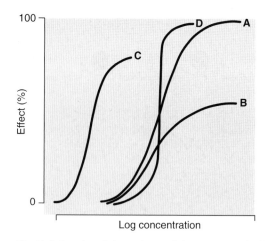

Fig. 9 Full and partial agonists and the concepts of efficacy and potency. Drug A is a full agonist while drug B is a partial agonist. Drugs A and B are equipotent even though A is more efficacious, while drug C has greater potency than either A or B. Drug D has similar potency to drug A and is equally efficacious, but it has a steeper dose–response curve.

refers to the relative concentration (or dose) of a drug needed to produce a given response. In Figure 9, drugs A and B are equipotent even though A is more efficacious; drug C has greater potency than either A or B (i.e. drug C achieves the same effect at a lower dose). The *shape* of the curve also has clinical significance: drugs A and D have similar E_{max} and EC_{50} values, but drug D has a much steeper curve; this may have clinically important consequences if undesirable effects (such as coma) are seen at the higher concentrations. Drug D may have a narrow therapeutic window.

Antagonists

Antagonists bind to receptors *without* stimulating them; by occupying the receptors they prevent access by agonists. Competitive antagonists (for example, beta-blockers; Ch. 3) form bonds with receptor molecules that are rapidly reversible, just like those of the agonist. As the antagonist concentration rises, progressively more receptors become occupied; however, the effects of a competitive antagonist may be abolished by increasing the agonist concentration so that the agonist competes with the antagonist for the binding site (Fig. 10). Non-competitive antagonists (e.g. omeprazole) form bonds with the receptor, usually at sites other than the 'natural' agonist binding site, that are near irreversible; in some cases, they may be covalent. When covalent bonding occurs, the inhibition of effect cannot be overcome entirely no matter how high the agonist concentration is raised (Fig. 11). The duration of action of such

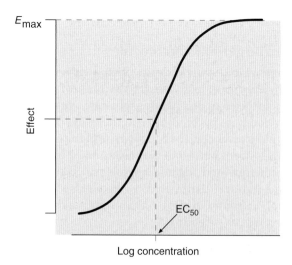

Fig. 8 A dose–response curve.

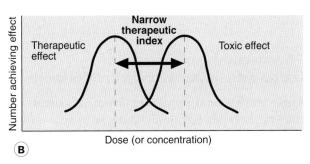

Fig. 10 Competitive antagonist. Curve A is the agonist effect in the absence of antagonist. Curve B is its effect in the presence of a fixed concentration of antagonist. The antagonist effect is abolished at high concentrations of agonist.

Fig. 12 Therapeutic window. **A**. A broad therapeutic index, where there is a wide gap between the desired effect and toxic effects. **B**. A narrow therapeutic index.

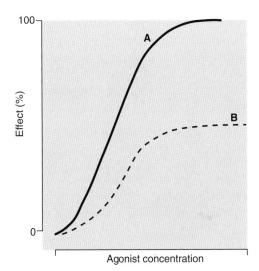

Fig. 11 Non-competitive antagonist. Curve A is the agonist effect in the absence of agonist. Curve B is its effect in the presence of a fixed concentration of antagonist. The antagonist effect cannot be overcome entirely, in contrast to the competitive antagonist.

the dose needed to produce the desired effect in 50% of the population and that needed for the undesired effect is termed the therapeutic window or index. Drugs with wide therapeutic windows (such as penicillins, β_2-agonists and thiazide diuretics) are generally safe and easy to use. Those with narrow therapeutic windows (such as digoxin, theophyllines, lithium and phenytoin) can be difficult to use unless plasma concentrations are measured relatively frequently: this is called therapeutic drug monitoring.

How drugs work at the 'level' of the intact animal

antagonists is determined by the rate of receptor turnover.

Therapeutic window

Clinicians use drugs to achieve a particular result, which is termed therapeutic. If the dose of any drug is increased sufficiently, unwanted or toxic effects invariably develop. In a given population, the dose of drug required to produce a desired effect varies, usually yielding a bell-shaped curve when plotted, a so-called normal distribution; the same is usually true for undesired effects (Fig. 12). The 'gap' between

Clinical sketch

A patient with infective endocarditis is treated with high-dose penicillin and gentamicin. The concentration of penicillin is not monitored, but that of gentamicin is monitored frequently.

Comment: infective endocarditis is fatal if improperly treated. Penicillin has a very large therapeutic window and, so long as the patient is not allergic, serious toxicity from penicillin is unusual. In contrast, the therapeutic index of gentamicin is very small: unless concentrations are carefully monitored, patients develop ototoxicity and nephrotoxicity.

A 30-year-old man has been abusing heroin for many years. Gradually, the dose needed to achieve the desired effect has increased. He is found dead in the street.

Comment: there is downregulation of opiate receptors in individuals who take the drug for long periods, and greater doses are needed to achieve euphoria (tolerance). Unfortunately, heroin (diamorphine) is also a respiratory depressant, and there is less tolerance to this effect.

Pharmacodynamic causes of interindividual variation in drug response

There are two main pharmacodynamic reasons for the variation between individuals in their response to drugs.

Variation in concentration of endogenous agonists

The concentration of endogenous agonists, such as catecholamines, can vary between individuals and within the same person. Predictably therefore, specific antagonists or agonists administered against this varying background produce variable responses.

Variation in receptors

Continued stimulation/inhibition of living systems tends to induce compensatory processes, and the area of receptor–agonist/antagonist interactions is no exception. Consequently, individuals continually exposed to an agonist/antagonist predictably require larger doses to achieve a given effect than would a drug-naïve subject. For example, people continually exposed to gamma-aminobutyric acid (GABA) agonists (such as benzodiazepine sedatives) need bigger doses to achieve an effect. This tolerance is thought, in part, to result from a decrease in receptor numbers, or downregulation. The opposite may also occur; in patients on long-term beta-blocker therapy, it is thought that catecholamine receptor numbers are increased – upregulation. This explains the tendency to a marked rise in blood pressure if the drug is stopped suddenly (rebound hypertension). In addition to changes in the numbers of a receptor, changes can also occur in receptor sensitivity to an agonist. Sensitivity can decrease with constant exposure although it is not fully understood how this occurs. There may also be genetic variation in the sensitivity of a receptor to a drug, with individual patients showing varying responses, e.g. responses of β-adrenoceptors.

Self-assessment on Chapter 1: questions

Multiple choice questions

1. Regarding drug receptors:
   a. A drug usually binds to only one receptor type
   b. Cellular responses to receptors that are ion channels are usually fast
   c. Cellular responses are slow if the mode of action involves modification of DNA transcription
   d. G-proteins amplify the effect of receptor stimulation
   e. Receptors are continually being synthesised and destroyed by the cell

2. Antagonists:
   a. Do not themselves bind to receptors but interfere with the binding of agonists
   b. Bind to receptors but do not stimulate them
   c. May bind covalently to receptors
   d. Usually bind to receptors for very short periods (fractions of a second)
   e. If competitive, can be overcome by increasing the agonist concentration

3. The following statements describe pharmacodynamic concepts:
   a. All drugs act by binding to cell macromolecules
   b. Drug A is said to be more potent than drug B if drug A's maximal effect is greater than that of drug B
   c. A partial agonist is a drug that binds to a receptor without stimulating it
   d. The expression therapeutic index refers to the difference between the concentration of a drug required to produce its effects and that required to produce toxicity
   e. Drug A is said to be more efficacious than drug B if drug A produces its maximum effect at a lower concentration than drug B

4. The following statements describe pharmacokinetic concepts:
   a. Only the unbound (free) drug fraction has pharmacological effects
   b. All drug metabolism takes place in the liver
   c. All drugs must first be metabolised before they can be excreted
   d. Only the unionised drug fraction may cross intact cell membranes
   e. Drug metabolites invariably lack pharmacological effects

Case history questions

Case history 1

A 40-year-old man is on salbutamol for his asthma. His doctor finds that he is hypertensive and starts him on atenolol.

1. How do salbutamol and atenolol work?
2. Is this good prescribing?
3. What will the likely outcome be to this man's hypertension and asthma?

Case history 2

You are the expert witness for the prosecution in a case of alleged medical negligence. A young woman on a low-dose combined oral contraceptive pill went on holiday to Greece with her boyfriend. She had read that many people catch gastroenteritis in this destination and sought advice from her doctor. He prescribed doxycycline and advised her to take this throughout her 3-week stay. Upon her return, she became concerned that she might be pregnant and did a pregnancy test: it was positive.

1. What might have happened?
2. Do you think she has a case?
3. What concerns might there be for the fetus?

Short note questions

Write short notes on the following:

1. A new drug is being developed and its manufacturers want to know its oral bioavailability:

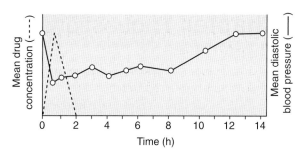

Fig. 13 Plasma concentration of the antihypertensive drug and changes in blood pressure.

a. What clinical reasons are there for determining oral bioavailability?

b. Should bioavailability be tested only with fasted subjects? If your answer is no, explain why.

c. How would you go about measuring bioavailability in a group of 12 healthy subjects?

2. An antihypertensive drug is given to 12 volunteers; the concentration of the drug is measured in the plasma, and its effects on blood pressure are recorded. As seen in Figure 13, the drug had a very short half-life (about 30 minutes) and was detectable for only 2 hours. However, as can also be seen in Figure 13, the effect on diastolic blood pressure was maximal 30 minutes after dosing and returned to predose values after 12 hours. Give two possible explanations for these findings.

3. Consider the following model of drug disposition: water is flowing into a washbasin at a rate of 10 L/min; there is a plug, but it has a 5 mm diameter hole in it.

a. just after the tap is switched on, is the rate of flow through the hole equal to, greater than or less than that from the tap?

b. If the tap is left running at 1 L/min, what will eventually happen to the level of water in the basin?

c. If the tap is left running at 1 L/min but the diameter of the hole is halved, what will happen to the level of water in the basin?

d. If the rate of flow is now gradually reduced, what will happen to the level of water in the basin?

e. In this model, is clearance best represented by the rate of flow through the drain, or by the diameter of the hole?

4. A new drug is found to be eliminated entirely by renal excretion, with no prior metabolism. Its renal clearance (found from plasma and urine concentration data) in an experiment on six healthy subjects is found to be about 200 ml/min; the mean glomerular filtration rate of the six volunteers is about 125 ml/min. What do these data tell you about the mode of excretion of the drug?

Extended matching items questions

Theme: Basic terminology in pharmacology

A. Absorption

B. Apparent volume of distribution

C. Area under the curve

D. Bioavailability

E. Clearance

F. Distribution

G. Enzyme induction

H. Enzyme inhibition

I. Excretion

J. Half-life

K. Metabolism

L. Pharmacodynamics

M. Pharmacogenetics

N. Pharmacokinetics

O. Solubility

P. Therapeutic window

For each of the following descriptions, select the most appropriate term from the list above.

1. The study of the genetic variability between individuals underpinning drug concentration and response.

2. A constant value with the units of measurement being volume per unit time (L/h).

3. The fraction of the dose administered proceeding in an unaltered state from the site of administration to the systemic circulation.

4. A reflection of the total exposure of the body to a drug, the units of measurement being g/L per unit time (h).

5. Carbamazepine reducing the efficacy of theophylline in a patient with chronic-obstructive pulmonary disease.

6. The difference in the dose (and concentration) needed to produce a therapeutic effect in 50% of the population and that dose (and concentration) needed to produce a toxic effect.

7. Ketoconazole increasing the likelihood of toxicity of an anti-arrhythmic drug in a patient with cardiac disease.

8. A pharmacokinetic variable, with the unit of measurement expressed in hours (h).

Self-assessment on Chapter 1: answers

Multiple choice answers

1. a. **False.** We often classify a drug by the type of receptor relevant to its pharmacological effect, but drugs probably bind to far more cell macromolecules than documented. Some of these interactions produce adverse effects, but many produce no obvious effect.

   b. **True.** The influx of ions induced by receptor activation rapidly changes conditions within the cell.

   c. **True.** Such a mechanism explains the slow response to corticosteroids.

   d. **True.** Once activated, many G-proteins remain active for longer than the receptor is occupied by the drug; the second message is dependent upon active G-protein, not occupied receptors, so the signal is amplified.

   e. **True.** Receptors have a variable lifespan; the cells can up- or downregulate receptor numbers by increasing/decreasing their rate of synthesis/destruction.

2. a. **False.** Antagonists bind to receptors without stimulating them; they therefore occupy receptors that would otherwise be occupied by agonist. This has the effect of reducing the effect of the agonist.

   b. **True.**

   c. **True.** Non-competitive (irreversible) antagonists may do this; there are few clinically used examples, e.g. the alpha-antagonist phenoxybenzamine.

   d. **True.** Competitive antagonists (the group in most common clinical use) usually bind for milliseconds and hence can be displaced by raising the concentration of the agonist.

   e. **True.** As agonist concentrations rise, receptor occupancy by agonist molecules becomes more likely at any given moment. Eventually the effect of the antagonist may be nearly completely overcome.

3. a. **False.** Some drugs act via physical effects, for example osmotic diuretics.

   b. **False.** This is the definition of efficacy.

   c. **False.** A partial agonist binds to a receptor and stimulates it; however, the maximal achievable response is lower than that seen with a full agonist. A partial agonist is also a partial antagonist!

   d. **True.**

   e. **False.** This is the definition of potency.

4. a. **True.** Only the unbound fraction is available to diffuse across membranes to reach its site of action.

   b. **False.** Other sites include lung, gut wall, plasma and kidney.

   c. **False.** Some polar compounds, such as gentamicin and digoxin, are excreted unchanged.

   d. **True.** The unionised fraction is lipid soluble and therefore can pass through the membrane.

   e. **False.** Many drugs act entirely via the effects of their metabolites, for example enalapril and zidovudine.

Case history answers

Case history 1

1. Salbutamol is an agonist at β_2-adrenoceptors while atenolol is a β-adrenoceptor antagonist with greater affinity for β_1- than for β_2-adrenoceptors. Even so, its use here carries the strong risk of antagonising the effects of the salbutamol.

2. This is very poor prescribing. In essence, the atenolol is being used for the long-term prevention of cardiovascular risk, such as stroke. There are many alternative drugs that could have been used. Increasingly, beta-blockers are less frequently used for the treatment of hypertension.

3. Salbutamol will have no deleterious effects on control of blood pressure but atenolol will quite possibly worsen the patient's asthma.

Case history 2

1. Oral contraceptive steroids are given in very low dose to avoid adverse effects; reliance is

placed on enterohepatic circulation. The tetracyclines, by killing gut bacteria, interrupt this circulation and can cause drug failure.

2. The court will decide but, on the face of it, she does. The doctor ought to have been aware of the interaction (see Appendix 1 of the BNF) and should have advised her to use alternative contraceptive precautions. Moreover, there was a dubious case for the antibiotic in any case – this was advised to be taken prophylactically, to prevent illness, and this has little evidence base.

3. Tetracyclines cross the placenta and may damage developing bone and teeth.

Short note answers

1. a. The new drug must have been shown to have desired pharmacological effects in vitro and also probably in an animal model to get this far. However, unless the drug gets into the human body, it cannot produce its effects. Bioavailability can vary markedly between species, and even between individuals; this is of obvious importance in deciding dose.

   b. Food can affect bioavailability, and this needs to be examined since the drug will, in due course, be in general use. In many cases, food reduces bioavailability, for example penicillins, cephalosporins, rifampicin, isoniazid and captopril, but in some cases it is increased (e.g. propranolol, metoprolol, griseofulvin and hydralazine).

   c. This is usually determined from the area under the curve (AUC) of the drug after oral dosing divided by that (in the same subject, but on a different occasion) after i.v. dosing. So in Figure 14, the two AUC values for drug A are about the same: this drug has a bioavailability of about 1.0. Drug B, however, has a much smaller AUC when it is given orally, and also a lower bioavailability.

2. a. This could be a prodrug, which produces its effects through an unidentified metabolite; as shown in Figure 15, the metabolite may have a much longer half-life than the parent compound.

   b. The drug could be a non-competitive antagonist, which binds irreversibly to its

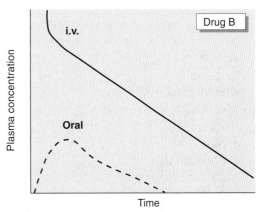

Fig. 14 Measuring bioavailability. Values for 2 days, A and B, given as an oral dose (---) or as an i.v. dose (—).

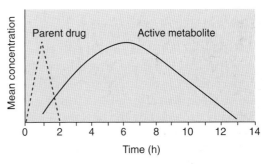

Fig. 15 Plasma concentration for parent drug (---) and active metabolite (—).

receptor. Drug effects would be terminated by receptor turnover, rather than drug elimination from the plasma.

3. This may seem a poor model for drug disposition, but the two have much in common. Soon after the tap is switched on, the rate of drainage from the basin is much less than the rate of entry, and water accumulates in the basin until the two are equal. Analogous with this is the period

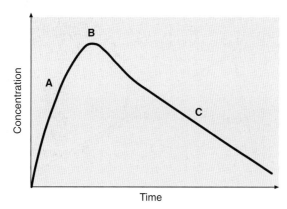

Fig. 16 Clearance of a drug.

immediately after drug dosing (phase A in Fig. 16): the rate of drug absorption exceeds that of elimination, and the plasma concentration rises. Because the rate of elimination is proportional to drug concentration, a time will come when the two are equal (point B in Fig. 16). In the model, narrowing the hole in the plug will reduce the rate of drainage, causing further accumulation of water in the basin until a new equilibrium is reached. The diameter of the hole represents the constant termed clearance. Finally, if the tap is gradually turned off over the next half hour or so, the level of water in the basin will fall. The same happens to a finite drug dose: as the proportion of the dose unabsorbed falls, the rate of absorption also falls, so that this is gradually exceeded by the rate of elimination (phase C in Fig. 16).

4. About 25% of the cardiac output (therefore about 1.2 L/min^{-1}) goes to the kidneys, and of this about 10% is filtered by the glomerulus (the glomerular filtration rate; GFR). The maximum clearance of a drug by this route is, therefore, equal to the GFR; in

fact most drugs have much lower filtration rates since only unbound drug can be filtered. The renal clearance of this new drug *exceeds* the GFR; the likeliest explanation is that it is extensively *secreted* by the renal tubules.

Extended matching items answers

Theme: Basic terminology in pharmacology

1. M. This is pharmacogenetics. We are gradually understanding more about the influence of genes on drug dose–concentration–response relationships. Of course the environment is also important.

2. E. Clearance is the volume of plasma completely 'cleared' of the drug per hour.

3. D. This is bioavailability. For an intravenous dose the bioavailability is 100% or 1.0.

4. C. The area under the curve (AUC) refers to the area under the concentration versus time curve for a drug.

5. G. This is an example of enzyme induction. The efficacy of theophylline is reduced because the drug concentrations are reduced.

6. P. The therapeutic window is of significant importance in prescribing and using drugs safely, as it influences the risk : benefit ratio of the drug. Drugs with a narrow therapeutic index include digoxin and phenytoin.

7. H. This is an example of enzyme inhibition. Ketoconazole is a potent enzyme inhibitor. If it inhibits the enzymes metabolising the anti-arrhythmic then higher concentrations of this second drug will result. Toxicity can then be a problem. This can be serious. Most anti-arrhythmics not only treat arrhythmias but can also cause arrhythmias.

8. J. Half-life: the time taken for the drug concentration to fall to half its original value, measured in units of time (h).

The autonomic nervous system

2.1	**Structure and function**	**21**
2.2	**Cholinergic drugs**	**23**
2.3	**Drugs acting on the sympathetic nervous system**	**25**
	Self-assessment on Chapter 2: questions	28
	Self-assessment on Chapter 2: answers	30

Overview

Many drugs have their effects, or adverse effects, by working on the autonomic nervous system. In this chapter the basic anatomy and physiology of the system is described, along with the classes of drug that affect it.

The autonomic system can be separated into sympathetic and parasympathetic divisions and the roles of these are described.

2.1 Structure and function

Learning objectives

At the end of this section you should be able to:
- describe the anatomical layout of the sympathetic and parasympathetic systems
- list the neurotransmitter substances released by preganglionic and postganglionic fibres of both systems
- describe the classification, relevant structure and function of the various receptors found in both systems
- describe the mechanisms that terminate neurotransmitter 'activity'.

Many drugs produce their effects by working on the autonomic system, including, for example, many antihypertensives and bronchodilators, and the same mechanisms explain the adverse effects of many others, for example some neuroleptics and the antiarrhythmics. The autonomic nervous system regulates visceral functions, such as cardiac output, gut motility, endocrine and exocrine gland function and blood vessel tone, and is not under conscious control. It is separated on anatomical and physiological grounds into *sympathetic* and *parasympathetic* divisions. It is useful to think of stimulation by the sympathetic division inducing conditions for *flight or fight*, such as increased heart rate and stroke volume, dilatation of the pupils, increased blood sugar, cutaneous vasoconstriction and contraction of sphincters, while stimulation by the parasympathetic system usually, but not always, has the opposite actions.

Structure of the sympathetic system

The sympathetic system is controlled by centres in the hypothalamus and brainstem. 'Outflow' from the brain is via the *descending reticular system* of synapsing neurones. Nerve fibres finally leave the spinal cord with the nerve roots, between T1 and L2, and pass into the *sympathetic trunk* where most synapse. The 'first order neurones' are referred to as *preganglionic. Postganglionic* fibres then pursue a lengthy course (Fig. 17), finally reaching such structures as the heart, blood vessels, bronchi, pupillary muscle and gut. One exception to this general pattern is innervation of the adrenal medulla, where first-order neurones travel directly to the organ and synapse with modified neurones in the medulla, which secretes adrenaline (epinephrine) into the circulation.

Structure of the parasympathetic system

The parasympathetic system is also controlled within the hypothalamus and brainstem, by a series

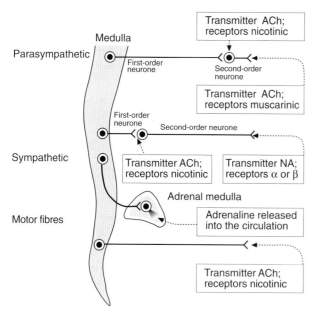

Fig. 17 Anatomy of the autonomic nervous system. ACh, acetylcholine; NA, noradrenaline (norepinephrine).

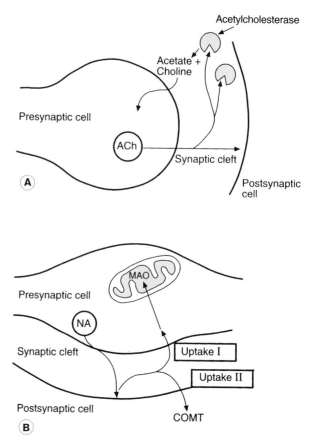

Fig. 18 Metabolism of neurotransmitters. **A**. Removal of acetylcholine (ACh) from the cholinergic synaptic cleft, which terminates its activity. **B**. In adrenergic synaptic clefts, noradrenaline (NA; norepinephrine) is absorbed into the cells where it is metabolised by monoamine oxidase (MAO) or by catechol-*O*-methyltransferase (COMT).

of specific nuclei. Preganglionic fibres leave the CNS with the cranial nerves (especially the vagus nerve) and sacral nerve roots. Unlike sympathetic ganglia, those of the parasympathetic system are very close to their destination, and postganglionic fibres are short (Fig. 17).

Function

Neurotransmitters

The term neurotransmitter is given to any molecule released by neurones that causes depolarisation of the membrane of another cell (another neurone, a muscle fibre or a gland). There are antagonists to specific receptors, described below.

Preganglionic neurotransmitters. Neurones of both parasympathetic and sympathetic systems release acetylcholine, as do somatic nerve fibres.

Postganglionic neurotransmitters. Second-order neurones of the parasympathetic system release acetylcholine. In contrast, fibres of the sympathetic system release noradrenaline (norepinephrine). There are two exceptions to this: (a) the sympathetic transmitter at sweat glands is acetylcholine, and (b) certain postganglionic sympathetic fibres release dopamine, for example those to the renal/splanchnic vasculature.

Termination of neurotransmitter action

The action of acetylcholine in synaptic clefts is terminated very rapidly by the local enzyme acetylcholinesterase (Fig. 18).

The action of noradrenaline (norepinephrine) is partly terminated by diffusion away from the cleft but mainly by cellular absorption. Absorption into the presynaptic cell (*uptake 1*) leads to metabolism of noradrenaline (norepinephrine) by mitochondrial monoamine oxidase (MAO). Absorption into the postsynaptic cell (*uptake 2*) leads to metabolism by catechol-*O*-methyltransferase (COMT) (Fig. 18).

Receptors

Receptors are divided into groups based on the neurotransmitter involved. They can be further subdivided by their response to agonists and knowledge of these subgroups and the effects of their stimulation has been used in the design of drugs for a desired effect.

Cholinergic receptors

Receptors on postganglionic fibres and effector cells differ in their structure, and this explains the selectivity of many of the drugs dealt with below.

Postganglionic receptors. In both sympathetic and parasympathetic divisions, receptors on the postganglionic cell membranes, as well as responding to acetylcholine, can be stimulated by the agonist nicotine. They are, therefore, termed *nicotinic*. The receptor is an ion channel for Na^+ and K^+, and activation of the receptor causes depolarisation of the postganglionic fibre.

Receptors on effector cells of the parasympathetic system. These are found in such tissues as smooth muscle and glands. They can be stimulated by muscarine and are, therefore, termed *muscarinic*. The cellular events that occur after stimulation of muscarinic receptors are complex: intracellular cyclic GMP levels rise, inositol phospholipid turnover accelerates and adenyl cyclase is inhibited, but the role of each second messenger is not established.

Adrenergic receptors

The adrenergic receptors (adrenoceptors) respond to catecholamines.

The α_1-adrenoceptors. These are *postsynaptic* and are found especially on smooth muscle. At a cellular level, stimulation causes release of inositol trisphosphate and an increase in intracellular Ca^{2+}. At an organ level, stimulation causes contraction of smooth muscle.

Clinical sketch

A man in his early sixties is prescribed doxazosin for hypertension. Although this does not appear to work very well in lowering his blood pressure the patient also has benign prostatic hypertrophy and has found that his symptoms of hesitancy and frequency have diminished. Consequently he wants to carry on taking the drug.

Comment: doxazosin is an antagonist at α_1-adrenoceptors. Its effect on these receptors in blood vessel walls in causing vasodilatation is utilized in the treatment of hypertension, although these drugs are not regarded as first line. However, there are also such receptors in the prostate and this class of drugs is indicated for benign prostatic hypertrophy.

The α_2-adrenoceptors. *Outside the CNS*, these are *presynaptic*, occurring at peripheral adrenergic nerve terminals. At a cellular level, stimulation causes inhibition of adenyl cyclase and reduction of intracellular cyclic AMP; this leads to inhibition of release of further noradrenaline (norepinephrine) from the terminal. Stimulation of α_2-adrenoceptors, therefore, acts as 'feedback' control of noradrenaline (nor-

epinephrine) release. In contrast, *inside the CNS*, α_2-adrenoceptors are *postsynaptic*, and are the main adrenoceptors of the CNS components of the sympathetic system.

The β_1-adrenoceptors. These are mainly located in the heart. At a cellular level, stimulation causes activation of adenyl cyclase and an increase in intracellular cyclic AMP. At an organ level, stimulation produces an increase in heart rate (positive chronotropic effect) and contractility (positive inotropic effect).

The β_2-adrenoceptors. These are widely distributed, but sites of particular importance include the smooth muscle of blood vessels, bronchi and uterus. The cellular mechanisms are the same as for β_1-adrenoceptors. At an organ level, stimulation of β_2-adrenoceptors produces smooth muscle relaxation.

Clinical sketch

A drug company representative comes to see you about a new cardioselective beta-blocker for use in patients with angina. He tells you that it is perfectly safe to use in patients with asthma.

Comment: theoretically, selective β_1-adrenoceptor antagonists are less likely to cause bronchoconstriction but in practice the degree of selectivity is not sufficient to categorically say that these drugs would be 'safe' in asthma.

Dopamine receptors. These are most numerous within the CNS, but they are also important in control of renal blood flow. Stimulation produces renal vasodilatation.

2.2 Cholinergic drugs

Learning objectives

At the end of this section you should be able to:
- distinguish drugs that are true agonists from those that block acetylcholine metabolism (anticholinesterases)
- outline the organ-specific effects of cholinergic agonists and their clinical uses
- appreciate that the anticholinergics in therapeutic use all act at the muscarinic receptor, and that there are no antinicotinics in common use
- list some antimuscarinic drugs and describe their clinical uses
- list the organ-specific effects of atropine.

A woman develops a painful red eye. The ophthalmologist diagnoses acute closed-angle glaucoma and plans surgery to correct this. To reduce the intraocular pressure immediately, pilocarpine eye drops are prescribed.

Comment: pilocarpine is a direct-acting cholinergic agonist. It causes pupillary constriction, thereby opening up the angle between the iris and the cornea. This enhances drainage of the aqueous humour.

Cholinergic agonists

True cholinergic agonists have their effect by a direct interaction with the cholinergic receptor; indirect agonists act by prolonging the life of acetylcholine.

True agonists

Pilocarpine is a muscarinic agonist applied topically to cause pupillary constriction (miosis) in the treatment of glaucoma (Fig. 19).

Bethanechol is another muscarinic agonist. It can be used to increase smooth muscle tone in the bladder when treating postoperative urinary retention. Bethanechol is contraindicated in patients with asthma, bradycardia and urinary/gut outflow obstruction.

Indirect agonists

Anticholinesterases act by inhibiting acetylcholinesterase, thereby prolonging the duration of acetylcholine action (see Ch. 8).

Cholinergic antagonists (anticholinergics)

Cholinergic antagonists can be classified as antimuscarinic or antinicotinic, depending on the subgroup of receptor affected. Only antagonists acting at muscarinic receptors are in common clinical use.

Antimuscarinic drugs

Clinical sketch

A 60-year-old man is admitted to hospital with an acute inferior myocardial infarction. Shortly after transfer to the coronary care unit he becomes bradycardic with a heart rate of 40 beats per minute and a blood pressure of 85/50 mmHg. The doctor's first-line treatment is an intravenous injection of atropine.

Comment: this is a common clinical problem and inferior myocardial infarctions can be associated with arrhythmias such as this. Atropine is used in the first instance to try and speed up the heart rate – atropine reduces vagal tone, increases sinus node automaticity and speeds conduction through the atrioventricular node.

The classical example of an antimuscarinic drug is *atropine*, a naturally occurring alkaloid that is a non-selective reversible muscarinic antagonist. All the other examples described below have structural similarities with atropine. The effects of atropine on various organs is as follows:

- eye: pupillary dilatation (mydriasis)
- CNS: in standard doses it causes mild sedation and in high doses, agitation, seizures, hallucinations and coma; anti-parkinsonian effects (see Ch. 6) can result from its action in basal ganglia
- gut: reduced secretion and motility, causing constipation
- heart: tachycardia (the vagus nerve is blocked)
- bronchi: bronchodilatation

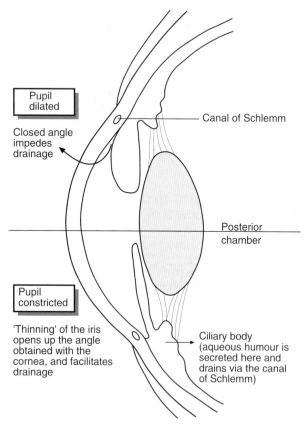

Pupil dilated

Closed angle impedes drainage

Canal of Schlemm

Posterior chamber

Pupil constricted

'Thinning' of the iris opens up the angle obtained with the cornea, and facilitates drainage

Ciliary body (aqueous humour is secreted here and drains via the canal of Schlemm)

Fig. 19 Use of miotics in closed-angle glaucoma.

- bladder: relaxation of the walls, which may lead to urinary retention
- sweat glands: reduced secretion.

> **Clinical sketch**
>
> A man develops parkinsonism from the neuroleptic drugs that he takes for schizophrenia; he takes trihexyphenidyl for this (see Ch. 6). He becomes depressed and takes an overdose of trihexyphenidyl. On admission, he is confused and has a narrow-complex tachycardia of around 160 beats/min; his blood pressure is low.
>
> *Comment: trihexyphenidyl is very like atropine, and causes these features in overdose. Acetylcholine 'agonists', such as physostigmine, may be helpful.*

Muscarinic receptors in these sites vary slightly in their drug affinities and this has led to a system of classification as subgroups. Detailed knowledge of this classification is of limited value, but the point to remember is that some drugs bind better at some muscarinic receptors than others, and this explains their selectivity.

Examples of antimuscarinic drugs

Atropine. Atropine is given intravenously (i.v.) to increase heart rate in patients with symptomatic bradycardias and during cardiac arrest caused by asystole or pulseless electrical activity. It may also be used topically in iritis as a mydriatic agent, to prevent the formation of adhesions between the iris and the cornea. Derivatives such as *tropicamide* are more commonly used in this setting.

Pirenzipine. This is a second-line drug for peptic ulcer (Ch. 11).

Trihexyphenidyl. Used for parkinsonism (see Ch. 6).

Ipratropium. Unlike the other examples, this molecule is polar and poorly absorbed from most sites. It is used topically for asthma.

Adverse effects

Adverse effects are dose related and include dryness of the mouth, urinary retention, constipation, raised intraocular pressure, tachycardia and confusion. In severe poisoning, there may be tachyarrhythmias, coma and seizures. Some drugs used for other indications have antimuscarinic side-effects, notably tricyclic antidepressants (Ch. 6), neuroleptics (Ch. 6) and disopyramide and quinidine (Ch. 3).

Contraindications

Glaucoma. Antimuscarinic agents induce mydriasis, which narrows the angle between the iris and the cornea, thereby reducing drainage of aqueous humour into the canal of Schlemm (Fig. 19).

Prostatic hypertrophy. Urinary retention is worsened.

> **Clinical sketch**
>
> A woman with closed-angle glaucoma presents with severe asthma; her doctors wonder whether it would be safe to use nebulised ipratropium.
>
> *Comment: glaucoma is a relative contraindication to the use of this atropine-like drug. However, exacerbation of glaucoma is uncommon, and the benefits may exceed the risks in a case such as this.*

Antinicotinic drugs

Antagonists at skeletal muscle nicotinic receptors (which are not part of the autonomic system) are widely used in anaesthesia as muscle relaxants (Ch. 8). Autonomic antinicotinic drugs (the 'ganglion blockers') were used in the past for hypertension but are now obsolete.

2.3 Drugs acting on the sympathetic nervous system

> **Learning objectives**
>
> At the end of this section you should be able to:
> - list the main adrenergic agonists and describe the effects of each agonist on specific tissues and the whole animal
> - list the receptor subtypes that each agonist binds to
> - describe the clinical uses of adrenergic agonists.

Adrenergic agonists (sympathomimetics)

Different endogenous and synthetic sympathomimetics have different affinities for the subtypes of adrenoceptors. From these, their effects can be predicted.

Noradrenaline (norepinephrine) binds to α_1-, α_2- and β_1-adrenoceptors. Injected i.v., noradrenaline (norepinephrine) tends to cause marked *vasoconstriction* and an increase in myocardial contractility:

blood pressure therefore rises. Although a positive chronotropic effect would be expected, this is usually overcome by vagal homeostatic mechanisms.

Adrenaline (epinephrine) binds to α_1-, α_2-, β_1- and β_2-adrenoceptors. The net effect of an i.v. injection of adrenaline (epinephrine) is usually unchanged vascular resistance (vascular resistance increases markedly in some vascular beds, while decreasing in others; this reflects local distribution of receptor types), increased myocardial contractility, increased heart rate, increased systolic blood pressure and little or no change in diastolic pressure.

Clinical sketch

A young woman sees an allergy specialist because she had a severe allergic reaction to peanuts while on holiday. She required admission to hospital because of breathing difficulties. The allergy specialist recommends she carries an adrenaline (epinephrine)-containing syringe and needle pen device with her at all times.

Comment: this sounds like anaphylaxis and can be life-threatening. Adrenaline (epinephrine) is an important treatment in these circumstances, and although this should not be entered into lightly, if the patient is able to give herself the drug at the earliest sign of a severe reaction, then this could be life-saving.

Clinical sketch

A young man is admitted to hospital with acute severe asthma. He is given regular salbutamol nebulisers and his condition improves. However, he complains of palpitations and he is quite clearly tachycardic. The doctors also want to monitor his blood potassium closely.

Comment: salbutamol is used in asthma because of its β_2 activity in causing bronchodilation. However, at high concentrations, almost certainly achieved with nebulisers, the drug also attaches to β_1-receptors and hence can cause a tachycardia. Stimulation of β-receptors also pushes potassium into cells and hence hypokalaemia can be a problem.

Isoprenaline binds to β_1- and β_2-adrenoceptors. The net effect of an i.v. injection is increased heart rate, increased myocardial contractility and decreased vascular resistance; blood pressure may fall. Isoprenaline injection is subject to limited bioavailability.

Dobutamine. This is selective for β_1-adrenoceptors, it causes increased heart rate and contractility. Blood pressure rises. Like dopamine, dobutamine at high concentration activates α_1-adrenoceptors, causing unwanted vasoconstriction.

Salbutamol. This is selective for β_2-adrenoceptors. It causes relaxation of vascular and bronchial smooth muscle. At higher concentrations, salbutamol becomes less selective, binding to β_1-adrenoceptors, which causes tachycardia.

Ephedrine. A non-selective sympathomimetic with a similar spectrum to adrenaline (epinephrine).

Therapeutic uses

Anaphylaxis. This syndrome of shock (secondary to vasodilatation) and bronchospasm in response to an allergen (Ch. 10) is treated with subcutaneous epinephrine (adrenaline), which induces bronchodilatation, vasoconstriction and raises blood pressure.

Clinical sketch

A man is admitted to the coronary care unit after a massive myocardial infarction. He is in sinus rhythm (rate of 100 beats/min) and is well hydrated but his blood pressure is unrecordable and his urine output is very low. The doctors start a constant rate infusion of dobutamine.

Comment: dobutamine is a β_1-agonist, which increases myocardial contractility. It can help in 'cardiogenic shock', as described here.

Asthma. Inhaled β_2-agonists such as salbutamol are drugs of first choice (Ch. 10).

Cardiogenic shock. This is caused by an acute reduction in myocardial contractility, usually after a massive myocardial infarction. Dobutamine, by its β_1-effects, increases stroke volume and heart rate and improves the perfusion of vital structures; however, if the concentration rises too high, dobutamine causes vasoconstriction through α-agonist activity. The use of such drugs is generally confined to high-dependency settings with a significant amount of haemodynamic monitoring.

Cardiac arrest. Adrenaline (epinephrine) may be given i.v. during attempts at resuscitation as part of Advanced Life Support protocols. It basically enhances the efficiency of cardiopulmonary resuscitation (chest compressions).

Reduction of local blood flow. The local anaesthetic lidocaine is formulated in combination with adrenaline (epinephrine) for certain procedures. Local vasoconstriction reduces the rate of removal of the anaesthetic from the site and prolongs its effect, while at the same time reducing blood loss. This drug combination must not be used when anaesthetising extremities (e.g. fingers) because of the risk of gangrene.

Nasal decongestants. Ephedrine is given orally to reduce nasal congestion; it is often present in proprietary cough mixtures.

Drug interactions

Non-selective, older, monoamine oxidase inhibitors (MAOI) are still sometimes used for depression (see Ch. 6). Ingestion of sympathomimetics (usually in cough mixtures) may cause severe hypertension.

Adrenergic antagonists (alpha- and beta-blockers)

Adrenergic antagonists, also known as alpha-blockers and beta-blockers, are considered in Chapter 3.

Two

Self-assessment on Chapter 2: questions

Multiple choice questions

1. The following statements are true:
   a. Salbutamol given i.v. causes tachycardia
   b. Dobutamine i.v. is indicated for shock secondary to gastrointestinal haemorrhage
   c. Isoprenaline i.v. causes bronchodilatation
   d. Noradrenaline (norepinephrine) i.v. causes bronchodilatation
   e. Dobutamine i.v. dilates renal arterioles

2. The action of noradrenaline (norepinephrine):
   a. Is terminated by its uptake from the synapse
   b. Is potentiated by inhibitors of monoamine oxidase B
   c. Is potentiated by tricyclic antidepressants
   d. Includes vasodilatation in some arteriolar beds
   e. Is potentiated by cocaine

3. Atropine:
   a. Is a direct agonist at autonomic acetylcholine receptors
   b. Slows the heart rate
   c. Causes a dry mouth
   d. Bronchodilates
   e. Raises intraocular pressure

Case history questions

Case history 1

A 6-year-old girl is brought to casualty because of collapse at home. She had been playing unsupervised in a local wood and had been well previously. She is semiconscious and confused, her pupils are dilated, her skin is dry and her pulse rate is 200 beats/min.

1. What might be the cause of her problem?
2. What should be done?
3. How is the autonomic nervous system involved?

Case history 2

A farmer is brought as an emergency after an accident with crop-spraying equipment, during which he was copiously sprayed with insecticide. He is salivating profusely and has difficulty breathing; his pulse rate is 40 beats/min.

1. What is the mechanism of the poisoning?
2. What should be done?

Case history 3

A 70-year-old man takes disopyramide (see Ch. 3) as prophylaxis against cardiac arrhythmias. He also has parkinsonism for which his doctor has put him on benztropine (see Ch. 6). He becomes constipated and, within 2 days of starting the latter drug, he is admitted in acute retention of urine.

What has happened?

Short note question

Write short notes on the relevance of the autonomic nervous system to clinical pharmacology and therapeutics, using clinical examples to illustrate your answer.

Extended matching items questions

Theme: autonomic agonists and antagonists

A. Atropine
B. Bisoprolol
C. Carvedilol
D. Dobutamine
E. Adrenaline (epinephrine)
F. Noradrenaline (norepinephrine)
G. Phenoxybenzamine
H. Pilocarpine
I. Propranolol

J. Prazosin

K. Salbutamol

L. Verapamil

From the list above, select the drug which best matches each of the receptor activities described below.

1. β_1-adrenoceptor antagonist.

2. Non-selective β-adrenoceptor antagonist.

3. Non-selective β-adrenoceptor antagonist with α_1 blockade.

4. α_1-, α_2- and β_1-adrenoreceptor agonist.

5. α_1-, α_2-, β_1 and β_2-adrenoceptor agonist.

6. α_1-adrenoceptor antagonist.

7. β_1-adrenoceptor agonist.

8. β_2-adrenoceptor agonist.

9. Muscarinic antagonist.

10. Muscarinic agonist.

Self-assessment on Chapter 2: answers

Multiple choice answers

1. a. **True.** Salbutamol has higher affinity for β_2- than for β_1-adrenoceptors; however, binding to the latter does occur, causing tachycardia.
   b. **False.** Dobutamine dilates splanchnic vessels, including those to the stomach/duodenum and could worsen bleeding.
   c. **True.** Isoprenaline binds to both β_1- and β_2-adrenoceptors.
   d. **False.** Noradrenaline (norepinephrine) has little activity at β_2-adrenoceptors.
   e. **False.** Dobutamine is a specific β_1-agonist and has little effect on splanchnic vessels.

2. a. **True.** Noradrenaline (norepinephrine) is taken up presynaptically (uptake I) and postsynaptically (uptake II).
   b. **False.** Monoamine oxidase A metabolises noradrenaline (norepinephrine) and 5-HT, while monoamine oxidase B metabolises dopamine.
   c. **True.** Tricyclic antidepressants inhibit uptake I.
   d. **False.** Noradrenaline (norepinephrine) binds to α_1-, α_2- and β_1-adrenoceptors.
   e. **True.** Cocaine interferes with uptake of noradrenaline (norepinephrine) from the synapse; unlike lidocaine, cocaine need not be formulated with adrenaline (epinephrine) for this reason.

3. Atropine:
   a. **False.** Atropine is an antagonist at these receptors.
   b. **False.** The vagus nerve carries acetylcholinergic parasympathetic fibres to the sinoatrial node, and stimulation slows the heart rate. By blocking this, atropine is positively chronotropic.
   c. **True.** Parasympathetic fibres are secretomotor to the salivary glands.
   d. **True.** See Chapter 10.
   e. **True.** By causing pupillary dilatation, atropine closes the angle between the cornea and the iris, opposing drainage of aqueous humour and raising intraocular pressure.

Case history answers

Case history 1

1. This patient has features of anticholinergic poisoning; she may have eaten deadly nightshade berries or fungi. She is confused because the alkaloid has crossed her blood–brain barrier.

2. Her airway should be protected and her stomach emptied (even if poisoning was some time ago as anticholinergics delay gastric emptying). Supportive care with attention paid to maintenance of breathing and the circulation, and termination of seizures (usually with diazepam), is indicated. The National Poisons Information Service should be contacted. Anticholinesterases (Ch. 8) may be useful to potentiate acetylcholine: physostigmine is then the drug of first choice since it crosses the blood–brain barrier.

3. Secretomotor fibres to her salivary and sweat glands have been blocked, as have parasympathetic fibres of the vagus.

Case history 2

1. Organophosphorus insecticides are potent and long-acting anticholinesterases: overactivity at parasympathetic receptors is responsible for the clinical features, and his breathlessness may be caused by bronchospasm.

2. Contaminated clothes should be removed, and he should be washed in copious amounts of water as the compound can cross the skin. Bronchospasm should be treated according to asthma guidelines (Ch. 10), and he should be given frequent doses of i.v. atropine for its antimuscarinic effects. Pralidoxime is a specific antidote capable of regenerating active cholinesterase by releasing it from covalent binding to the insecticide.

Case history 3

Benztropine is an antimuscarinic, and disopyramide also has antimuscarinic side-effects. Both tend to increase the tone of the bladder sphincter, decrease the tone of the bladder wall and cause urinary retention. Both can also cause constipation. In addition, disopyramide can occasionally *cause* tachyarrhythmias through its antimuscarinic activity (though this complication has not happened here). This is an example of a pharmacodynamic interaction.

Short note answer

Many drugs produce their effects by working on the autonomic system, and the same mechanisms explain the adverse effects of many others. Dealing with such drugs (which include antihypertensives, antiarrhythmics, bronchodilators, neuroleptics) as agonists and antagonists at autonomic receptors allows better understanding of their therapeutic use, and adverse effects.

1. Define what you mean by agonists and antagonists.

2. Deal with cholinergic receptors.
   a. *Nicotinic agonists*: none in regular clinical use; mention 'indirect agonists', i.e. the anticholinesterases
   b. *Nicotinic antagonists*: none in regular clinical use (ganglion blockers are obsolete)
   c. *Muscarinic agonists*: for example, pilocarpine, which causes pupillary constriction and is used in glaucoma, or bethanechol, which causes increased muscle tone in the bladder
   d. *Muscarinic antagonists*: for example, atropine (also list several other antimuscarinics and their uses). Give the adverse effects of antimuscarinic drugs. Mention drugs that either achieve their effect through antagonism of muscarinic receptors (e.g. pirenzipine, benztropine and ipratropium) or produce adverse effects by the same mechanism (e.g. quinidine, disopyramide, tricyclic antidepressants).

3. Deal with adrenergic receptors: cover the effects of stimulation of α_1-, α_2-, β_1- and β_2-adrenoceptors and describe their anatomical locations.

4. Describe the clinical use of the agonists salbutamol, adrenaline (epinephrine), noradrenaline (norepinephrine), isoprenaline, dobutamine and dopamine.

5. Describe the clinical use of the antagonists propranolol, atenolol, prazosin and phenoxybenzamine.

Extended matching items answers

1. B. Bisoprolol. Used in the treatment of ischaemic heart disease and hypertension.

2. I. Propranolol. Can be used in the management of hypertension, but more frequently used nowadays for the symptomatic management of hyperthyroidism.

3. C. Carvedilol. Increasingly used in the treatment of heart failure.

4. F. The profile is characteristic of noradrenaline (norepinephrine). Used in intensive care for conditions such as septic shock.

5. E. The profile characteristic of adrenaline (epinephrine).

6. J. Prazosin. Used in the treatment of hypertension and benign prostatic hypertrophy.

7. E. Dobutamine. Can be helpful in cardiogenic shock.

8. K. Salbutamol. Used in the treatment of asthma (and hyperkalaemia because of its effects on potassium).

9. A. Atropine.

10. H. Pilocarpine.

Drugs in cardiovascular disease 1: prevention

3.1	Clinical aspects and cardiovascular risk factors	33
3.2	Hypertension	34
3.3	Hyperlipidaemia	41
	Self-assessment on Chapter 3: questions	44
	Self-assessment on Chapter 3: answers	47

Overview

Major risk factors for cardiovascular and cerebrovascular disease may be non-modifiable (age, gender, family and personal history) or modifiable (smoking, hyperlipidaemia, hypertension and diabetes). These factors will combine to put a person at high or low risk of cardiovascular or cerebrovascular events. Patients are considered to be at high risk if they have established ischaemic heart disease, a combination of risk factors that makes their risk of a cardiovascular event greater or equal to 30% over 10 years, severe hypertension or hyperlipidaemia. For these patients drug treatment may be necessary to lower the risk. The major classes of drug to treat hypertension are: thiazide diuretics, beta-blockers, drugs acting on the renin–angiotensin–aldosterone system and calcium-channel blockers. The major drugs used to treat hyperlipidaemia are the 3-hydroxy-3-methylglutaryl-CoA reductase inhibitors ('statins').

3.1 Clinical aspects and cardiovascular risk factors

Learning objectives

At the end of this section you should be able to:

- list the major non-modifiable and modifiable risk factors
- understand the interaction of these factors to produce overall cardiovascular risk
- identify patients at high risk of cardiovascular disease
- advise on general and specific measures to decrease that risk.

Clinical sketch

A 57-year-old man has smoked 40 cigarettes a day for the past 40 years. His blood pressure is 186/106 mmHg and his total cholesterol to serum HDL ratio is 5. He has recently been diagnosed as suffering from type 2 diabetes mellitus.

Comment: this man illustrates how risk factors accumulate in individual patients to put them at high risk of a cardiovascular event. Work out this patient's cardiovascular risk (i.e. the risk of a cardiovascular event over the next 10 years) from the risk tables in Figure 20.

Cardiovascular disease (such as angina, myocardial infarction) and cerebrovascular disease are among the most common causes of death. The presence of cardiovascular risk factors puts a person at higher or lower risk of these conditions. These risk factors may be non-modifiable (e.g. age, gender, family or personal history) or modifiable (smoking, hyperlipidaemia, hypertension). Diabetes mellitus is a further risk factor that is partially modifiable by better control of the diabetes. Many of these risk factors are asymptomatic until they cause disease, and so it may be wise to screen apparently healthy people to detect them.

In general, many risk factors can be treated by lifestyle changes that could be almost universally recommended (better diet, stopping smoking, more exercise). Some modifiable risk factors may require pharmacological intervention (hyperlipidaemia, hypertension and, for some patients, stopping smoking – see Ch. 18).

In deciding whether to treat these conditions, it is generally helpful to consider the patient's overall risk. In patients with more non-modifiable risk factors or with established cardiovascular disease, it is important to treat the modifiable risks more aggressively.

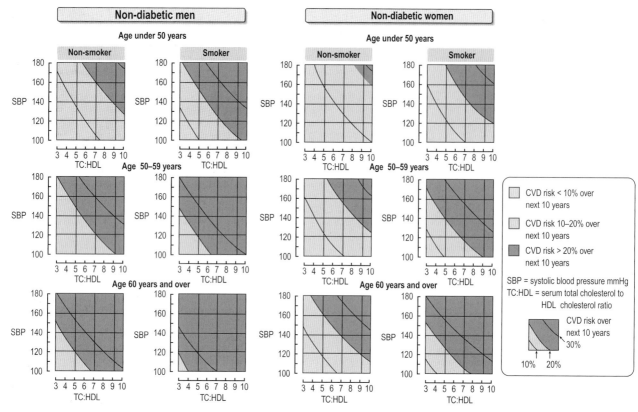

Fig. 20 Coronary risk prediction charts. These charts are used to estimate risk of coronary heart disease (CHD: non-fatal myocardial infarction and coronary death) for individuals who have not developed symptomatic CHD or other major, atherosclerotic disease. SBP, systolic blood pressure (mmHg); TC:HDL, ratio JOF serum total cholesterol to high density lipoprotein cholesterol. (With permission from Heart 2005, 91: v1–v52.)

Primary prevention is intended to stop the disease from becoming established, e.g. in a patient with many risk factors. Secondary prevention is limiting further damage in patients who already have the disease (e.g. patients who have had a myocardial infarction).

Level of risk

Patients are at high risk of coronary and cerebrovascular disease if they have:

- a previous history of ischaemic heart disease
- evidence of end-organ damage caused by hypertension (e.g. cardiac enlargement)
- diabetes mellitus
- multiple risk factors giving an overall risk of 20% or more of having a cardiovascular event over the next 10 years.

The relative risk of an event can be calculated from epidemiological data. An easy way to assess risk in practice is a series of graphs based on this epidemiological data (see Fig. 20). These graphs do not apply to patients who have already had ischaemic heart disease and may not apply well to some very high-risk populations such as Asians resident in the UK.

Sometimes a single risk factor is so important or severe that it requires treatment on its own, even if the patient's overall risk is less than 20%.

3.2 Hypertension

Learning objectives

At the end of this section you should:

- be able to identify patients whose blood pressure requires treatment
- be able to advise on general measures
- be able to describe each of the four major classes of antihypertensive drug and give examples
- be able to describe how these drugs might be used in practice
- know the management of hypertensive emergencies.

Clinical sketch

A 72-year-old woman has a blood pressure of 180/84 mmHg. Her doctor is aware of this but is reluctant to treat her because this blood pressure is normal for her age.

Comment: blood pressure does tend to rise with increasing age, but this is associated with an increased risk of stroke, which can be reduced by treating the hypertension. This pressure is definitely not 'normal' for her age although it is fairly common. The target in such a patient will be a systolic of less than 140 mmHg. This may be difficult to achieve without causing unacceptable adverse effects and this must be balanced against the potential benefits to the patient of successfully lowering her blood pressure to this target. This patient has lone systolic hypertension, once not considered a cardiovascular risk but now known also to be associated with an increased risk of stroke.

Hypertension refers to high blood pressure, which can damage blood vessels and predispose to the development of atheromatous disease. In severe cases, it can also cause heart and renal failure. Treating hypertension reduces mortality and morbidity from these conditions, particularly from cerebrovascular disease but also from ischaemic heart disease.

Causes of hypertension

The cause of hypertension is usually unknown ('primary' or 'essential' hypertension), but about 5–10% of cases are secondary, resulting from alcohol abuse, coarctation of the aorta, phaeochromocytoma (a tumour that secretes catecholamines), primary hyperaldosteronism (often due to Conn's syndrome – an excess of aldosterone secretion from either an adenoma or bilateral adrenal hyperplasia), Cushing's syndrome (excessive glucocorticoids, either endogenous or iatrogenic), or renal disease (including renal artery stenosis).

Diagnosis

Blood pressure is a continuous variable and the point at which it becomes 'hypertension' is a little arbitrary. The British Hypertension Society guidelines for when to start treatment are shown in Figure 21. These take account of both the severity of the blood pressure alone and also the overall cardiovascular risk.

Blood pressure should usually be measured on three or more occasions, while the patient is sitting comfortably, over a period of several weeks before a decision is made to treat, although very high blood pressure with complications may require immediate treatment. Systolic blood pressure is more important than diastolic.

Treatment

Urgent lowering of blood pressure is rarely necessary (but see below, Box 1, Hypertensive emergencies). Non-pharmacological treatment should be the first approach in mild to moderate hypertension, including weight loss, alcohol and salt restriction, perhaps behavioural therapy, and mild exercise. Other cardiovascular risk factors, such as smoking, hyperlipidaemia, etc., should also be considered. If these measures fail to improve the blood pressure substantially over a period of months, or sooner in patients with more severe hypertension or more risk factors, drug therapy should be considered.

The target blood pressure is usually a systolic pressure of less than 140 mmHg, or a fall of at least 10 mmHg, and a diastolic pressure of not more than 85 mmHg, but these figures, like the level at which to begin treatment, depend on consideration of the patient's risk factors – diabetic patients, for instance, should be treated to achieve 130/80 mmHg or less.

Drugs in hypertension

There are four major classes of drug used in the treatment of hypertension:

- thiazide and other diuretics
- beta-blockers
- drugs that affect the renin–angiotensin–aldosterone system
- calcium-channel blockers.

Thiazides and other diuretics

Diuretics promote the excretion of water. They can act at different sites in the nephron and in different ways. There are three major groups:

- thiazides
- loop diuretics
- potassium-sparing diuretics.

Thiazides

Thiazides act by inhibiting the absorption of Na^+ in the distal convoluted tubule. Water is lost with the Na^+. More Na^+ reaches the distal tubule, where it is exchanged for K^+, and the thiazides also cause K^+ loss. Magnesium is also lost, while Ca^{2+} is retained

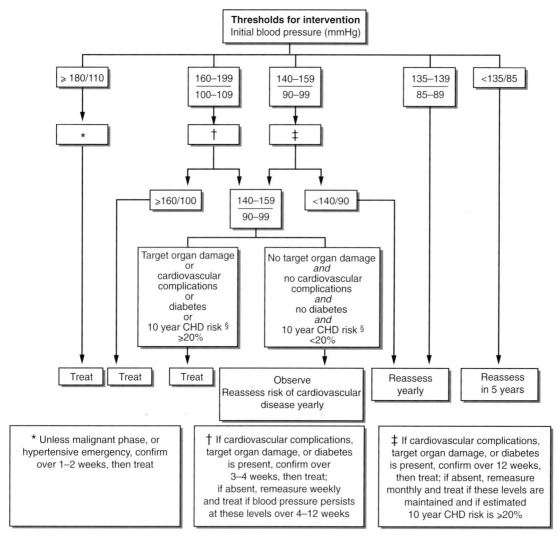

§ Assessed with risk chart for cardiovascular disease

Fig. 21 The British Hypertension Society guidelines on when to start treatment in hypertension (Journal of Human Hypertension (2004) 18:139–185).

(Fig. 22). The major effect in hypertension, however, is a vasodilatory effect, and little effect comes from the diuresis.

The maximal hypotensive response to thiazides is reached at relatively low doses, In the past, thiazides were used in excessively high doses with no better antihypertensive effect and a higher incidence of adverse effects.

Example. Bendroflumethiazide is well absorbed after oral administration and causes a diuresis in about 1–2 hours which lasts for up to 12 hours.

Therapeutic uses
- hypertension
- congestive cardiac failure.

Adverse effects
- dehydration: a risk in all diuretic use, especially in the elderly
- hypokalaemia: usually mild and not requiring treatment
- hyponatraemia
- hyperuricaemia/gout (due to impaired clearance of uric acid)
- impaired glucose tolerance/diabetes mellitus
- hypercholesterolaemia: in short-term therapy, but probably not seen in long-term use
- impotence
- hypercalcaemia.

Contraindications
- gout
- renal disease.

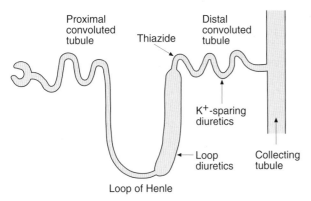

Proximal convoluted tubule

Thiazide

Distal convoluted tubule

K⁺-sparing diuretics

Loop diuretics

Collecting tubule

Loop of Henle

Fig. 22 Sites of action of diuretics.

Loop diuretics

Loop diuretics (*furosemide* or *bumetanide*) are not effective antihypertensives if used alone. They are useful in hypertension only in combination with other drugs or in renal failure. They are discussed in the section on heart failure in Chapter 4.

Potassium-sparing diuretics

Potassium-sparing diuretics are a chemically diverse group that, unlike other diuretics, retain potassium (K⁺). They act in the distal convoluted tubule where K⁺/Na⁺ exchange occurs and are only weak diuretics. Their major use now is in heart failure (see Ch. 4) but they are also effective in treating or preventing hypokalaemia caused by thiazides or loop diuretics, and in some cases of hypertension due to hyperaldosteronism. In the past, K⁺ supplements were widely used, but very high doses are required, reducing patient compliance. It is not often necessary to prevent or treat diuretic-induced hypokalaemia, but if this is required, K⁺-sparing diuretics should be used.

Examples. *Spironolactone* is an aldosterone antagonist. Aldosterone causes Na⁺ retention and K⁺ loss, and spironolactone does the reverse. It can be used in treating hypertension caused by primary hyperaldosteronism (Conn's syndrome). It is also used in heart failure and in other conditions with fluid retention.

Triamterene and *amiloride* interfere with Na⁺/K⁺ exchange.

All are administered orally.

Adverse effects
- hyperkalaemia
- gynaecomastia (spironolactone only).

Drug interactions

The action of thiazides and loop diuretics is inhibited by non-steroidal anti-inflammatory drugs. Lithium (Ch. 6) excretion may be reduced by diuretics and this can lead to serious toxicity.

Potassium-sparing diuretics can interact with K⁺ supplements or angiotensin-converting enzyme (ACE) inhibitors to cause dangerous hyperkalaemia.

Loop diuretics can be combined with K⁺-sparing diuretics to reduce K⁺ loss, or with ACE inhibitors in heart failure or hypertension.

Beta-blockers

The beta-blockers competitively block the β-adrenoceptors in the heart and thereby reduce the noradrenaline- (norepinephrine) and adrenaline (epinephrine)-induced production of cyclic AMP. The β-adrenoceptors in the heart are mostly β₁-adrenoceptors but β₂-adrenoceptors are also present. Beta-blockers can be non-selective (act on both types of receptor) or selective (mainly affect β₁-adrenoceptors).

Beta-blockers improve oxygen availability by:

- decreasing oxygen demand
  — slowing the heart
  — reducing its force of contraction
- increasing oxygen supply by lengthening diastole, during which most blood flow in the coronary arteries occurs.

They are, thus, effective in treating angina (see Ch. 4) and also lower blood pressure in patients with angina and in other patients. The exact mechanism of this lowering of blood pressure is not known.

Beta-blockers must be avoided (even the relatively selective β₁-blockers) in patients dependent on β-stimulation, e.g. asthmatics.

Some beta-blockers have partial agonist (stimulating) activity (also known as intrinsic sympathomimetic activity) at the β-adrenoceptor in addition to beta-blocking properties. These drugs may cause less bradycardia and peripheral vasoconstriction than other beta-blockers.

When blocked by prolonged use of a beta-blocker, the β-adrenoceptor may undergo upregulation, i.e. the number and sensitivity of the receptors increase. This may make sudden withdrawal of beta-blockers dangerous in patients with ischaemic heart disease, as the patient may suffer a rebound worsening of angina.

Examples. Beta-blockers may be lipophilic (penetrate lipids and cell membranes well and are metabolised by the liver) or hydrophilic (do not penetrate lipids and membranes so well and are excreted unchanged by the kidney rather than metabolised). The three beta-blockers most widely used are:

propranolol: a lipophilic non-selective beta-blocker
atenolol: a hydrophilic β₁-selective blocker
metoprolol: a lipophilic β₁-selective blocker.

Therapeutic uses
- hypertension
- angina pectoris
- myocardial infarction (both acute treatment and to reduce risk of recurrence)
- antiarrhythmic
- heart failure (see Ch. 4)
- anxiety (reduces manifestations of anxiety such as tremor).

Chapter 4 gives more details of therapeutic uses.

Adverse effects
- bradycardia, including heart block
- bronchospasm
- peripheral vasoconstriction: cold hands and feet
- fatigue, depression, vivid dreams (especially the lipophilic drugs).

Contraindications
- asthma or any obstructive airway disease
- Raynaud's phenomenon or peripheral vascular disease
- heart block of any degree

Drugs affecting the renin–angiotensin–aldosterone system

The renin–angiotensin–aldosterone system (Fig. 23) is vital in maintaining blood volume and renal blood supply. In some hypertensives, this system is relatively overactive. ACE inhibitors are particularly effective in hypertension if used with a diuretic; this increases dependence on the renin–angiotensin system, which is then blocked. Angiotensin II has other effects in tissues, resulting in new tissue formation. In some situations this may be harmful.

ACE inhibitors

ACE inhibitors prevent the formation of angiotensin II, preventing its vasoconstrictor effects as well as decreasing aldosterone production and fluid retention. ACE also breaks down a number of inflammatory peptides, such as bradykinin, and the potentiation of these may contribute to its antihypertensive effect.

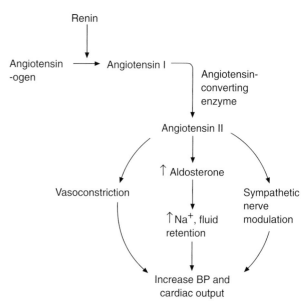

Fig. 23 The renin–angiotensin–aldosterone axis.

Examples
Captopril is given orally and is cleared by the kidney. It is given two or three times per day.
Enalapril is also given orally. It is a prodrug and is activated to the active compound, enalaprilat, by the liver. It is cleared by the kidneys. Enalapril is given once per day.
Ramipril is given orally, usually twice per day.

Therapeutic uses
- hypertension
- cardiac failure: ACE inhibitors clearly reduce mortality (Ch. 4)
- after myocardial infarction
- reducing progression to renal failure in diabetic patients with microalbuminuria (whether hypertensive or not).

These last two uses may relate to preventing inappropriate new tissue development.

Adverse effects
- severe hypotension: especially in renal artery stenosis, or in patients with heart failure, on the first dose, or in patients on high-dose diuretics; these patients may be highly dependent on raised renin and angiotensin concentrations. Starting doses should be very low and gradually increased. The dose of diuretic should be reduced as much as possible before starting ACE inhibitors
- hyperkalaemia: because K⁺-losing effects of aldosterone are blocked

- impairment of renal function: through decrease in renal perfusion and intrarenal haemodynamics
- cough: very common but not usually serious, probably occurs through potentiation of bradykinin
- angioedema: more serious and possibly also caused by potentiation of bradykinin
- occasionally worsening of asthma. Use with caution in these patients.

Contraindications
- renal artery stenosis, which is often asymptomatic but should be suspected in a patient with hypertension and peripheral vascular disease
- other forms of renal disease: ACE inhibitors should be used cautiously because they may precipitate a reduction in renal function.

Drug interactions
- with K^+-sparing diuretics or K^+ supplements: a risk of dangerous hyperkalaemia.

Angiotensin II receptor antagonists

Drugs can block the receptor at which angiotensin II acts rather than blocking its production. Their effects are broadly similar to those of ACE inhibitors, but because they will not affect bradykinin, cough is rare. They are predominantly used at present in the management of hypertension but may be increasingly used for the management of heart failure and diabetic nephropathy.

Examples
Losartan (short acting); *valsartan* (longer acting).

Calcium-channel blockers

In cardiac muscle or vascular smooth muscle, a change in membrane potential causes Ca^{2+} to enter the cell through voltage-dependent calcium channels. Calcium is essential in the interaction between actin and myosin filaments causing muscle contraction. Calcium-channel blockers inhibit the voltage-dependent calcium channels, and reduce Ca^{2+} entry. They reduce smooth muscle contraction and cause vasodilatation and hence are useful in hypertension and in angina. They also reduce the force of contraction of the heart, and slow the heart rate in vitro. They have no effect on skeletal muscle, which is less dependent on exogenous Ca^{2+}.

Examples. There are three types of calcium-channel blocker, which bind to different but related receptor sites on the calcium channel and have different effects in different tissues.

Dihydropyridines. This group (e.g. *nifedipine*, *amlodipine*) mainly cause intense arterial vasodilatation and lower the blood pressure and the afterload (i.e. the load against which the heart must eject blood) on the heart. If short-acting drugs are used, the vasodilatation can cause a sympathetic reflex, which increases the heart rate and force of contraction. Amlodipine is long acting, while nifedipine is short acting but administered in modified release preparations to mimic a long-acting drug. They are well absorbed orally and metabolised by the liver.

Verapamil. Unlike nifedipine, verapamil tends to have more effect on the heart, slowing the heart and reducing force of contraction, and less effect on the peripheral circulation. It also slows conduction through the atrioventricular (AV) node (where the action potential is largely dependent on Ca^{2+}) and has a special role in treating supraventricular tachycardia. Verapamil is usually given orally or can be given intravenously in treating supraventricular tachycardias. It is metabolised by the liver, and there is extensive first pass metabolism.

Diltiazem has more effect on the heart than nifedipine, and more effect on the peripheral circulation than verapamil. Diltiazem is metabolised by the liver.

Therapeutic uses. All the calcium-channel blockers are used for hypertension and angina. Nifedipine is also used for Raynaud's phenomenon and verapamil is also used for supraventricular tachycardia.

Adverse effects. These mainly result from smooth muscle relaxation and vasodilatation.

nifedipine: facial flushing and ankle swelling, headaches and dizziness
verapamil: headaches and dizziness, constipation, heart block and bradycardia
diltiazem: constipation, ankle oedema, flushing, headache.

Drug interactions. Nifedipine can be combined with beta-blockers in angina or hypertension; rarely, the combination may precipitate heart failure. The combination of verapamil with beta-blockers can be dangerous (especially if verapamil is given i.v.) and causes severe hypotension and bradycardia.

Other drugs used in hypertension

Other drugs used in hypertension include alpha-blockers and some drugs used in special circumstances, which are considered below. Some drugs are largely obsolete: they include hydralazine, an arterial vasodilator, and methyldopa, which still has a role in treating hypertension in pregnancy.

Three

Alpha-blockers

The alpha-blockers (e.g. *prazosin, doxazosin*) vasodilate by blocking the α_1-adrenoceptor in peripheral blood vessels. Adverse effects include postural hypotension (particularly a risk after the first dose), headache, urinary frequency and tachycardia. There is some concern that these drugs may not reduce mortality despite lowering blood pressure.

Choice of drug in hypertension

All the four major classes have been shown to reduce mortality from stroke and, in some cases, from myocardial infarction. In general, most believe that the key to reducing events is lowering the blood pressure adequately rather than using any particular class of drugs.

In the past, the general approach was the use of 'stepped care': i.e. step 1, a thiazide or a beta-blocker; step 2, a thiazide and a beta-blocker; step 3, a thiazide, a beta-blocker and a vasodilator. This approach is still often applied but today a more 'tailored care' approach is favoured, i.e. tailoring the choice of drug to the individual patient taking into account the total risk factor profile.

There is debate over whether patients who fail to respond to the first antihypertensive drug should have a second drug added to the first or substituted instead of the first.

Clinical sketch

A patient presents with high blood pressure which is sustained on repeated readings. The doctor initiates treatment with bendroflumethiazide and although this lowers blood pressure slightly, it is still unsatisfactory. The doctor then adds in a second drug, atenolol, which again achieves some lowering of blood pressure, but this remains unsatisfactory. The doctor adds in a third drug, a calcium-channel blocker, amlodipine. Satisfactory blood pressure is achieved on this.

Comment: many patients need multiple drug therapy to achieve satisfactory blood pressure levels. This increases the risk of adverse effects. Some patients may have apparently uncontrollable hypertension, not because their blood pressure is genuinely poorly controlled but because the patient may be poorly compliant with antihypertensive medications, or because the patient has the phenomenon of white coat hypertension, i.e. the blood pressure goes up whenever it is measured. Failure to recognise this condition can lead to overtreatment. It is best detected by 24 hour ambulatory blood pressure monitoring.

Thiazides. The oldest drugs, the thiazides, have particularly strong evidence and are inexpensive, which is important considering the large numbers of hypertensive patients. They are therefore the first choice for most patients, especially the elderly. However, they are not suitable for patients with hypercholesterolaemia, renal disease or gout.

Beta-blockers. These are also a reasonable first choice, especially in younger patients or patients with angina pectoris. They are not suitable for patients with asthma, heart failure or peripheral vascular disease. There is some evidence that they are less effective than the other classes in reducing major cardiovascular events.

ACE inhibitors. First choice in diabetics but best avoided in renal disease; they need close monitoring of renal function.

Calcium-channel blockers. These tend to have a higher rate of adverse effects, but this is improved by the use of slow-release preparations. Useful in patients with angina, hyperlipidaemia or renal disease. Expensive.

Alpha-blockers. These are considered a second-line drug in patients who do not tolerate other drugs; possibly suitable particularly for hyperlipidaemics or patients with urinary hesitancy.

Combinations. No more than 50–60% of patients will respond to any one drug; many patients will need more than one. Appropriate combinations include thiazide plus beta-blocker; thiazide plus ACE inhibitor; beta-blocker plus calcium-channel blocker; ACE inhibitor and calcium-channel blocker. A logical scheme of combining drugs with some supportive evidence is given in the ABCD rule, where A stands for ACE inhibitors or angiotensin II receptor blockers, B for beta-blockers, C for calcium channel blockers and D for diuretics. It is broadly thought that A and B drugs act in a similar manner, while C and D drugs also act by similar mechanisms. It is logical therefore that if an AB drug does not work as first line, one should try instead a CD drug (and vice versa). If one wishes to achieve added effects, one should combine an AB drug with a CD drug in the first instance.

In coexisting disease. Some patients who have hypertension and other diseases might be considered more suitable for certain drugs:

- with asthma or chronic obstructive pulmonary disease (COPD): diuretics or calcium-channel blockers
- with heart failure: diuretics and ACE inhibitors

- with angina: beta-blockers or calcium-channel blockers
- with diabetes mellitus: ACE inhibitors.

Monitoring

Patients treated for hypertension need regular monitoring of their blood pressure and for adverse effects and review of their cardiovascular risk. Patient education on the need for antihypertensives and on the use of their medication is very important.

Treatment of hypertension in special circumstances

Box 1 outlines the treatment of hypertensive emergencies.

Box 1 Hypertensive emergencies

Emergency lowering of blood pressure is only indicated in patients with hypertensive encephalopathy, or hypertension-induced renal or heart failure. These conditions are nowadays unusual.

Very high blood pressure readings alone in the absence of these conditions do not warrant emergency blood pressure reduction, which may be dangerous by reducing cerebral or coronary perfusion.

If emergency treatment is needed, the patient should be admitted to hospital for rest and very careful monitoring.

Oral therapy with beta-blockers, ACE inhibitors or calcium-channel blockers may be adequate in most cases. In rare cases where parenteral therapy is necessary, *sodium nitroprusside* is given by i.v. infusion, but only in an intensive care ward. Sodium nitroprusside is a very powerful arterial and venous vasodilator. It acts very rapidly and has a very short duration of action: blood pressure rises within a minute of the infusion being stopped. It allows control of the blood pressure while other slower-acting drugs are introduced. If used for prolonged periods (>24 hours), cyanide, a toxic metabolite, may form. *Labetalol*, a combined alpha- and beta-blocker, can also be given i.v.

Resistant hypertension

Failure to respond to triple therapy with standard drugs should be fully investigated to exclude secondary hypertension. Poor compliance with treatment or 'white coat' hypertension are common and may give the appearance of resistance.

Minoxidil is used in resistant hypertension. It is a vasodilator that causes fluid retention and tachy-

cardia and for that reason should be used only with diuretics and a beta-blocker. A peculiar side-effect is the stimulation of male pattern hair growth, and hence it is generally avoided in women.

Hypertension in pregnancy

This is covered in Chapter 19.

3.3 Hyperlipidaemia

Learning objectives

At the end of this section you should be able to:
- identify patients who require treatment for hyperlipidaemia
- describe the drugs used in the treatment of hyperlipidaemia and their practical use.

Hyperlipidaemia refers to high levels of fats in blood. There are two major fractions of fats in blood: cholesterol and triglycerides.

Cholesterol is derived from the diet and also manufactured in all cells but mainly by the liver. It is essential for the formation of lipid membranes, steroid hormones and many other vital bodily functions. Triglycerides are used as an energy source.

Clinical sketch

A 62-year-old man had a myocardial infarction but has now recovered. His serum cholesterol is 5.8 mmol/L despite diet. His medications include aspirin and atenolol. He wonders if his cholesterol should be treated.

Comment: this is secondary prevention, i.e. the treatment of a patient who has already had an event to try to prevent further events. Patients who have had an event have already shown themselves to be at very high risk, and the risk tables do not apply to such patients. The risk tables only apply to primary prevention. Other examples of patients worthy of secondary prevention include patients with established angina or peripheral vascular disease. Such patients need rigorous lowering of their serum cholesterol, ideally to a serum cholesterol of less than 5 mmol/L. This is likely to require the prescribing of a drug such as simvastatin.

Absorbed cholesterol is taken from the intestine in chylomicrons to the liver. Cholesterol and triglyceride are then transported in the blood from the liver in association with lipoproteins, as very low density lipoproteins (VLDL). VLDL are broken down by lipoprotein lipase in peripheral tissues to low density lipoproteins (LDL). LDL carry cholesterol to the cells, and these are cleared by specific receptors on the cells and especially in the liver. LDL cholesterol is particularly associated with atheroma and cardiovascular disease. High density lipoproteins (HDL) carry cholesterol from the tissues back to the liver (reverse transport) and seem to be protective against atheroma. The ratio of LDL cholesterol to HDL cholesterol is used in measuring cardiovascular risk.

Triglycerides are less important than cholesterol in causing atherosclerosis. High triglyceride concentrations are associated with pancreatitis.

Some forms of hypercholesterolaemia are inherited either as a single gene (usually severe), or more commonly as polygenic traits (less severe). Hypercholesterolaemia may occur as an isolated abnormality or in association with rises in triglycerides. Isolated hypertriglyceridaemia can also occur.

The exact cholesterol concentration requiring treatment depends on the patient's overall cardiovascular risk. In high-risk patients, such as those who have established ischaemic heart disease, treating a total cholesterol level above 3.5 mmol/L would be appropriate, while in otherwise healthy patients, patients might be better treated on the basis of their overall cardiovascular risk (cholesterol $\geq$3.5 and a risk $\geq$20% over 10 years). All diabetic patients are considered to be at high risk. The target cholesterol is the lower of:

- in high risk patients: $\leq$3.5 mmol/L or a 25% reduction in total cholesterol (whichever is lower), or a 30% reduction in LDL
- for other patients: $\leq$5.0 mmol/L or a 25% reduction in total cholesterol (whichever is lower), or a 30% reduction in LDL.

Some advocate administering statins to patients at high risk without any subsequent monitoring of the cholesterol, on the grounds that it allows statins to be prescribed to large numbers of patients easily, without the time-consuming barrier of excessive monitoring and will reduce cardiovascular risk regardless of the final concentration of cholesterol attained.

In patients with a family single gene inherited hyperlipidaemia, more aggressive treatment should be undertaken even in the absence of other risk factors. These patients often have very high cholesterol levels (>8.0 mmol/L).

Lowering cholesterol concentrations by some drugs reduces mortality from ischaemic heart disease either in secondary prevention or in high-risk patients in primary prevention. It may also reduce the risks of stroke although this is less certain.

Underlying diseases that may cause hyperlipidaemia, such as hypothyroidism or liver disease, should be excluded. At least two readings of cholesterol should be obtained over 2–3 months.

Treatment

The first line of treatment for hyperlipidaemia should always be diet, although in many patients this will be ineffective, sometimes because of poor compliance. Drug therapy may be needed in patients who do not respond to diet alone after several months. Drugs may take several weeks to achieve their effects and frequent changes of drug are not advised.

Drugs in hypercholesterolaemia

The statins: 3-hydroxy-3-methylglutaryl-CoA reductase inhibitors

3-Hydroxy-3-methylglutaryl (HMG)-CoA reductase is an enzyme that controls the rate-limiting step in the synthesis of cholesterol in the liver. If inhibited, the hepatocyte cannot manufacture cholesterol and responds by increasing its uptake of LDL from the blood. This does not interfere with the production of steroid hormones. Drugs that inhibit this enzyme are the most effective cholesterol-lowering drugs and reduce plasma LDL by as much as 50% depending on the dose used. In patients treated with these drugs, the relative risk of cardiovascular disease falls by about 25–30%. They are usually very well tolerated.

These drugs are very effective and are proven to reduce the risk of death and cardiovascular events in high risk patients.

Examples

Simvastatin and *atorvastatin*, both taken once a day. Simvastatin has the best evidence base and is far less expensive.

Therapeutic use

Hypercholesterolaemia, with or without hypertriglyceridaemia, which may also be lowered.

Adverse effects
- headache
- abdominal pain
- transient minor elevations of liver function tests or of creatine phosphokinase are common and

usually resolve spontaneously despite continued therapy

- myositis (rare but can be severe)
- simvastatin (but not atorvastatin) can interfere with the metabolism of warfarin.

Other drugs

Ezetimibe inhibits the intestinal absorption of cholesterol. It can be used alone or in combination with statins. It can cause gastrointestinal disturbances.

Nicotinic acid lowers both cholesterol and triglyceride concentrations by inhibiting synthesis. It also increases HDL cholesterol. Its use is limited by its adverse effects, in particular vasodilatation and facial flushing. It can be used alone or with statins.

Fibrates (e.g. *gemfibrozil*, *bezafibrate*, *fenofibrate*) mainly lower triglycerides, and to a lesser extent LDL cholesterol, while increasing HDL cholesterol. Their exact actions are unclear but may include inhibition of HMG-CoA reductase (see above) and activation of lipoprotein lipase. They are heavily protein bound and this may interfere with other drugs, e.g. warfarin. They are proven to lower mortality from ischaemic heart disease, though in general are less effective and not as well tolerated as statins.

Their adverse effects include myositis, gastrointestinal upset and increased gallstone formation.

Three

Self-assessment on Chapter 3: questions

Multiple choice questions

1. Drugs used in treating hypertension include:
   a. Diuretics
   b. Levodopa
   c. Oral nitrates
   d. ACE inhibitors
   e. Naproxen

2. In hypertension:
   a. A curable cause is found in most cases
   b. Treatment reduces the risks of stroke
   c. The choice of drug is often dictated by the patient's overall condition
   d. Non-drug therapy has no role
   e. A blood pressure reading of 210/120 mmHg with no complications requires urgent i.v. therapy

3. Calcium-channel blockers:
   a. Are negatively inotropic
   b. Are all highly selective for vascular smooth muscle
   c. Can cause oedema
   d. Sublingual nifedipine may be used in hypertensive crisis
   e. Are proven to reduce the risk of stroke when used to treat hypertension

4. With regard to hypercholesterolaemia:
   a. Patients with an average serum cholesterol are not at risk of myocardial infarction
   b. Lowering serum cholesterol by drugs improves life expectancy
   c. Hyperthyroidism may cause hypercholesterolaemia in patients without overt ischaemic heart disease
   d. Cholesterol is a vital part of cell membranes
   e. High HDL cholesterol is associated with an increased risk of atherosclerosis

5. Considering the drugs used to treat hyperlipidaemia:
   a. Simvastatin inhibits drug-metabolising enzymes
   b. Gemfibrozil may cause gallstones
   c. Simvastatin has a long safety record and can be recommended as first-line therapy
   d. Statins can be used for mixed hyperlipidaemia
   e. Ezetimibe increases the metabolism of LDL

6. The following drugs are correctly paired with their adverse effects:
   a. Gemfibrozil and abdominal pain
   b. Beta-blockers and cold hands
   c. Verapamil and diarrhoea
   d. Simvastatin and Addison's syndrome (adrenocortical failure)
   e. Thiazides and hypothyroidism

Case history questions

Case history 1

A 54-year-old man is a non-insulin-dependent diabetic and obese. He smokes 20 cigarettes per day. His blood pressure is 160/100 mmHg and his serum cholesterol is 6.4 mmol/L.

1. What is his risk of a cardiovascular event over the next 10 years?
2. What advice should he be given about his lifestyle?
3. What drug therapies might be considered for his hypertension?
4. What target would you set for his blood pressure control?
5. What drug therapies might be considered for his hypercholesterolaemia?
6. Should he be on any other drugs?

Case history 2

A 55-year-old woman is found to have a blood pressure of 180/110 mmHg on several occasions. No cause is found, although she is obese.

1. She asks why she should be bothered about her blood pressure; what will you tell her?
2. What other cardiovascular risk factors need to be considered?

3. What drug therapy might be considered as a first line?

Her blood pressure is still not controlled.

4. What factors might you need to reconsider?
5. What drug therapy might be tried next?

Case history 3

A 45-year-old man who has had a myocardial infarction is found to have a serum cholesterol of 6.4 mmol/L.

1. Is this cause for concern?

His triglycerides are normal and the LDL cholesterol is the fraction raised. He is given a low-cholesterol diet but his serum cholesterol does not improve over the next 3 months.

2. What treatment should be considered now?
3. What adverse effects should he be warned of?
4. What other drugs might he need to take?
5. Will lowering the patient's serum cholesterol substantially reduce the risk of further episodes of ischaemic heart disease?

Short note questions

Write short notes on the following:

1. Describe the management of a patient presenting to his GP with a blood pressure of 170/110 mmHg, with no other symptoms or signs of organ damage.
2. Two patients are found to have a serum cholesterol of 6.0 mmol/L and total cholesterol to HDL ratio of 4.2. The first is a 52-year-old man who has angina and smokes. The second is a 36-year-old woman who is normotensive (systolic blood pressure of 128 mmHg) and a non-smoker. She is not diabetic. How would you treat each of these two patients?

Extended matching items questions

Theme: Treatment of hypertension

Options
A. Doxazosin
B. Irbesartan
C. Hydralazine
D. Bendroflumethiazide
E. Diazepam
F. Amiodarone
G. Moxonidine
H. Minoxidil
I. Atenolol
J. Diltiazem
K. Isosorbide mononitrate
L. Enalapril
M. Nifedipine
N. Methyldopa

For each of the patients numbered 1–4 below, all of whom have mild hypertension, select the *most* appropriate drug therapy to lower the blood pressure from options A–N above. Each option may be used once, more than once or not at all.

1. A 40-year-old woman who has asthma and who uses salbutamol and beclometasone inhalers.
2. A 50-year-old man who has been an insulin-dependent diabetic for 30 years and who has significant proteinuria.
3. A 70-year-old man with a previous history of gout.
4. A 60-year-old woman, a heavy smoker despite your advice, who also has COPD (chronic obstructive pulmonary disease) and angina.

Patients 5–8 are treated for hypertension. In each case, they have suffered an adverse drug effect. Select from options A–N above which drugs might have caused the adverse effects described and which drugs would be suitable alternatives.

5. A 57-year-old woman with wheeze and coughing.
6. A 58-year-old woman with ankle swelling. She also has asthma.

7. A 70-year-old man who has developed type 2 diabetes mellitus.

8. A 30-year-old woman with severe headache.

For patients 9 and 10 below, their blood pressure has been uncontrolled on their first line drug therapy, the dose of which has been optimised. From the list of options, select a suitable drug either to combine with their existing therapy or to substitute for it.

9. A 60-year-old man whose BP is 170/96 despite enalapril.

10. A 48-year-old woman whose BP is 160/94 despite amlodipine.

Self-assessment on Chapter 3: answers

Multiple choice answers

1. a. **True.** Thiazides are the main diuretics used but in patients with resistant hypertension or renal disease, loop diuretics are used.
   b. **False.** Levodopa is used to treat Parkinson's disease (see Ch. 6). Methyldopa is sometimes used to treat hypertension.
   c. **False.** Oral nitrates have little effect in hypertension.
   d. **True.** This is their most common use.
   e. **False.** Naproxen is a non-steroidal anti-inflammatory drug, many of which can cause fluid retention and exacerbate hypertension.

2. a. **False.** Only in 5–10% of cases is an underlying and treatable cause found.
   b. **True.** This is the main justification for treating hypertension.
   c. **True.** This is the essence of 'tailored care'.
   d. **False.** Although how effective non-drug therapy is, is often debated.
   e. **False.** Blood pressure is often overtreated in this situation. Oral therapy is probably adequate.

3. a. **True.** They reduce the force of contraction and may cause cardiac failure. Nifedipine may increase the force of contraction by sympathetic reflex; however, if the patient is taking beta-blockers, this is prevented and the negative inotropic effects of nifedipine may become more apparent.
   b. **False.** Hence adverse effects such as constipation, caused by smooth muscle relaxation in the gastrointestinal tract.
   c. **True.** Due to venodilatation. This oedema is resistant to diuretics which should not be used to treat it. If it is a problem, change to a different antihypertensive.
   d. **False.** This was a popular treatment that lowered the blood pressure but can cause stroke or myocardial infarction because of the speed with which the blood pressure falls. Urgent treatment in hypertension is rarely necessary, so oral preparations are best used (including long-acting preparations of nifedipine).
   e. **True.** For some specific calcium-channel blockers (e.g. nitrendipine, a derivative of nifedipine) and presumably also for other calcium-channel blockers.

4. a. **False.** Cholesterol is only one risk factor and, in the UK, the average concentration is associated with ischaemic heart disease.
   b. **True.** Both in secondary prevention and in high-risk patients.
   c. **False.** Hypothyroidism causes hypercholesterolaemia.
   d. **True.**
   e. **False.** High HDL cholesterol concentrations seem to be protective against ischaemic heart disease. High LDL cholesterol concentrations are associated with increased risk. The ratio of HDL to LDL cholesterol is the favourite measure of cholesterol for assessing cardiac risk.

5. a. **True.** It can interfere with the metabolism of warfarin – an effect not found with pravastatin.
   b. **True.** A well-recognised adverse effect.
   c. **True.** Simvastatin has an established safety record and is proved to reduce overall mortality in hypercholesterolaemic patients with ischaemic heart disease.
   d. **True.** Not all statins are licensed for this use.
   e. **False.** It blocks absorption of cholesterol in the brush border of the small intestine.

6. a. **True.** Because of gastrointestinal upsets and gallstones.
   b. **True.** They block vasodilatory β_2-adrenoceptors (even the β_1-adrenoceptor selective drugs).
   c. **False.** On the contrary, constipation may be a problem.
   d. **False.** If simvastatin blocks cholesterol synthesis, it might be expected to have an effect on cholesterol-based hormonal production, such as cortisol. In fact, this is not a problem.
   e. **False.** There is no association.

Case history answers

Case history 1

1. His risk of an ischaemic event over the next 10 years is very high – probably of the order of 30–40%. The risk graphs should not be used for patients with established cardiovascular disease, or any diabetic patients, all of whom should be considered at high risk and worthy of aggressive treatment of all his risk factors.

2. He needs to stop smoking, lose weight and ensure good control of his diabetes.

3. The antihypertensive drug of first choice in this man would be an ACE inhibitor but thiazides or beta-blockers would be a reasonable alternative. Beta-blockers might be avoided if he requires insulin. There is uncertainty over whether calcium-channel blockers should be used in diabetics. Some studies have suggested that calcium-channel blockers cause poorer outcomes than other drugs in diabetics, but other studies have rejected this view.

4. The blood pressure target for this man is 130/80 mmHg. This is a rigorous target and most patients will require combination therapy to achieve it.

5. His hyperlipidaemia is probably of a mixed type, i.e. both raised triglycerides and cholesterol, so either a statin (simvastatin is best for this) or a fibrate would be reasonable.

6. There are many other drugs that could be considered in this case: aspirin for reduction of risk of cardiovascular events, nicotine replacement therapy to help him stop smoking, and of course medication may be required to control his diabetes.

Case history 2

1. Blood pressure at this level increases her risk of stroke and myocardial infarction substantially – probably by a factor of about 2. Her absolute risk of a cardiovascular event (i.e. either stroke or myocardial infarction) is probably around 10–15% over the next 10 years. So she can be told that drug therapy can be expected to reduce risks of such events.

2. The other risk factors that might be considered are her cholesterol, her family history and her menopausal state: the risk of cardiovascular disease rises after the menopause, and it is not certain that hormone replacement therapy can prevent this rise (see Ch. 12).

3. There are several reasonable choices: thiazides, beta-blockers, calcium-channel blockers or ACE inhibitors are the most widely used. Thiazides or beta-blockers are the first choice both on grounds of the weight of evidence for their use and also of cost.

4. Is she complying with drug and other treatment? Does she have white coat hypertension? Could she have secondary hypertension? Has the blood pressure been measured properly, e.g. large cuff in an obese patient? Always ask about adverse effects of drugs, which a patient may not volunteer but which may result in poor adherence to the prescribed drugs.

5. One would consider adding a second drug, e.g. thiazides with a beta-blocker, or a trial of substitution, for instance swapping a thiazide for a beta-blocker or vice versa.

Case history 3

1. Yes: this cholesterol is raised and is probably a contributory factor in such a young patient having an infarct. If persistently elevated above 3.5 mmol/L, it should be treated with drug therapy. Other risk factors such as smoking etc. should also be considered. Note that this is secondary prevention, i.e. the patient has already had an event. The guidelines in Figure 21 do not apply to these patients, who need more aggressive treatment of all risk factors.

2. Drug treatment with simvastatin or pravastatin should be the first choice.

3. Serious but rare adverse effects include hepatitis and myositis. More common and less severe are headache and abdominal pain, and sometimes (simvastatin) nightmares.

4. A patient like this will probably also be on low-dose aspirin, a beta-blocker and possibly an ACE inhibitor.

5. Yes, and it will reduce mortality risk (by around 30%).

Short note answers

1. The management of this patient should follow the broad guideline laid out in Figure 21. The patient should have the blood pressure

measurement repeated on a number of occasions over 1 month, but if it is found to be sustained the patient is going to need treatment. Non-pharmacological treatment is indicated, such as weight loss, increased exercise and also addressing general cardiovascular risk factors, such as smoking etc. If the patient needs antihypertensive therapy, this should be tailored to the particular patient's needs. You should list some of the more commonly used drugs and which kinds of patient you would or would not use them in.

2. The first patient is a case for secondary prevention where rigorous lowering of his cholesterol is required. The second patient is a case of possible primary prevention and her data can be put into the risk tables. This demonstrates that, in fact, she is at fairly low risk of a cardiovascular event; therefore, at present she would not be a priority for cholesterol-lowering therapy, the risks of which might outweigh the benefits for her. (The 10-year risk for cardiovascular event in the first patient is of the order of 45–50%.)

Extended matching items answers

1. D is best but M is also acceptable. Of the main classes of antihypertensive, this patient is clearly unsuitable for a beta-blocker. ACE inhibitors are not ideal in asthmatics either, although they might be used with caution: their potentiation of bradykinin might exacerbate asthma, and their propensity to cause cough (especially in women, where it occurs in about 15–20%) can give rise to diagnostic problems. Thiazides are effective, inexpensive, have the longest experience and are proven to prevent stroke. Consequently, they are an ideal first choice. A long-acting calcium-channel blocker would also be a reasonable choice, e.g. sustained-release nifedipine or possibly diltiazem. The other listed antihypertensives should be reserved drugs for patients who fail to respond to the first line suggested.

2. L is the best choice. ACE inhibitors have been shown to reduce proteinuria in diabetics and this seems to slow developing nephropathy. This effect seems to be over and above any benefit in slowing nephropathy achieved just by lowering the blood pressure. Angiotensin receptor antagonists such as irbesartan (B) would probably have a similar effect, although this is the subject of ongoing trials at present. Calcium-channel blockers have a weaker and less certain effect. Beta-blockers should probably be avoided in insulin-taking diabetics: they could mask some of the early symptoms of hypoglycaemia. Neither beta-blockers nor thiazides are shown to benefit proteinuria.

3. I would be best but L or M are also reasonable. Clearly a thiazide would not be a good choice here as it would be likely to exacerbate his gout. Other reasonable alternatives are, therefore, calcium-channel blockers, ACE inhibitors and beta-blockers. This case and the others illustrate the importance of tailoring the medication to the patient's profile.

4. M or J would be best. Here we are using an antihypertensive which also has antianginal actions to try to achieve better control of two problems. Lowering the blood pressure alone might improve the angina but it seems reasonable to try to improve both with specific medication if possible. Beta-blockers would probably be the most effective for both but are excluded by her COPD. Isosorbide mononitrate is widely used in angina but has no useful antihypertensive effect.

5. This could be the result of beta-blockers (I) or possibly ACE inhibitors (L). There are many other options open but best would be a thiazide diuretic (D) or possibly a calcium-channel blocker of the nifedipine (M) or amlodipine type.

6. This could be the same patient as in 5 but a year later! The ankle swelling is probably due to nifedipine (M). Given her asthma, the diuretic is the best choice (D) but if an ACE inhibitor was not the cause of her wheeze and coughing before, then cautious use of enalapril (L) would be reasonable.

7. The drug best described as causing type 2 diabetes is D. However, here is an association between hypertension and diabetes, and diabetes can develop on any drug as an association if not as cause and effect. If the patient was on a thiazide, it would make sense to stop it and to switch to a drug such as enalapril (L) or irbesartan (B). Several other drugs would be reasonable choices also.

8. Many drugs can cause headache, which could also be an effect of poorly controlled BP. However, the most likely candidates are the calcium-channel blockers, M or J. Alternatives would include any of the other major classes of antihypertensives e.g. B, I or L.

9. Following the ABCD rule here, a good choice would be a CD drug, e.g. D or M. Loop diuretics could also be used with enalapril; used alone, loop diuretics (e.g. furosemide) are poor antihypertensives because they cause secondary hyperaldosteronism which acts as a counter-regulatory mechanism to retain fluid and push up BP. However, in the presence of an ACE inhibitor the counter-regulatory effects are blocked, and ACE inhibitors with loop diuretics are a very effective antihypertensive combination (also widely used in heart failure, see Ch. 4).

10. The ABCD rule would suggest using I (atenolol) or L (enalapril) or B (irbesartan) in this case, either as a substitute or as an add on. Do not forget, when faced with a patient who apparently does not respond to one or more drugs, to ensure that you are not actually dealing with poor adherence to medication or with a 'white coat' effect.

Drugs in cardiovascular disease 2: treatment

4.1	Ischaemic heart disease	51
4.2	Cardiac failure	54
4.3	Cardiac arrhythmias	59
	Self-assessment on Chapter 4: questions	62
	Self-assessment on Chapter 4: answers	66

- know the emergency management of acute coronary syndromes including myocardial infarction
- be able to list the drug therapy that might be used in a patient after recovery from acute myocardial infarction.

Overview

This chapter reviews the drugs used in the treatment of established heart disease. The most common such disease is ischaemic heart disease, which presents as angina or with acute coronary syndromes including myocardial infarction. Angina is treated with drugs that decrease the workload of the heart. Acute myocardial infarction is also treated with such drugs, together with thrombolytic agents to remove the clot that has blocked a coronary artery. Cardiac failure is the end result of a number of processes damaging the heart muscle, such as ischaemic heart disease or hypertension. It is mainly treated by 'offloading' the heart using ACE inhibitors, and by reducing fluid overload by using diuretics. Cardiac arrhythmia may complicate ischaemic heart disease but may also occur for other reasons. Drugs used to treat such arrhythmias are often negatively inotropic and may themselves cause arrhythmias.

4.1 Ischaemic heart disease

Learning objectives

At the end of this section you should:
- be able to explain the pathophysiology of atheromatous disease, angina and acute coronary syndromes including myocardial infarction
- be able to describe the drugs used in the treatment of angina pectoris and how these drugs are used in practice
- be able to describe the drugs used in the treatment of acute myocardial infarction and acute coronary syndromes

Ischaemic heart disease is usually caused by atherosclerosis, with narrowing of the coronary arteries. Risk factors are described in Chapter 3. The most frequent manifestations of ischaemic heart disease are sudden death, angina pectoris or myocardial infarction.

Angina pectoris

Angina pectoris ('stable' angina) occurs when there is an imbalance between the oxygen supply (reduced by the narrowed vessels caused by atheroma or, rarely, in some patients, by spasm of a coronary artery) and oxygen demand (typically during exercise) and presents most commonly as an intermittent chest pain of short duration (Fig. 24). It is typically provoked by exertion or stress and is eased by rest.

Management of stable angina

The management of stable angina involves:

1. Treating a single acute attack:
   — rest
   — *glyceryl trinitrate* (GTN) tablets or spray
   — medical attention for patients whose attacks do not respond within minutes to a first or second GTN tablet (see below).
2. Prophylactic therapy: this should be taken regularly and involves four types of drug:
   — beta-blockers
   — calcium-channel blockers
   — oral nitrates
   — nicorandil.

Decreased by:
Coronary artery
disease
Anaemia

Increased by:
Exercise
Tachycardia
Hypertension

Increased by:
Nitrates
Calcium-channel blockers
Beta-blockers

Decreased by:
Nitrates
Calcium-channel blockers
Beta-blockers

Fig. 24 The balance of oxygen demand and supply in the heart.

Each drug acts in a different way and they can often usefully be combined in the same patient. In general for patients with exercise-induced angina, a beta-blocker should be first choice.

3. Aspirin is also used, provided there are no contraindications, to reduce the risk of serious thrombotic complications. In patients who have had a previous myocardial infarction, aspirin has been shown to reduce the risks of further infarcts.
4. Correct risk factors where possible.
5. Many patients may benefit from interventions to relieve blockages in coronary vessels. Selection of patients for this depends on investigation, including treadmill exercise testing and angiography.

Clinical sketch

A patient with angina is treated initially with a regular beta-blocker and GTN as required. His angina gradually deteriorates and a calcium-channel blocker is added. This leads to initial improvement, but again over a period of 12 months there is a deterioration and a long-acting oral nitrate is added.

Comment: antianginal drugs are often used in combination, although the evidence that such combinations are more effective than single or at the most two drugs is weak. Patients with angina that is difficult to control (and many would advocate all patients) should have angiography to see if they are suitable for angioplasty or surgery. Patients also need their cardiovascular risk factors assessed and treated and this patient should probably also be on aspirin and, if his cholesterol is raised, on a lipid-lowering agent.

Acute coronary syndromes

The term acute coronary syndrome refers to a range of syndromes of acute myocardial ischaemia, including unstable angina, Non-ST Segment Elevation Myocardial Infarction (NSTEMI), and ST Elevation Myocardial Infarction (STEMI). The diagnosis is based on the clinical features of the chest pain, the presence or absence of significant ECG changes, or evidence of myocardial necrosis. In each case the pathology is similar: a plaque becomes eroded or ruptures, releasing its contents into the bloodstream and provoking a clotting cascade.

If the cascade proceeds to the point of a fibrin and platelet clot completely obstructing a major artery, the result is a full thickness myocardial infarction in the territory supplied by that artery. This is usually associated with severe chest pain, ST elevation on the ECG and a rise in enzymes leaked from cardiac muscle cells. Cardiac troponins are sensitive indicators of such myocardial necrosis.

If the result is a platelet plug which does not completely obstruct the artery, platelet emboli may fly off from the clot to block small vessels further down. The result may be again chest pain, but without a clear ST elevation on the ECG. There may still, however, be a rise in the troponins confirming a degree of myocardial cell damage. In simple unstable angina, there is usually an unstable plaque but little sign of myocardial damage on either the ECG or via measurement of cardiac troponins. Clinically, the patient experiences angina at rest for the first time, or an increase in the severity or frequency of attacks with little or no provocation over a short period of time. Obviously there is some degree of overlap between these clinical syndromes.

Myocardial infarction

Apart from loss of myocardium (which may lead to heart failure), the patient is also at risk from potentially fatal arrhythmias. Prompt action may reduce the loss of myocardium and improve survival.

Management of an acute myocardial infarction with ST elevation on ECG

Management is described in Box 2.

1. Sublingual glyceryl trinitrate (it may be a severe attack of angina, and not a myocardial infarction)
2. Pain relief – use i.v. opiates (usually with an antiemetic)
4. Aspirin (if there is no contraindication) orally
5. Thrombolytic drugs (if there is no contraindication) (see Ch. 5)
6. Other treatments can also decrease mortality but are less widely used, including i.v. beta-blockers.

Clinical sketch

A 70-year-old man gets chest pain on exertion. This has been diagnosed as angina but has been stable for some time. One day he gets severe chest pain while sitting down, which is typical of his angina. He uses his GTN spray, which gives transient relief but the pain recurs within a matter of a few minutes. He uses the GTN spray again, but gets little relief. The pain persists and he feels short of breath and unwell.

Comment: this patient had previously stable angina but it now seems to be unstable, since it is occurring at rest. It has also failed to respond to GTN spray. This patient should seek medical attention immediately, either by contacting his GP or by going to the local A&E department, possibly by ambulance. He may have an acute coronary syndrome and he may require urgent hospital admission, investigation and stabilisation.

Treatment after myocardial infarction

All of the following drugs have been proven to reduce mortality after myocardial infarction; they are often used in combination:

- beta-blockers
- ACE (angiotensin-converting enzyme) inhibitors
- aspirin
- clopidogrel
- lipid-lowering therapy (statins have the best evidence).

NSTEMI and unstable angina

Because there is little fibrin in the platelet clot in these conditions, there is no role for thrombolysis with fibrinolytic drugs. Instead the emphasis is on reducing platelet aggregation as well as easing the patient's symptoms. Antiplatelet agents are used: the extent of antiplatelet therapy is increased in patients with higher levels of risk of proceeding to a full ST elevation MI. Aspirin alone may be used in the lowest risk patients, aspirin and clopidogrel in higher risk patients, and glycoprotein IIb/IIIa receptor inhibitors (e.g. tirofiban, eptifibatide) in high-risk patients or patients with NSTEMI identified by raised troponins. These patients are all treated also with low-molecular-weight heparins. These drugs are discussed in Chapter 5. Other treatment is to initiate prophylactic antianginals immediately, especially beta-blockers. Patients whose pain does not settle quickly may need an invasive procedure to make an anatomical diagnosis and relieve blockages with balloon procedures in angioplasty.

Drugs to treat ischaemic heart disease

Nitrates

At a cellular level, nitrates are converted in the body to nitric oxide (NO), which combines with sulphydryl (–SH) groups to form nitrosothiols. These activate the enzyme guanyl cyclase to produce the second messenger cyclic GMP. Cyclic GMP causes smooth muscle relaxation and vasodilatation (Fig. 25).

In the body, nitrates dilate blood vessels in three areas: the venous circulation, which decreases venous return and the preload on the heart; the arterioles, reducing peripheral resistance and the afterload (both of these reduce the stress on the myocardial wall and lower oxygen demand); and the coronary arteries, especially if there is coronary spasm (this improves oxygen supply). The reduction in preload is probably the major effect.

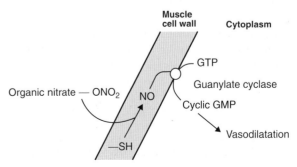

Fig. 25 The actions of nitrates.

Nitrate tolerance

Many patients become tolerant to the antianginal effects of nitrates if they receive them for prolonged periods (>24 hours) as a result of depletion of the essential –SH groups. When prescribing, a nitrate-free period should be built into the regimen. For example, *isosorbide dinitrate* taken at 8 a.m. and 2 p.m. provides cover for daytime exertion and leaves the patient free of nitrates overnight, preventing tolerance. The best regimen must be worked out for each patient.

Examples

Glyceryl trinitrate is well absorbed when given sublingually; if taken orally, it is broken down by first pass metabolism in the liver. GTN is volatile, and the tablets should be kept in a sealed dark container; tablets from an opened container will lose their effect after about 4 weeks. A GTN spray is more expensive but keeps longer. It acts very rapidly after sublingual use, within 1–2 minutes, and the effects last for 30–60 minutes. It can also be given i.v. or in the form of GTN ointment or transdermal patches as it can be absorbed through the skin. All patients with angina should carry either GTN tablets or spray with them at all times to treat any acute attacks.

Isosorbide dinitrate is taken sublingually, orally or i.v. It is absorbed more slowly but has a longer action. It is partly metabolised by the liver to isosorbide mononitrate, and both the dinitrate and mononitrate contribute to its effects. Its half-life is 2–4 hours. Isosorbide mononitrate can also be given orally. It is not metabolised by the liver, and so more reliable plasma nitrate concentrations are obtained after mononitrate than dinitrate – this is usually of little practical importance.

Therapeutic uses

- angina pectoris – acute treatment and prophylaxis
- congestive cardiac failure (see below).

Adverse effects

These result from vasodilatation and include headache (from vasodilatation of cerebral blood vessels) and facial flushing (very common).

Nicorandil

Nicorandil has dual actions, partly nitrate-like and partly those of a potassium-channel opener (similar effects to a calcium-channel blocker). It is as effective as other drugs in monotherapy.

Other drugs

See Chapter 3 for:

- beta-blockers
- calcium-channel blockers
- ACE inhibitors.

See Chapter 5 for:

- aspirin
- low-molecular-weight heparin
- thrombolytic agents.

4.2 Cardiac failure

Learning objectives

At the end of this section you should:
- be able to list the causes of heart failure
- be able to describe the pathophysiology of heart failure including the role of the renin–angiotensin–aldosterone system
- know the drugs used in the treatment of heart failure and the use of these drugs in practice.

Cardiac failure is usually the result of damage to the myocardium, from ischaemic heart disease, myocarditis or cardiomyopathy. Other causes include poorly controlled hypertension or damage to the valves of the heart, fluid overload, metabolic disease such as thyrotoxicosis, or drugs. Cardiac failure may result in poor perfusion of tissues or vital organs (forward failure) and congestion of the lungs or periphery with excessive fluid (backward failure, causing pulmonary or peripheral oedema). Treatment of acute pulmonary oedema is described in Box 3.

Box 3 Treatment of acute pulmonary oedema

- Oxygen, usually in high concentration
- Morphine with antiemetic i.v.
- Loop diuretic i.v.
- Sublingual or i.v. nitrates should be used to reduce preload. Some advocate their immediate use in all patients, others as a reserve if no rapid response to other therapies
- If hypotensive and still in pulmonary oedema, consider possible cardiogenic shock – may need positive inotropes to stimulate the heart (e.g. dobutamine)
- Consider underlying causes, e.g. ischaemic heart disease, arrhythmia, valvular disease, etc.

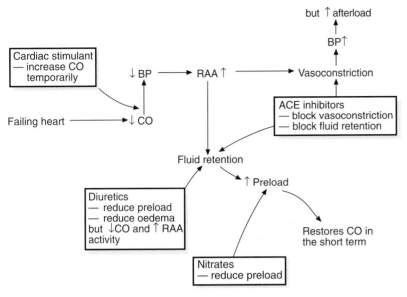

Fig. 26 Treating heart failure. BP, blood pressure; CO, cardiac output; RAA, renin–angiotensin–aldosterone axis.

Table 1 New York Heart Association classification of heart failure

Grade	Description	Typical drugs
I	Left ventricle dysfunction detectable but asymptomatic	ACE inhibitor
II	Dyspnoeic on mild to moderate exertion	ACE inhibitor and diuretic
III	Dyspnoeic on mild exertion	ACE inhibitor and diuretic and spironolactone
IV	Dyspnoeic at rest	ACE inhibitor and diuretic and spironolactone

Reduced perfusion of vital organs prompts counter-regulatory mechanisms to restore perfusion. The sympathetic nervous system causes peripheral vasoconstriction and stimulates the heart directly. The renin–angiotensin–aldosterone system, a physiological means of controlling blood pressure and fluid balance, is activated. Renin is secreted by the juxtaglomerular apparatus in the kidney in response to a fall in renal perfusion. Renin converts angiotensinogen, a protein produced by the liver, to angiotensin I, and ACE converts this to the active angiotensin II. Angiotensin II acts at specific receptors (AT receptors) to cause direct vasoconstriction, raising blood pressure (Fig. 26). It also stimulates release of aldosterone from the adrenal gland, which in turn promotes Na^+ and fluid retention and enhances the actions of the sympathetic system by promoting noradrenaline (norepinephrine) release.

In decreased perfusion due, for instance, to bleeding all of these, which restore circulating blood volume and increase blood pressure, are very useful. But in cardiac failure in the long term they increase the strain on the failing heart and are ultimately detrimental. Heart failure therefore tends to be progressive. The New York Heart Association classification of heart failure and drugs likely to be used at each stage are shown in Table 1.

Treatment of chronic cardiac failure involves reducing fluid retention with diuretics and reducing the preload or afterload on the heart by using vasodilators, particularly the ACE inhibitors, which will also block the renin–angiotensin–aldosterone system (Fig. 26). Drugs that increase the force of contraction of the heart (positive inotropic drugs) have only a minor role and may be harmful.

A male patient aged 75 has previously had a myocardial infarction. He now finds that he gets progressively shorter and shorter of breath when he exerts himself. His ankles tend to swell. He feels generally tired, but has no chest pain.

Comment: the commonest cause of cardiac failure in the western world is ischaemic heart disease, leading to left ventricular dysfunction. The aim of treating acute myocardial infarction is to prevent loss of myocardium; however, as more patients survive myocardial infarctions and grow older, the incidence of heart failure is rising. This patient is probably suffering from cardiac failure, particularly given his previous history of myocardial infarction, but we cannot exclude other causes of pulmonary disease as the cause of his symptoms. He should have an echocardiogram. He will probably need treatment with an ACE inhibitor and a diuretic. When stable, he will also benefit from a beta-blocker unless there are other contraindications to this.

The patient presents to hospital with palpitations and shortness of breath. On examination he is found to be in atrial fibrillation.

Comment: atrial fibrillation is probably the commonest pathological cardiac arrhythmia. It can compromise cardiac function in two ways. First, the loss of the atrial 'push' (which may account for 20–25% of total cardiac output) and, second, and more important, the

rapid heart rate can lead to poor filling of the left ventricle with even more loss of cardiac output. Treatment should be, if possible, to get the patient out of atrial fibrillation (this may require electrical cardioversion). If this is not possible or feasible then controlling the rate with digoxin or with beta-blockers would be the usual treatment. The patient will need a loading dose of digoxin over 24–48 hours in hospital followed by a lower maintenance dose. The patient should also be considered for warfarin therapy to reduce the risk of embolic phenomena from the atrial fibrillation. The cause of the atrial fibrillation should be investigated and treated if necessary.*

The patient is treated with a standard dose of digoxin (and warfarin, see Ch. 5) and his atrial fibrillation comes under control. Subsequently he develops chronic renal failure with a decrease in his creatinine clearance. He presents at the A&E department with a heart rate of 30 beats/min.

Comment: digoxin is cleared by filtration. In patients with impaired renal function, accumulation of digoxin with adverse effects such as profound bradycardia can occur. The maintenance dose needs to be reduced in patients with impaired renal function. It is important to monitor plasma concentrations of digoxin and adjust the dose as well, but the patient response is always more important than plasma concentration.

Drugs to treat congestive cardiac failure

The main types of drug used are:

- diuretics
- ACE inhibitors
- nitrates
- beta-blockers
- inotropic drugs.

Diuretics

Thiazides may be used alone in mild heart failure. For moderate to severe heart failure, loop diuretics will be used. In very severe heart failure with extensive resistant oedema, thiazides (especially metolazone) may be used cautiously with loop diuretics to achieve a very profound diuresis.

Loop diuretics

The loop diuretics act by inhibiting the resorption of Cl^- in the ascending limb of the loop of Henle. This causes loss of Cl^- and its main cation, Na^+, and water follows the electrolytes.

The response to loop diuretics is dose related. They have a greater diuretic effect than the thiazides.

When used i.v. in acute pulmonary oedema, the loop diuretics also cause venodilatation and reduce preload before diuresis can start. Like the thiazides, the loop diuretics cause K^+ loss, but unlike them, they also cause Ca^{2+} loss.

Examples. Furosemide or *bumetamide* act within 10 minutes of an i.v. dose. After oral administration, their effects peak at about 1 hour and last about 4–6 hours.

Therapeutic uses
- congestive heart failure
- oedema for other reasons
- hypertension (only in combination with other drugs or if renal failure present; Ch. 3).

Adverse effects
- hypokalaemia
- renal impairment: resulting from dehydration and from prerenal failure and a direct toxic effect on the kidney
- ototoxicity, i.e. deafness (furosemide only).

Drug interactions. These are as for thiazides (Ch. 3).

Potassium-sparing diuretics

The K$^+$-sparing diuretics are a chemically diverse group that, unlike other diuretics, retain K$^+$. They act in the distal convoluted tubule where K$^+$/Na$^+$ exchange occurs and are only weak diuretics. Their major use is in treating or preventing hypokalaemia caused by thiazides or loop diuretics. In the past, K$^+$ supplements were widely used, but very high doses are required, reducing patient compliance. It is often not necessary to prevent or treat diuretic-induced hypokalaemia, but if this is required, K$^+$-sparing diuretics should be used. This is not usually necessary and may be dangerous (possible severe hyperkalaemia) in patients taking ACE inhibitors as well as diuretics.

Examples. *Spironolactone* and *eplerenone* are aldosterone antagonists. Aldosterone causes Na$^+$ retention and K$^+$ loss, and spironolactone does the reverse.

Triamterene and *amiloride* interfere with Na$^+$/K$^+$ exchange.

All are administered orally.

Therapeutic uses. *Spironolactone*:

- severe congestive heart failure (usually with loop diuretics and with ACE inhibitors): in these patients it reduces mortality probably by ensuring the maximum blockade of the renin–angiotensin–aldosterone system
- primary hyperaldosteronism (Conn's syndrome)
- ascites resulting from liver disease
- diuretic-induced hypokalaemia.

Triamterene/amiloride:

- diuretic-induced hypokalaemia
- oedema.

Adverse effects
- hyperkalaemia
- gynaecomastia (spironolactone only).

Drug interactions. Combinations with K$^+$ supplements or ACE inhibitors may lead to dangerous hyperkalaemia.

Other diuretics

Osmotic diuretics (e.g. *mannitol*) are filtered by the glomerulus and retain water in the tubule by their osmotic effects, causing diuresis. They are rarely used, but when they are, it is most often to lower intracranial pressure and in glaucoma. The carbonic anhydrase inhibitor *acetazolamide* causes mild diuresis and severe hyperkalaemia. It is used to treat glaucoma.

ACE inhibitors and angiotensin receptor blockers

The ACE inhibitors are described in Chapter 3. In heart failure, they have been shown to reduce mortality by about 25%, to ease symptoms and to reduce hospitalisation. They should be used in all grades of heart failure if tolerated. Even in the mildest failure, they reduce the risk of further deterioration. The angiotensin receptor blockers are similar but not quite as effective and they can be used in patients who cannot tolerate ACE inhibitors, particularly those who suffer with a troublesome cough.

Nitrates

Nitrates are venodilators and, therefore, reduce preload on the heart. This is very effective in acute heart failure where i.v. isosorbide dinitrate may be used. In chronic heart failure, nitrates may be used as venodilators but the combined arterial and venous vasodilatation achieved by ACE inhibitors is more effective.

Beta-blockers

Some beta-blockers (*carvedilol*, *bisoprolol* and *metoprolol*) have been shown to reduce mortality and hospitalisations when given to patients with stable heart failure (i.e. not within 2–3 months of any deterioration or hospital admission). They may do this by protecting the myocardium from excessive sympathetic stimulation, from ischaemia or from arrhythmias. Beta-blockers are negatively inotropic so they must be used cautiously under expert guidance.

Inotropic drugs

The inotropic drugs are cardiac stimulants. *Digoxin* is discussed below. Other positive inotropes such as dobutamine (stimulates β_1-adrenoceptors) can be used in acute cardiogenic shock (i.e. severe acute heart failure with hypotension). Attempts to use other positive inotropes (e.g. milrinone) in the long term have been abandoned as they increased mortality.

Digoxin and other digitalis glycosides

At a cellular level, the digitalis compounds block the exchange of intracellular Na$^+$ for extracellular K$^+$ by inhibiting Na$^+$/K$^+$-ATPase in the cell membrane; this increases intracellular Na$^+$ and encourages its

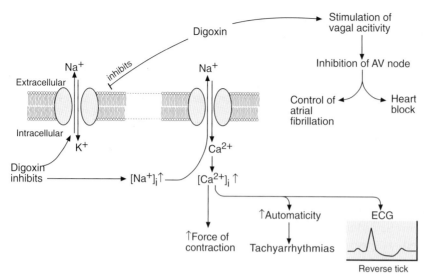

Fig. 27 Actions of digoxin. AV, atrioventricular.

exchange for Ca^{2+}, raising intracellular Ca^{2+} and causing a positive inotropic effect (Fig. 27). These effects cause characteristic changes in the electrocardiograph (ECG) ('reverse tick').

In the body, digitalis compounds also stimulate the vagus and increase vagal tone. This is its mode of action in its main clinical use, which is to slow the heart in atrial fibrillation. The positive inotropic effect may be useful in heart failure, even if the patient is in sinus rhythm.

Examples. Digoxin can be given orally (well absorbed) or parenterally and is excreted unchanged by the kidneys. Its half-life is 1.5 days but is greatly prolonged in renal impairment. Digoxin has a narrow therapeutic range, and it is useful to monitor plasma digoxin levels. If a rapid effect is required and because of the long half-life, it is useful to give a loading dose initially, followed by a maintenance dose daily.

Digitoxin has a longer half-life, about 6 days, and is metabolised by the liver.

Therapeutic uses
- atrial fibrillation (to slow the ventricular response)
- congestive heart failure (even in patients in sinus rhythm).

Adverse effects
- note hypokalaemia or hypercalcaemia increases the risk of digitalis toxicity
- hypothyroidism or old age increases sensitivity to standard doses
- gastrointestinal effects: anorexia, nausea, vomiting, occasionally diarrhoea
- neurological effects: malaise, fatigue, depression, confusion, insomnia, altered colour vision (yellow/green predominance)
- cardiovascular effects: any cardiac arrhythmia may occur, especially ventricular bigeminy and bradycardias including complete heart block; the ECG may show first-degree heart block at an early stage, but serious arrhythmias may occur without warning
- others: gynaecomastia.

Contraindications
- acute myocardial ischaemia (may increase oxygen demand)
- disease of the atrioventricular (AV) node (may cause heart block)
- renal impairment (especially digoxin)
- before electrical cardioversion (may precipitate heart block in the presence of digoxin toxicity).

Drug interactions
- diuretics may cause hypokalaemia and worsen digoxin toxicity
- verapamil, amiodarone and quinidine all increase plasma digoxin levels by reducing its clearance.

Treatment of digoxin toxicity. Treatment depends on severity: in very severe overdose, hyperkalaemia and hyponatraemia can occur because of the cellular effects.

1. Withdraw drug
2. Correct low serum K^+ by i.v. administration
3. Treat ventricular arrhythmias

4. Digoxin-specific antibodies will bind to and inactivate digoxin and can be used in life-threatening cases (very expensive).

4.3 Cardiac arrhythmias

Many minor cardiac arrhythmias often do not require treatment; for example, atrial or ventricular ectopics. Others are more serious and require treatment for termination or prevention. This may include correction of the underlying cause where possible; non-drug treatment, such as carotid sinus massage for supraventricular tachycardias; electrical cardioversion or pacemaking for serious supraventricular or ventricular arrhythmias; and drugs.

Antiarrhythmic drugs are usually classified according to the Vaughan Williams system, which is based on the changes in the action potential produced by drugs in isolated cardiac cells. Many drugs have mixed properties and do not fit neatly into any one class. The classification is of limited clinical value.

The action potential

The gradient of electrical charge across the membrane of a resting cardiac cell is −80 to −90 mV. This is maintained by movement of ions through specific ion channels in the membrane. Depolarisation and repolarisation of cardiac cells occurs in the following stages (Fig. 28):

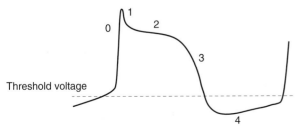

Fig. 28 The action potential in a Purkinje fibre. Cells from the atrioventricular node and other fibres show different patterns.

Phase 0: rapid depolarisation caused by entry of Na^+ through the 'fast' sodium channel

Phase 1: early repolarisation, caused by closing of the sodium channel and opening of potassium channels

Phase 2: a plateau where there is a balance between K^+ exit and Ca^{2+} entry; the Ca^{2+} entry is through the opening of 'slow' channels

Phase 3: the late repolarisation phase caused by further K^+ exit and closing of the calcium channels

Phase 4: the slow depolarisation phase; the resting potential is restored and Na^+ and K^+ concentrations are restored by exchange pumps. There is a slow entry of Na^+ into the cell, decreasing the potential difference until the threshold potential is reached and a new action potential is triggered.

Classes of antiarrhythmic drug

Class I

Class I drugs block the rapid Na^+ current and slow phase 0. There are three subgroups: Ia, which delays repolarisation and lengthens the action potential; Ib, which accelerates repolarisation and shortens the action potential; and Ic, which has no effect on action potential duration but affects Purkinje tissue to slow conduction and prolong the QRS complex.

Class Ia. Disopyramide is the most commonly used in Europe. Disopyramide is used to treat atrial and ventricular arrhythmias. It may be given orally (as prophylaxis) or i.v. (for treatment). Its adverse effects include anticholinergic effects (urinary retention, blurred vision, dry mouth) and a negative inotropic effect, leading to hypotension or heart failure. It may precipitate cardiac arrhythmias in some patients.

Class Ib. Lidocaine (also used as a local anaesthetic, see Ch. 8) is given i.v. (poorly absorbed orally and subject to first pass metabolism) to treat acute ventricular arrhythmias such as ventricular tachycardia, especially after myocardial infarction as it is particularly effective in ischaemic tissue. It is rapidly metabolised by the liver with a half-life of 2 hours during prolonged infusion. Single bolus doses have a much shorter duration of action (5–10 minutes) because of redistribution. Its toxic effects include drowsiness, paraesthesia and convulsions. It has little negative inotropic or proarrhythmic effect. Mexiletine is similar but is active after oral administration.

Class Ic. *Flecainide* is used orally or i.v. for atrial or ventricular arrhythmias. It is proarrhythmic and negatively inotropic, and it is usually reserved for very serious arrhythmias. It may also cause dizziness, headache and rashes.

Class II

The class II drugs are the beta-blockers, which have little effect on intracellular electrical activity except to slow phase 4. They may be given i.v. or orally, especially for atrial or exercise-induced arrhythmias. See above for adverse effects and other uses. *Sotalol* is a beta-blocker, the most widely used as an antiarrhythmic, but this is largely used because of its class III effects (see below).

Class III

The class III drugs prolong the action potential by inhibiting repolarisation (phase 3). *Amiodarone* is used to treat atrial and ventricular arrhythmias. It also has Na^+-blocking effects (class I). It has little negative inotropic effect but it lengthens the QT interval. It is difficult to use because it has an exceedingly long half-life of 25–110 days, and because of its adverse effects: These include:

- proarrhythmia
- pneumonitis and pulmonary fibrosis
- hypo- or hyperthyroidism
- peripheral neuropathy
- hepatitis.

Minor effects include:

- corneal microdeposits of the drug (may cause halos around lights)
- photosensitivity of the skin and skin pigmentation.
- drug interactions, with decreased metabolism of warfarin, increased digoxin concentration.

Sotalol is both a beta-blocker (class II) and a class III drug

Class IV

The calcium antagonists (verapamil and diltiazem mainly, but not dihydropyridines) are effective in AV nodal arrhythmias, where the action potential largely results from Ca^{2+} entry rather than Na^+ entry. Verapamil is used i.v. or orally to treat supraventricular arrhythmias.

Other drugs used in cardiac arrhythmias

The following three drugs do not fit into the classification given above.

Atropine. The anticholinergic drug atropine is used acutely in severe symptomatic bradycardias, as it blocks vagal tone. If long-term treatment is required, an electronic pacemaker is used.

Digoxin. Used for atrial fibrillation (see above).

Adenosine. This purine nucleoside acts on specific adenosine receptors in the sinoatrial node and causes bradycardia. It is used i.v. to treat supraventricular arrhythmias. It has no negative inotropic effects (unlike verapamil) and a very short half-life (less than 2 seconds) and so adverse effects are likely to be only transient; they include wheezing (asthma is contraindication), flushing and hypotension.

Clinical sketch

A patient with recurrent ventricular tachycardia is treated with *amiodarone*. This controls his arrhythmia, but he complains of progressive shortness of breath.

Comment: in this case the pathology underlying the arrhythmia (e.g. ischaemic heart disease) may have given rise to heart failure. Alternatively, long-term amiodarone therapy is associated with pulmonary fibrosis. It can be difficult to sort out which is responsible in a patient like this and the patient will need further investigation. Such dilemmas are not unusual in patients with multiple problems.

Drug of choice in arrhythmias

The antiarrhythmic drug of choice depends on speed of response required, presence of other conditions, including heart failure etc. Remember non-pharmacological methods (vagal stimulation manoeuvres, electrical cardioversion) may be more appropriate, depending on the circumstances:

- supraventricular tachycardia (not caused by Wolff–Parkinson–White): the aim is to convert back to sinus rhythm. Adenosine or verapamil for treatment, sotalol or verapamil for prophylaxis
- arrhythmias caused by Wolff–Parkinson–White: amiodarone, disopyramide, flecainide
- atrial flutter: the aim is to convert back to sinus rhythm (use disopyramide or flecainide or amiodarone), or alternatively to atrial fibrillation (use digoxin) which is easier to control. Drugs are generally unsatisfactory in this condition.

- atrial fibrillation: for acute atrial fibrillation, disopyramide or amiodarone or flecainide to cardiovert back to sinus rhythm. If unsuccessful, or if the atrial fibrillation is of long standing, use digoxin or beta-blocker to control the rate; (remember anticoagulation; Ch. 5). Maybe use digoxin or beta-blocker short term until the patient is well anticoagulated and then attempt electrical cardioversion.
- ventricular tachycardia: lidocaine, amiodarone.

Four

Self-assessment on Chapter 4: questions

Multiple choice questions

1. Drug combinations used in the treatment of angina include:
   a. Glyceryl trinitrate and salbutamol
   b. Digoxin and verapamil
   c. Nifedipine and isosorbide dinitrate
   d. Diazepam and atenolol
   e. Metoprolol and nifedipine

2. The following drugs are safe to use in patients with congestive cardiac failure:
   a. Bisoprolol
   b. Carbenoxolone
   c. Enalapril
   d. Amoxicillin
   e. Morphine

3. A patient with an acute myocardial infarction should usually be given:
   a. Thrombolytic therapy
   b. Paracetamol
   c. Diamorphine
   d. Nitrates
   e. Diazepam

4. With regard to the use of nitrates:
   a. Tolerance occurs only to the adverse effects and not to the antianginal effect
   b. Nitrates may have a diuretic effect
   c. Glyceryl trinitrate is given to relieve angina rapidly
   d. The major adverse effects of nitrates are predictable from their pharmacological action
   e. Liver metabolism rapidly terminates the action of all nitrates

5. Beta-blockers:
   a. May be used to treat tachycardia in patients with hypovolaemic shock or acute pulmonary oedema arising from cardiac failure
   b. Atenolol cannot precipitate asthma
   c. Downregulation of adrenoceptors may occur in patients who take propranolol long term
   d. Lipophilic beta-blockers are more likely to cause CNS adverse effects

   e. Plasma concentrations are closely related to clinical activity

7. Drugs that may worsen cardiac failure include:
   a. Corticosteroids
   b. Calcium-channel blockers
   c. Nitrates
   d. Indometacin
   e. Digoxin

8. In congestive heart failure:
   a. Secondary hyperaldosteronism is a feature
   b. Fluid retention is a physiological response to a fall in cardiac output
   c. Positive inotropic drugs are the major treatment
   d. Diuretics prevent activation of the renin–angiotensin–aldosterone system
   e. Thiazides and loop diuretics may have vasodilator effects

9. In diuretic treatment:
   a. Thiazides may cause hypercholesterolaemia
   b. Hyperkalaemia is a common adverse effect of thiazides and loop diuretics
   c. High-dose thiazides are appropriate in severe hypertension
   d. Furosemide acts mainly in the distal convoluted tubule
   e. Potassium-sparing diuretics are the first choice in treating congestive cardiac failure

10. Digoxin:
   a. May be safely used in standard doses in patients with a glomerular filtration rate of 10 ml/min
   b. May cause tachyarrhythmias or bradyarrhythmias
   c. May cause hyponatraemia and hyperkalaemia in overdose
   d. May cause ST elevation on an ECG
   e. If given with diuretics, the serum K^+ should be monitored

11. ACE inhibitors:
   a. Are specific and only block breakdown of angiotensin

b. Are effective vasodilators

c. Improve life expectancy of patients with congestive cardiac failure

d. May increase intrarenal blood flow

e. Cough is the most common adverse effect

12. The following statements are correct:

a. Many antiarrhythmics span several classes of the Vaughan Williams classification

b. Lidocaine is excreted unchanged by the kidney

c. Many antiarrhythmics have negative inotropic effects

d. If administered orally at a steady dose, amiodarone reaches a steady plasma concentration after about 25 days

e. Adenosine is used to treat supraventricular tachycardias

Case history questions

Case history 1

A 65-year-old man presents to an A&E department with a history of severe central chest pain for 2 hours and typical ECG changes of an acute inferior myocardial infarction.

1. What drugs should he be given in the absence of any contraindication?

2. What contraindications would make you hesitate about giving each of these?

The patient suddenly develops an acute bradycardia.

3. What drug might you give to correct this?

The patient subsequently has an uncomplicated course.

4. What drug therapy would be appropriate for him to continue taking at home after discharge?

5. What advice might you give him?

Case history 2

A 60-year-old man who smokes and who has a history of chronic obstructive pulmonary disease (COPD) is diagnosed as having angina on exertion.

1. What drug therapy might he be given?

2. What advice might he be given?

3. What is nitrate tolerance and how can it be avoided?

He is also found to be hypercholesterolaemic, with a cholesterol of 8.6 mmol/L.

4. How would you treat this initially?

His serum cholesterol fails to respond to your first treatment.

5. What would you consider next?

He uses nebulised high-dose salbutamol for his COPD but notices that this tends to bring on an attack of angina.

6. Why might this be?

Case history 3

A 45-year-old woman develops recurrent supraventricular tachycardias. She is treated with several drugs over a period unsuccessfully, and then given amiodarone, which seems to control the arrhythmias.

1. What blood tests should be considered before she starts on amiodarone?

2. If she starts taking it at the usual maintenance dose, how long will it be before the plasma concentrations of the drug reach steady state?

3. She is also taking warfarin because of a previous pulmonary embolism: does starting amiodarone pose any problems, and if so, how can the problems be managed?

4. Why was amiodarone not the first choice of antiarrhythmic drug?

Case history 4

A 70-year-old man develops dyspnoea and oedema and is found to have mild congestive cardiac failure.

1. What drug or drugs might he be started on?

He is also found to be in atrial fibrillation and this is assumed to be chronic.

2. How should this be treated?
3. If he does not respond adequately to your first choice of treatment for his heart failure, what drug or drugs might be added in later?
4. If he develops acute pulmonary oedema, how should this be treated?

He complains of knee pain and is prescribed indometacin.

5. Why might this be unwise?

Short note questions

Write short notes on the following:

1. The drug therapy that a patient might take for secondary prevention after a myocardial infarction.
2. The use of ACE inhibitors in cardiovascular disease.

Extended matching items questions

Theme: treatment of ischaemic cardiovascular disease

Options
A. Atenolol, aspirin, simvastatin
B. Amiodarone
C. Isosorbide mononitrate, enalapril, glyceryl trinitrate
D. Verapamil
E. Isosorbide mononitrate, glyceryl trinitrate
F. Atenolol

For each of questions 1–6, below, choose the most appropriate answer from options A–G above. Each option may be used once, more than once, or not at all.

1. Which therapy would be appropriate to reduce the rate of contraction of the left ventricle?
2. Which therapy would be appropriate to decrease oxygen demand on the heart?
3. Which therapy would be appropriate to facilitate secondary prevention of further episodes after myocardial infarction?
4. Which therapy would be appropriate to increase oxygen supply to the heart?
5. Which therapy would be appropriate for angina pectoris?
6. Which therapy would be appropriate when there is a requirement for sulphydryl groups for drug function?

Theme: treatment of arrhythmias

Options
A. Digoxin
B. Flecainide
C. Lidocaine
D. Sotalol
E. Atropine
F. Adenosine
G. Amiodarone

For each of questions 1–6, below, choose the most appropriate answer from options A–G, above. Each option may be used once, more than once, or not at all.

1. Which of these drugs might be used to control rate in chronic atrial fibrillation?
2. Which of these might be used to control paroxysmal atrial fibrillation?
3. Which is the first line treatment for ventricular tachyarrhythmias immediately after acute myocardial infarction?
4. Which might be used to treat bradycardia after myocardial infarction?
5. Which drug can cause pulmonary toxicity?
6. Which drug can be used to treat acute supraventricular tachycardia?

Theme: treatment of congestive cardiac failure

Options

A. Spironolactone

B. Bumetanide

C. Enalapril

D. Irbesartan

E. Metolazone

F. Bisoprolol

G. Digoxin

H. Nitrates

For each of questions 1–6, below, choose the most appropriate answer from options A–H, above. Each option may be used once, more than once, or not at all.

1. Which drug or drugs reduce activity in the angiotensin–renin–aldosterone axis?

2. Which drug or drugs increase activity in the renin–angiotensin–aldosterone axis?

3. Which are the drugs of choice in acute pulmonary oedema?

4. Which drug or drugs may cause potassium retention?

5. Which drug or drugs can cause bronchospasm?

6. Which drug or drugs will cause vasodilatation?

Self-assessment on Chapter 4: answers

Multiple choice answers

1. a. **False.** Glyceryl trinitrate is appropriate, but salbutamol is a β_2-agonist.

   b. **False.** Digoxin may increase oxygen demand and worsen ischaemic heart disease. It has no role in angina unless there is also atrial fibrillation. Verapamil is useful in angina and is sometimes combined with digoxin to control difficult cases of atrial fibrillation (because of its effects at the AV node).

   c. **True.** Both of these drugs are used in angina and act by different mechanisms and so can be usefully combined.

   d. **False.** The use of diazepam, a sedative, is inappropriate: it will have no effect on myocardial oxygen balance. Atenolol is valuable in angina. Beta-blockers are sometimes used in anxiety states because they reduce the somatic manifestations (tachycardia, tremor, etc.).

   e. **True.** Both drugs are used in angina and can be combined in more severe cases.

2. a. **True.** Beta-blockers reduce myocardial remodelling which is harmful, and reduce the risks of arrhythmias in patients with cardiac failure. However, they should only be given to stable patients in whom other therapies such as ACE inhibitors, diuretics have been optimized first.

   b. **False.** Carbenoxolone is structurally related to aldosterone and may cause fluid retention.

   c. **True.** Enalapril should be used with diuretics as standard therapy in most cases of cardiac failure.

   d. **True.** But some penicillins have a large Na^+ load, e.g. carbenicillin, and should be avoided in cardiac failure.

   e. **True.** Morphine is used for its vasodilatating and sedative effects in addition to diuretics and vasodilators in acute left ventricular failure.

3. a. **True.** Standard treatment unless there is a clear contraindication. A patient who has recently had streptokinase could be given alteplase.

   b. **False.** This would be inadequate as analgesia and has no antiplatelet action. Aspirin in contrast has been proven to improve mortality.

   c. **True.** Pain relief is very important, and strong opiates are the drugs of choice.

   d. **True.** Usually in the form of a GTN spray, but some would give them i.v.

   e. **False.** The patient may understandably be anxious, but this is better treated by pain relief and reassurance.

4. a. **False.** Tolerance occurs to both, although often more to the adverse effects; hence the need for a nitrate-free period when prescribing nitrates.

   b. **False.** Nitrates are effective in heart failure by reducing preload (venous vasodilatation).

   c. **True.** Standard treatment.

   d. **True.** Since nitrates are vasodilators, and the adverse effects are vasodilatatory in nature, this is a definition of a type A adverse effect (see Ch. 21).

   e. **False.** Although true for glyceryl trinitrate (GTN), this is not true for isosorbide mononitrate.

5. a. **False.** This is likely to kill a patient.

   b. **False.** Even the β_1-specific blockers such as atenolol block β_2-adrenoceptors to some extent.

   c. **False.** Upregulation, i.e. increased number and sensitivity of receptors, occurs.

   d. **True.** Because they cross the blood–brain barrier more readily.

   e. **False.** The clinical activity often lasts longer than might be anticipated from the plasma half-life. The relevant factor is the duration of receptor binding, which is difficult to measure; plasma concentration is only a surrogate for this, which works reasonably well for some drugs but not for beta-blockers.

7. a. **True.** May cause Na^+ retention.

   b. **True.** Negative inotropes.

   c. **False.** Frequently used to treat cardiac failure.

   d. **True.** Along with most non-steroidal anti-inflammatory drugs, it may reduce prostaglandin production in the kidney and hence cause fluid retention and reduce the effects of diuretics.

   e. **False.** Its positive inotropic effect may be of value in some patients but its most common use is in slowing the heart allowing it to be more efficient in cardiac failure related to atrial fibrillation.

8. a. **True.** May cause Na^+ and fluid retention. Secondary hyperaldosteronism may be worsened by diuretic therapy.

   b. **True.** Ultimately it becomes harmful in cardiac failure.

   c. **False.** A very minor part (if used at all) of therapy for most cases of heart failure.

   d. **False.** Diuretics may increase activation of the renin–angiotensin–aldosterone system.

   e. **True.** This accounts for some of the action of furosemide in acute pulmonary oedema and for the action of thiazides in hypertension.

9. a. **True.** Probably not a long-term effect.

   b. **False.** Hypokalaemia is common.

   c. **False.** More likely to cause adverse effects with little increase in hypotensive effects.

   d. **False.** Furosemide is a loop diuretic that works mainly in the ascending limb of the loop of Henle.

   e. **False.** Potassium-sparing diuretics are weak and loop diuretics are the first choice.

10. a. **False.** Digoxin is likely to have a very long half-life in a patient with such poor renal function, and the patient would be at risk of digoxin toxicity if usual doses were used.

    b. **True.** Almost any arrhythmia can result from digoxin: heart block or ventricular bigeminy are the most common.

    c. **True.** Because K^+ can no longer enter the cell nor Na^+ leave the cell as a result of the poisoning of the Na^+/K^+-ATPase.

    d. **False.** ST depression is the common change seen on ECG in a reverse tick pattern.

    e. **True.** Since diuretics may cause hypokalaemia, and hypokalaemia makes digoxin toxicity more likely.

11. a. **False.** Other peptides such as bradykinin are also affected.

    b. **True.** Hence their value in hypertension and cardiac failure.

    c. **True.** Hence should be widely used in these patients.

    d. **False.** May decrease intrarenal blood flow and cause renal impairment.

    e. **True.** Especially in women.

12. a. **True.** For instance amiodarone, which is mainly type III but also partially type I.

    b. **False.** Lidocaine is metabolised by the liver.

    c. **True.** This poses problems in managing many patients with cardiac disease.

    d. **False.** Steady state will occur after five half-lives – anything up to 500 days for amiodarone.

    e. **True.** Verapamil was in the past the most common first choice but adenosine is more widely used now.

Case history answers

Case history 1

1. Aspirin, glyceryl trinitrate (GTN), an opiate for pain relief, a thrombolytic such as streptokinase. Other drugs proved to be of benefit but less often used include beta-blockers, i.v. nitrates.

2. A history of active peptic ulceration, surgery or cerebrovascular accident within the previous 6 months, allergy to aspirin or streptokinase.

3. Atropine (not isoprenaline which would increase myocardial oxygen demands and might worsen his myocardial infarction).

4. GTN to be used as required, aspirin and a beta-blocker or an ACE inhibitor (and almost certainly a statin).

5. Lifestyle modification, graded exercise (perhaps as part of a rehabilitation programme), stopping smoking, management of acute angina, what to do in the event of further severe pain and what follow-up arrangements are made.

Case history 2

1. GTN to be used as required; prophylactic therapy: normally a beta-blocker would be the first choice in a patient with exercise-induced asthma. However, in this patient this might not be appropriate because of the COPD. Alternatives are, therefore, calcium-channel blockers and oral nitrates. Think of his cholesterol too, and maybe even nicotine replacement therapy.

2. Stop smoking, lifestyle modification, how to cope with attacks of chest pain.

3. Loss of efficacy of nitrates in treating angina, probably the result of depletion of sulfhydryl groups. Avoid by building a nitrate-free period into the drug regimen, e.g. overnight.

4. Diet, management of other risk factors for ischaemic heart disease, exclude liver and thyroid disease and perhaps screen his family. However, it is unlikely that a cholesterol this high will respond sufficiently to diet alone. Many would start a statin e.g. simvastatin now rather than wait.

5. Drug therapy with diet, e.g. simvastatin, and if this has been tried already, use higher doses and if still unsuccessful try adding a second line drug such as ezetimibe.

6. Salbutamol stimulates β_1- and β_2-adrenoceptors in the heart and may cause tachycardia, increasing myocardial oxygen demand and possibly precipitating angina.

Case history 3

1. Thyroid function tests (hyperthyroidism may cause arrhythmias and the tests may be affected by amiodarone therapy), electrolytes, liver function tests.

2. A long time! Usually quoted as five half-lives: in the case of amiodarone, this could be between 125 and 500 days. Hence a high loading dose is usually given for a short period to saturate the tissues, then a lower maintenance dose.

3. Amiodarone may prolong the duration of warfarin activity and increase INR (international normalised ratio). This is best managed by careful regular measurement of INR when amiodarone is introduced and adjustment of the dose of warfarin accordingly.

4. Amiodarone has too many serious long-term effects to be first choice; but this has to be judged patient by patient.

Case history 4

1. A diuretic, e.g. furosemide, in a low dose, possibly but not necessarily with a K$^+$-sparing diuretic. An ACE inhibitor would be useful in addition.

2. Digoxin and possibly warfarin (patients on diuretics taking digoxin will need careful monitoring of K$^+$ levels).

3. An ACE inhibitor if not already used (but stop a K$^+$-sparing diuretic if he has been on one), and possibly digoxin.

4. Intravenous opiate, furosemide and possibly nitrates, oxygen.

5. Indometacin may cause fluid retention and interfere with the effects of the diuretic. It may also not be necessary; why not use a simple analgesic?

Short note answers

1. These drugs include aspirin (for its antiplatelet effects), beta-blockers (proven to reduce mortality in the long term after myocardial infarction), an ACE inhibitor (proven also to reduce mortality after myocardial infarction, possibly by preventing morphological changes in the left ventricle), a lipid-lowering agent such as simvastatin (again proven to reduce mortality after myocardial infarction).

2. This should cover the use of ACE inhibitors in heart failure, hypertension and after myocardial infarction. A particularly good answer would also include their use in high-risk patients without such conditions such as patients with diabetes and ischaemic heart disease.

Extended matching items answers

Theme: treatment of ischaemic cardiovascular disease

1. D. This drug lowers the rate of contraction of the left ventricle and relaxes smooth muscle.

2. F. This (single) drug acts in stable angina by decreasing oxygen demand in the heart.

3. A. May all be used in secondary prevention after myocardial infarction (possibly in addition to other drugs).

4. F. This (single) drug acts in stable angina by increasing oxygen supply to the heart.

5. E. These drugs may both be used to treat angina pectoris.

6. E. These drugs both require the presence of sulphydryl (–SH) groups to function.

Theme: treatment of arrhythmias

1. A, D, maybe G. Usually digoxin or a beta-blocker such as sotalol. Amiodarone is occasionally used.

2. B, D or G. Digoxin may slow the ventricular response if the patient goes into atrial fibrillation, but does not reduce the likelihood of this change in rhythm, whereas sotalol and amiodarone will.

3. G. But lidocaine may also be used less commonly.

4. E.

5. G. Amiodarone can cause pneumonitis (sotalol and adenosine can cause bronchospasm, which might also be thought of as a form of pulmonary toxicity).

6. F is best but amiodarone or flecainide could also be used.

Theme: treatment of congestive cardiac failure

1. A, C, D. By a variety of mechanisms

2. B, E. By causing a diuresis, they will trigger counter regulatory mechanisms stimulating the renin–angiotensin–aldosterone axis.

3. B, H. Either alone or together. Also use morphine and oxygen.

4. A, C, D. Check electrolytes regularly. If using these together, be very cautious.

5. F or C. By different mechanisms.

6. C, D, H. All useful in reducing preload and afterload. A loop diuretic such as bumetanide also causes vasodilatation in acute pulmonary oedema but not in chronic use.

Drugs and the blood

5.1 **Coagulation and thrombosis**　　71

5.2 **Formation of blood**　　76

　　Self-assessment on Chapter 5: questions　　78

　　Self-assessment on Chapter 5: answers　　81

Overview

Thrombosis and embolism are important in the pathology of a range of diseases (e.g. myocardial infarction, venous thromboembolic disease). Drugs such as heparin and warfarin are used to treat and to prevent such conditions by preventing extension of the embolism or thrombosis, but carry a risk of causing bleeding. Antiplatelet agents have a weaker antithrombotic effect but may be particularly effective in conditions involving risk of arterial thrombosis (e.g. cerebrovascular disease or coronary heart disease). They are associated with less risk of bleeding. Formed thromboses can also be dissolved by thrombolytic drugs, for instance in the treatment of myocardial infarction.

Anaemia is caused by failure of formation of blood or blood loss. Iron, vitamin B_{12} and folic acid are all essential in blood formation and are used therapeutically in deficiency states.

5.1 Coagulation and thrombosis

Learning objectives

At the end of this section you should be able to:
- list conditions where thrombosis and embolism may be important
- explain how heparin and warfarin work and are used
- explain how they are monitored
- describe the common antiplatelet drugs
- describe thrombolytic drugs.

Thrombosis or clotting of the blood occurs as a result of the interaction of several clotting proteins in the blood. Many of these are produced by the liver and act as a cascade, amplifying their effect (Fig. 29). This is a vital mechanism in preventing blood loss after injury, but it can also happen in other circumstances where it is less desirable. For instance, a myocardial infarction is usually caused by a thrombus developing on a ruptured atheromatous plaque and blocking the coronary artery. A thrombotic stroke is similar. Thrombosis may form in one site and then move to block a blood vessel elsewhere; this is a called an embolus: for instance, patients with atrial fibrillation may develop thrombi in the non-contracting left atrium and are at high risk of a stroke. This can be reduced by anticoagulation.

Conditions where thrombi or emboli are harmful to patients are treated with anticoagulants, which are drugs that inhibit normal clotting.

Anticoagulant therapy

Indications for anticoagulation

The main indications for anticoagulant therapy are:

- treatment or prophylaxis of venous thromboembolic disease: deep venous thrombosis of the leg or pulmonary embolism
- atrial fibrillation, especially in the presence of structural heart disease, particularly poor left ventricular function or mitral stenosis
- mechanical prosthetic heart valve
- acute coronary syndromes (low molecular weight heparin (LMWH)).

Risk factors

Venous thromboembolic disorders occur as a result of a triad (Virchow's triad) of hypercoagulable state,

Intrinsic pathway
(e.g. triggered by collagen)

Extrinsic pathway
(e.g. triggered by factor III released from cell membrane)

XII ⟶ XIIa

XI ⟶ XIa

*VII ⟶ VIIa

*IX ⟶ IXa

Factor VIII
Ca^{2+}

Factor III
Ca^{2+}

X ⟶ Xa ⟵ X

(Prothrombin) *II ⟶ IIa (Thrombin)

Fibrinogen ⟶ Fibrin

*Factors where production is decreased by warfarin

Fig. 29 The coagulation cascade. The intrinsic and extrinsic pathways amplify the response of blood damaged tissue. They converge in the formation of thrombin and interact in other ways also. Clotting factors are activated sequentially, increasing the response. Heparin enhances interaction between thrombin and antithrombin III, and between antithrombin III and many of the factors in the intrinsic pathway. The proteins are given roman numbers and the activated form is the 'a' form.

vessel wall damage and stasis of blood. Not all may be present in the one patient but risk factors include

- immobility (e.g. after surgery or illness)
- malignant disease
- tissue damage (e.g. after surgery or myocardial infarction)
- genetic predisposition (e.g. factor V or prothrombin mutations)
- pregnancy or oestrogen therapy (see Ch. 12).

Contraindications to anticoagulation

None of the following contraindications is absolute – the risks must be weighed against the benefits:

- renal or liver disease
- peptic ulcer disease
- recent surgery or trauma
- other conditions that might cause a risk of bleeding (e.g. patient at risk of falling).

Heparin

Heparin is a naturally occurring mucopolysaccharide. It binds to antithrombin III and enhances its anticoagulant effect, inhibiting the formation of thrombin, factor Xa and other clotting factors. It is active in vitro as well as in vivo.

Heparin given parenterally, either subcutaneous (s.c.) or i.v. (usually as an infusion). It has a short half-life and is metabolised by the liver.

Low molecular weight heparins (e.g. dalteparin, enoxaparin)

The low molecular weight heparins (LMWH, e.g. dalteparin) are purified derivatives that have more consistent activity than common unfractionated heparin. Consequently, they require less monitoring. They have a longer duration of action than unfractionated heparin and are therefore more convenient (for instance, in the treatment of deep vein thrombosis LMWH can be given s.c. once or twice a day compared with a continuous i.v. infusion of unfractionated heparin, perhaps allowing home therapy rather than hospital admission). However, they are more expensive.

Therapeutic uses of heparin

Heparin is indicated:

- where immediate or short-term anticoagulation is required
- in acute coronary syndromes.

Clinical sketch

A 25-year-old woman presents with a swollen left leg while taking a combined oral contraceptive pill. She has also experienced some chest pain and shortness of breath. Her mother died of a pulmonary embolus following an operation 4 years earlier.

Comment: this patient requires immediate treatment and investigation. The history is strongly suggestive of a thrombosis in the deep veins of the leg, associated with a pulmonary embolus. The combined oral contraceptive pill can increase the risks of such events. There may be a familial predisposition, suggested by the history of her mother, which will need further investigation. This patient needs immediate investigation (ventilation/perfusion scanning or CT pulmonary angiography) and treatment. Treatment will involve withdrawing the oral contraceptive pill (and providing alternative suitable contraception); immediate treatment will be i.v. heparin or subcutaneous low molecular weight heparin followed by warfarin for a period, usually of 6 months in this instance.

Two years on, the same patient is now off the oral contraceptive and anticoagulation, but presents with chest pain and shortness of breath. Ventilation perfusion scanning again confirms the presence of a pulmonary embolus. She is treated immediately with LMWH.

Comment: this patient has now had two thromboembolic episodes and the usual advice would be that she should be treated with anticoagulation for life. This will require careful and regular monitoring and carries risks of bleeding, but in this case the benefits outweigh the risks.

Clinical sketch–cont'd

Three years later the same patient has been taking warfarin with no problems. However, she develops a respiratory tract infection and is prescribed erythromycin.

Comment: warfarin is the drug most commonly involved in serious drug interactions. It is metabolised by liver enzymes and if this metabolism is inhibited (for instance, by drugs such as erythromycin) its effects will be greatly intensified and this may lead to serious bleeding.

The duration of heparin therapy is determined by the indication. If it is to be followed by long-term oral anticoagulation, warfarin may be started immediately and heparin discontinued, usually within 72 hours.

Monitoring heparin

The degree of anticoagulation achieved is monitored by measuring the activated partial thromboplastin time (APTT), and the dose is adjusted, usually until the APTT is two to three times longer than a normal control. There is usually no need to monitor the degree of anticoagulation when s.c. heparin is used as prophylaxis. LMWHs do not usually require monitoring but if it is necessary, monitoring would be of activated factor Xa concentrations.

Adverse effects

- bleeding, locally at the site of injection or more distantly
- hypersensitivity may occur rarely (often skin reactions, some serious)
- thrombocytopenia may occur (regular platelet counts necessary for both types of heparin if used for more than 5 days)
- osteoporosis or hair loss in long-term use.

Reversal. In the event of bleeding caused by either heparin, it may be sufficient to stop the heparin. If a more urgent reversal is needed, *protamine* can be given i.v.; it binds to heparin and reverses its effects. If given in excessive dose, however, protamine may itself have anticoagulant effects.

Other injected anticoagulants

Heparinoids and fondaparinux act similarly to heparin. Hirudins can be given to patients with heparin-induced thrombocytopenia.

Oral anticoagulants

These competitively inhibit the formation of the vitamin K-dependent clotting factors (II, VII, IX, X).

Their onset of action is determined by the time required to clear those factors which are already formed, usually 48–72 hours to achieve their full effect. They are only active in vivo.

Warfarin is the most widely used. It is given orally, heavily protein bound (99%) and is metabolised by cytochrome P450 enzymes (especially CYP 2C9 but also others) of the liver. There is enormous variation in sensitivity to warfarin, in part determined by genetic factors because of its metabolism. Other factors are body weight, diet and patient compliance. Careful monitoring and individual dose adjustment is required. Drug interactions may occur either by protein displacement or especially by effects of other drugs on liver enzymes (see below).

Therapeutic uses

Warfarin is used for long-term anticoagulation. It is given initially as a loading dose and later as a maintenance dose.

Monitoring oral anticoagulants

Warfarin dose is adjusted according to its anticoagulant effect, measured by the prothrombin time, often expressed as the INR (international normalised ratio, in which internationally standardised reagents are used) and the dose adjusted to achieve the desired ratio to control values. For the treatment of thromboembolic disease this is usually 2–3, and for arterial disease, it is 3–4.5. The INR should be measured daily when therapy is initiated, but monthly in long-term use when the patient is stable.

Adverse effects

- bleeding: spontaneous or after minor trauma
- hypersensitivity
- teratogenetic: should not be given in the first trimester of pregnancy.

Drug interactions

Warfarin is probably the drug most commonly involved in serious drug interactions. Great caution is required when other drugs are coprescribed (see the clinical sketch on p. 72). Patients must be fully aware of the risks of drug interaction, with both prescribed drugs and with those that may be bought without prescription, and patients should carry an anticoagulant card.

- Drugs that inhibit cytochrome P450 enzymes will increase the effects of warfarin: cimetidine, erythromycin, ciprofloxacin, co-trimoxazole, metronidazole, fluconazole.

- Drugs which induce P450 enzymes will decrease the effects of warfarin: rifampicin, many antiepileptics.

These lists are not exhaustive. If a patient has been stabilised on warfarin while taking one of these drugs, its withdrawal may have serious consequences.

- Drugs that have an antiplatelet effect, such as aspirin, may enhance the anticoagulant effect of warfarin and should generally be avoided. This is a pharmacodynamic interaction.

Reversal of warfarin effects

The effects of warfarin can be reversed by administration of vitamin K. This can be given i.v. or orally, the dose and route determining whether the reversal is short term or long term. This will take several hours to act, and in urgent cases it may be necessary to replace the deficient clotting factors (usually by giving fresh frozen plasma or factor concentrate i.v.).

Other oral anticoagulants such as phenindione or acenocoumarol are occasionally used instead of warfarin.

Antiplatelet drugs

Platelets are important in the initiation of thrombosis. Platelets are activated by tissue damage and release thromboxane A$_2$, an arachidonic acid derivative that activates further platelets and promotes platelet aggregation, as well as causing vasoconstriction. The platelets block and narrow blood vessels and may precipitate the clotting cascade. Platelets are also activated by ADP (adenosine diphosphate), thrombin, and fibrinogen. Platelets aggregate by cross linking at a specialised receptor, the glycoprotein IIb/IIIa receptor. Drugs can block several of these steps so as to reduce platelet activity and reduce the risk of thrombosis.

Aspirin. Even in low doses, aspirin irreversibly inhibits cyclo-oxygenase, which is essential for the formation of thromboxane A$_2$. Aspirin also inhibits the formation of the antithrombotic prostaglandin prostacyclin, produced by the endothelium. The duration of effect on platelets is greater than that on endothelium (platelets have no nuclei and so cannot regenerate cyclo-oxygenase), so the balance is to prevent thrombosis.

Dipyridamole inhibits phosphodiesterase preventing formation of intraplatelet cAMP, and thereby inhibiting aggregation.

Clopidogrel blocks ADP receptors. It also impairs response of the platelet to collagen, fibrinogen and thrombin.

Glycoprotein IIa/IIIb receptor antagonists. These (e.g. *tirofiban*) are also an effective antiplatelet agent by inhibiting the final common pathway of platelet aggregation.

Therapeutic uses

The antiplatelet agents are particularly effective in conditions involving arterial thrombosis where platelets are more important, such as myocardial infarction or angina, and cerebrovascular accident or transient ischaemic attacks. They may have some, but less, effect in venous thrombosis where clotting factors are more important.

Aspirin as an antiplatelet agent

Aspirin is useful in a wide variety of rheumatological conditions and as an analgesic. (These effects are discussed in Ch. 7.) Aspirin is a highly effective and inexpensive antiplatelet drug. There is some controversy over the most appropriate dose of aspirin as an antiplatelet drug, since higher doses may cause more adverse effects and may increase the degree of inhibition of prostacyclin.

In acute coronary syndromes, aspirin reduces the risk of infarction in unstable angina, reduces the number of severe exacerbations in patients with stable angina and possibly slows disease progression. When given to patients with an acute myocardial infarction, it reduces mortality to a similar extent as thrombolytic therapy (see below). The combination of aspirin and thrombolytic drugs is more effective than either alone. When given to patients after myocardial infarction, aspirin reduces the risks of further ischaemic events.

In patients at high risk of cardiovascular or cerebrovascular events, aspirin should be used in addition to lipid-lowering therapy, unless there are contraindications.

In cerebrovascular disease, aspirin is also used to treat transient ischaemic attacks and as secondary prophylaxis to prevent further thrombotic cerebrovascular accidents.

After cardiovascular surgical procedures, aspirin also reduces the rate of closure of coronary artery grafts or of restenosis after coronary angioplasty.

Adverse effects of aspirin

Most important are gastric irritation and bleeding, and hypersensitivity.

Other antiplatelet drugs

Dipyridamole is an alternative to aspirin in cerebrovascular disease; it may also be used with aspirin, where the effects are additive. Adverse effects include gastrointestinal upsets and hypersensitivity.

Clopidogrel is used in high-risk patients to prevent cardiovascular events. It is an alternative to aspirin in cardiac disease; it may also be used with aspirin for greater effect, but also with increased risk of bleeding. Other adverse effects include gastrointestinal upsets and hypersensitivity. *Tirofiban* is used intravenously in some acute coronary syndromes (see Ch. 4), along with aspirin and with LMWHs. Adverse effect is bleeding.

Thrombolytic drugs

Thromboses are dynamic – they are breaking down (thrombolysis) at the same time they are forming, with a variable balance between the two processes. Thrombolysis occurs when a blood protein, plasminogen, is converted to plasmin, which breaks down fibrin. Thrombolytic drugs activate plasmin and push the balance towards thrombolysis (Fig. 30).

Therapeutic uses

Thrombolytic drugs are most commonly used in the treatment of myocardial infarction. If given early, they can break down the thrombus that has caused the infarct, unblocking the artery, allowing reperfusion and limiting the extent of the damage. This has been proven to reduce mortality from myocardial infarction substantially.

Thrombolytic drugs are also used in the treatment of acute thrombotic stroke (though they must be given within 3 hours of the onset of the stroke – alteplase only) or severe pulmonary embolism.

Fig. 30 The action of thrombolytic drugs.

Contraindications to thrombolytic therapy

- active peptic ulcer
- bleeding condition of any sort
- severe hypertension
- recent surgery or trauma.

Adverse effects

- bleeding
- allergy (streptokinase only).

Streptokinase

Streptokinase is produced from β-haemolytic streptococci. It may react with antibodies in patients previously exposed either to streptokinase or a recent streptococcal infection, leading to allergic reaction (1–2% of patients) or to unpredictable effectiveness. Streptokinase is given i.v. as a short infusion and its effects last about 3–4 hours.

Alteplase

Alteplase is a naturally occurring activator of plasminogen in humans, produced by genetic recombinant techniques. Since it is not 'foreign', it does not usually cause allergic reactions. Alteplase is as effective as, or possibly more effective than, streptokinase but may be associated with more haemorrhagic complications and is more expensive. It is given as a short i.v. infusion. Tenecteplase is similar but is given as a bolus rather than an infusion – this may make it suitable for use by medical or paramedical staff attending patients in their own homes.

> **Clinical sketch**
>
> A patient presents with acute myocardial infarction. The pain started 4 hours ago and there is marked ST elevation on the ECG. The patient had a myocardial infarction 2 years earlier which was treated with streptokinase.
>
> *Comment: this is an indication for urgent thrombolysis and antiplatelet therapy. The patient should be given aspirin. Patients given streptokinase may develop antibodies to the enzyme, which can render its antithrombotic effect erratic and undependable. For this reason, patients who have previously received streptokinase should generally receive alteplase for subsequent infarction. Alteplase is commonly given in combination with heparin.*

Antifibrinolytic drugs

Antifibrinolytic drugs can be useful in conditions where there is excessive bleeding. *Tranexamic acid* inhibits activation of plasminogen. It is used occasionally to try to stop uncontrolled bleeding, e.g. after dental extraction in haemophiliacs (in addition to clotting factors), after streptokinase overdose or in the treatment of severe menorrhagia.

5.2 Formation of blood

Anaemia is defined as a deficiency of haemoglobin, below the normal for the patient's age and sex. There are many causes, and each case needs careful investigation; anaemia itself is not an adequate diagnosis. This discussion is limited to those anaemias caused by deficiencies that can be corrected pharmacologically.

Bear in mind that as well as correcting anaemia, drugs can also cause anaemia:

- drugs that cause bleeding, e.g. non-steroidal anti-inflammatory drugs
- drugs that suppress the marrow, e.g. cytotoxic drugs or occasionally a severe adverse reaction to other drugs
- drugs that promote red cell breakdown, e.g. methyldopa or high-dose penicillin.

Iron-deficiency anaemia

In iron-deficiency anaemia there is either an inadequate intake of iron to meet physiological needs (e.g. in menstruation, in pregnancy or in elderly patients with a poor diet), or there is loss of iron (e.g. in patients with chronic bleeding).

Diagnosis
- anaemia is hypochromic microcytic
- serum iron and iron stores are low.

Treatment
Iron is well absorbed from the small intestine when there is an iron-deficient state. Oral iron salts are usually used, often for 3–4 months to ensure that the anaemia is corrected and stores replenished. Failure to respond to oral iron is usually because of poor compliance (see Ch. 19) but may occasionally be the result of malabsorption or of continued blood loss.

Ferrous sulphate. Adverse effects include constipation, epigastric pain and nausea. If these are intolerable, a reduced dose or an alternative preparation should be used. The stools usually darken in patients taking oral iron.

Iron dextran. Occasionally oral forms cannot be tolerated, and iron (iron dextran) can be given by i.v. infusion or by deep intramuscular (i.m.) injection. The major risk of the infusion is anaphylaxis.

Vitamin B_{12} deficiency

Vitamin B_{12} is necessary for the adequate formation of nucleic acids. Deficiency usually arises from an autoimmune disease affecting the gastric mucosa so that a cofactor necessary for the absorption of the vitamin is not produced. This is called pernicious anaemia. The body usually has extensive stores and the anaemia will not arise for some months or years. Diagnosis is by finding out if the:

- anaemia is hypochromic but macrocytic
- bone marrow contains megaloblasts.

In severe cases (sometimes even without severe anaemia), the spinal cord may also be damaged.

Treatment
Treatment is by i.m. vitamin B_{12} (*hydroxocobalamin*), avoiding the need for absorption from the gastrointestinal tract. Lifelong treatment will be required, usually with 3-monthly injections.

Clinical sketch

A 65-year-old woman presents with weight loss and a microcytic anaemia. The general practitioner prescribes ferrous sulphate, but the anaemia fails to respond.

Comment: anaemia alone is not a sufficient diagnosis. This patient may well have a malignancy that has caused the weight loss and probably blood loss leading to the microcytic anaemia. Replacing iron stores is not going to stop further bleeding. This patient needs full investigation on first presentation.

Folic acid deficiency

Folic acid is also a cofactor for nucleic acid production, and deficiency also causes a hypochromic macrocytic anaemia. Body stores of folic acid are very limited, and deficiency is usually quickly apparent. Deficiency arises from malabsorption, from inadequate diet or from excessive demand, e.g. in pregnancy or in patients with rapid cell turnover (severe psoriasis or haemolytic anaemia). Folic acid replacement is by mouth, with very high doses being used if malabsorption is the underlying problem.

Folic acid in pregnancy.

See Chapter 19.

Other causes of anaemia

Erythropoietin, a glycoprotein released by the kidney, stimulates the bone marrow to produce red blood cells. In renal disease and especially in patients on dialysis, it is deficient and the patient may become anaemic. Erythropoietin can now be synthesised (*epoetin*) and given parenterally as a replacement to treat such patients. Adverse effects are usually the result of its overuse, when an attempt is made to restore haemoglobin levels fully to normal. This may result in severe hypertension with encephalopathy and thrombosis. Most patients are asymptomatic with a haemoglobin of around 10 g/dl (100 g/L) and experience no adverse effects.

Granulocyte colony stimulating factors (GCSF), e.g. filgrastim, encourage white cell proliferation in the marrow and are increasingly used in patients with neutropenia, especially after anticancer chemo-therapy (see Ch. 15).

Five

Self-assessment on Chapter 5: questions

Multiple choice questions

1. Heparin:
   a. Can be taken orally
   b. Activity may be enhanced by drugs that are heavily protein bound
   c. By the subcutaneous route reduces the risk of thromboembolic disease in hospitalised patients
   d. Is antagonised by protamine
   e. Dosage is monitored by the international normalised ratio (INR)

2. Drugs that may interact with warfarin include:
   a. Phenytoin
   b. Metronidazole
   c. Clarithromycin
   d. Trimethoprim
   e. Gemfibrozil

3. Warfarin:
   a. Is active in vitro
   b. Can be antagonised by vitamin K
   c. Hypersensitivity is a common adverse effect
   d. Should not be given to pregnant women in the first trimester
   e. Is used to treat pulmonary embolism

4. Aspirin:
   a. Inhibits the production of both aggregatory and anti-aggregatory mediators
   b. Improves the prognosis in acute myocardial infarction
   c. Increases bleeding time
   d. In low doses may be safely given to patients with allergy to aspirin
   e. Is contraindicated in cerebrovascular disease

5. Thrombolytics:
   a. Depend on the presence of plasminogen
   b. Are contraindicated in patients with active peptic ulcer disease
   c. Dosage is adjusted according to bleeding time
   d. Activity of streptokinase may be decreased in patients with a recent streptococcal infection
   e. Bleeding is a potentially serious complication

6. In treating anaemia:
   a. Oral iron is often poorly absorbed by iron-deficient anaemics
   b. Patients with B_{12} deficiency may present with weakness of the legs
   c. Folate deficiency may occur because of gastrointestinal bleeding
   d. Erythropoietin is deficient in chronic renal disease
   e. Anaemia should always be treated in the first instance by blood transfusion

7. Drugs that may cause anaemia include:
   a. Indometacin
   b. Carbimazole
   c. Methotrexate
   d. Penicillin
   e. Morphine

Case history questions

Case history 1

A 57-year-old man develops an extensive deep venous thrombosis after discharge from hospital, where he has recently had a cholecystectomy. He also has pleuritic chest pain and breathlessness.

1. Should he be admitted to hospital?
2. What drug or drugs should he receive initially?
3. What drug should he receive for long-term management?
4. How is the dose determined?
5. What interactions must he be warned of?

Case history 2

A 25-year-old woman with menorrhagia and a poor diet presents with an iron-deficient anaemia.

1. How should the anaemia be treated?
2. What likely adverse effects of treatment should the patient be warned of?
3. If the patient fails to respond to treatment, what possible explanations should be considered?
4. When would i.v. therapy be considered?

Short note question

Compare and contrast warfarin and heparin as drugs.

Extended matching items questions

Theme: Drug selection

Options

A. Unfractionated heparin

B. Warfarin

C. Streptokinase

D. Dalteparin

E. Indometacin

F. Aspirin

G. Clopidogrel

H. Diclofenac

From the list of options above, select the most appropriate drug to use in each of the following scenarios.

1. Treatment of a pulmonary embolus occurring in a 25-year-old woman who is 36 weeks pregnant.

2. Long-term secondary prevention following a transient ischaemic attack in a 60-year-old man with widespread vascular disease.

3. Prophylaxis against thromboembolism in a 55-year-old woman patient with a metallic prosthetic mitral valve.

4. First line treatment in the treatment of an acute thromboembolic cerebrovascular accident in a 75-year-old woman with a history of smoking and hypertension.

5. Treatment of an acute inferior myocardial infarction with ST segment elevation on the ECG in addition to aspirin.

Theme: Adverse effects of anticoagulants

Options

A. Reye's syndrome

B. Diarrhoea

C. Intracranial haemorrhage

D. Hypotension

E. Gastrointestinal bleeding

F. Malabsorption

G. Teratogenicity

H. Osteoporosis

From the list of options above, select the best match for each of the following statements.

1. The risk of this condition increases when thrombolytic therapy is given with other anticoagulants.

2. Long-term treatment with low molecular weight heparin can cause this condition.

3. Streptokinase administration is frequently accompanied by this condition.

4. Aspirin-containing preparations should not be given to young children because of an association with this condition.

5. Aspirin is a common cause of this adverse drug reaction.

Theme: Patient management

Options

A. Heparin

B. International normalised ratio (INR)

C. Full blood count

D. Aspirin

E. Dipyridamole

F. Activated partial thromboplastin time (APTT)

G. Warfarin

H. Dalteparin

I. Vitamin K

J. Fresh frozen plasma

K. Protamine

L. Cimetidine

Select the most appropriate option from the list above for each of the questions below. Each option may be used once, more than once, or not at all.

1. A 30-year-old woman develops a deep vein thrombosis. She presents to the A&E department. Select the most appropriate drug to use for anticoagulation immediately. How will it be administered?

2. Select the most appropriate means of monitoring her anticoagulation.

3. The patient needs oral anticoagulation for 3 months afterwards. Select a suitable drug and identify how it will be monitored.

4. Identify two drugs from the list which might cause dangerous interactions with this drug.

5. Some weeks later, the patient is found to be dangerously over-anticoagulated and requires an antidote. Which drug or drugs will you administer?

6. Which drug is an antidote to excessive doses of heparin?

Theme: Thrombolytic drugs in coronary heart disease

Options

A. Aspirin

B. Indometacin

C. Dipyridamole

D. Tirofiban

E. Alteplase

F. Dalteparin

G. Warfarin

H. Tranexamic acid

I. Clopidogrel

J. Streptokinase

K. Phenindione

Select the most appropriate option from the list above for each of the questions below. Each option may be used once, more than once, or not at all.

1. Select a drug or drugs which act against cyclo-oxygenase to inhibit platelet activity

2. Select a drug or drugs which prevents cross-linking of platelets

3. Select a drug which increases plasmin activity and one which decreases plasmin activity

4. Which antiplatelet drugs might be used in combinations?

5. Which drug or drugs are most likely to cause hypersensitivity reactions?

6. Which drug or drugs can be administered subcutaneously?

Self-assessment on Chapter 5: answers

Multiple choice answers

1. a. **False.** Heparin must be used parenterally.
   b. **False.** Heparin is not itself protein bound and so is unaffected by other drugs in this way.
   c. **True.** Patients who are immobilised in hospital should be considered for subcutaneous heparin.
   d. **True.** Used in overdoses of heparin.
   e. **False.** The INR is used to monitor warfarin. The APTT is the correct test to monitor heparin. Clotting time is an alternative.

2. a. **True.** Liver enzyme induction.
   b. **True.** Liver enzyme inhibition.
   c. **True.** A liver enzyme inhibitor although this is often forgotten.
   d. **False.** No plasma protein binding or enzyme inhibition.
   e. **True.** Plasma protein displacement.

3. a. **False.** It is only active as a result of the inhibition of protein metabolism and so can only act in vivo and only after 1–2 days.
   b. **True.** Warfarin is a competitive antagonist for vitamin K.
   c. **False.** Bleeding is by far the most common adverse effect: hypersensitivity is rare.
   d. **True.** May be teratogenic.
   e. **True.** Although there are many other indications also.

4. a. **True.** Both prostacyclin (anti-aggregatory from the endothelium) and thromboxane A_2 (pro-aggregatory, from the platelets) are affected. In theory, low-dose aspirin inhibits thromboxane more, since platelets have no nuclei and cannot secrete new thromboxane-manufacturing enzymes.
   b. **True.** By as much as streptokinase in some trials.
   c. **True.** Prevents formation of platelet plugs.
   d. **False.** In hypersensitivity, the dosage is usually unimportant in triggering a reaction.
   e. **False.** It is widely used for this indication.

5. a. **True.** Thrombolytics activate plasminogen to plasmin, which then breaks down established clots.
   b. **True.** The risks would seem to outweigh the benefits.
   c. **False.** There is at present no way of adjusting the dose according to need, and all patients receive the same dose.
   d. **True.** Antistreptococcal antibodies may be present and inhibit streptokinase.
   e. **True.** The most common and serious adverse effect.

6. a. **False.** In the absence of a specific malabsorption syndrome, iron is very avidly absorbed by iron-deficient patients.
   b. **True.** Lack of vitamin B_{12} can cause damage to the spinal cord.
   c. **False.** Folate deficiency is the result of either an inadequate diet or excessive utilisation, e.g. in psoriasis, pregnancy, etc.
   d. **True.** Can now be given to such patients to correct their anaemia.
   e. **False.** Anaemia is a sign, not a diagnosis. Transfusion may interfere with investigations of the underlying cause as well as being potentially hazardous.

7. a. **True.** By gastrointestinal blood loss.
   b. **True.** By marrow suppression.
   c. **True.** By marrow suppression (folate antagonism).
   d. **True.** High-dose penicillins may cause haemolytic anaemia.
   e. **False.** This has never been recorded.

Case history answers

Case history 1

1. Yes. The clinical suspicion is that of a deep vein thrombosis associated with a pulmonary embolus. The risk of life-threatening pulmonary embolus warrants urgent admission to hospital.
2. Heparin should be given immediately, usually s.c. low molecular weight heparin.

3. Warfarin will usually be given after a deep venous thrombosis/pulmonary embolus to reduce the risks of recurrence or extension of the clot.

4. Dose of warfarin is determined by its effects on clotting, as measured by the INR (international normalised ratio).

5. Warfarin is commonly involved in serious drug interactions; there are many examples, including those with liver enzyme inducers and inhibitors (see Ch. 20).

Case history 2

1. Oral iron, usually ferrous sulphate, for several months, both to treat the anaemia and renew iron stores.

2. Constipation, darkening of the faeces and other gastrointestinal symptoms are the most common adverse effects of oral iron preparations.

3. The diagnosis should be reconsidered: if the patient genuinely has an iron-deficient anaemia, then could malabsorption be responsible? However, the most likely explanation for failure to respond is either continued heavy blood loss or poor compliance with the medication.

4. Intravenous iron is rarely necessary. May be needed in case of severe malabsorption or if the patient is unable to tolerate a variety of oral iron preparations.

Short note answer

The answer should consider:

1. Routes of administration (oral warfarin versus parenteral heparin)

2. Mechanisms of action (immediate versus more slowly developing effects on different clotting factors)

3. Potential adverse effects (most commonly bleeding for both)

4. Risks of interactions (greater for warfarin)

5. Clinical circumstances in which each is used (short-term anticoagulation for heparin, longer term for warfarin, and some examples of each would be appropriate).

Extending matching items answers

Theme: Drug selection

1. D. Warfarin is best avoided in pregnancy because of its teratogenic potential and problems with uncontrolled bleeding at the time of delivery. Low molecular weight heparin (e.g. dalteparin) is the best drug in these circumstances. In the setting of a massive life-threatening pulmonary embolism associated with cardiovascular collapse, then thrombolysis with streptokinase could be *considered*.

2. F. Aspirin is generally first line in these circumstances. Although also NSAIDs, diclofenac and indometacin do not have antiplatelet activity.

3. B. Metallic prosthetic valves carry a high risk of thromboembolism, particularly those in the mitral position. Warfarin is the best drug to use here because of the long-term indication.

4. F. Again, aspirin is first line here.

5. C. The patient should be given thrombolysis (with streptokinase here) as well as aspirin. Each confers its own benefit, but the effect is greater than the sum of each given alone. An example of a synergistic drug interaction.

Theme: Adverse effects of anticoagulants

1. C. Intracranial haemorrhage is a serious risk associated with both thrombolysis and oral anticoagulants such as warfarin. This is significantly increased when both are given together.

2. H. Osteoporosis is a problem of long-term therapy with all low molecular weight heparins.

3. D. Although bleeding is a problem most known about with streptokinase, hypotension in the immediate period of infusion is a much more common clinical problem.

4. A. Aspirin is associated with a rare metabolic abnormality of Reye's syndrome in young children and hence should not be given to this group. Analgesia or antipyresis with paracetamol or ibuprofen is safer.

5. E. The association of NSAIDs and gastrointestinal bleeding is well documented.

Aspirin is commonly administered and even at low dose can cause gastric irritation and bleeding. This is a potentially serious adverse drug reaction. As with all prescribing considerations, the risks and benefits of treatment need to be weighed in the balance.

Theme: Patient management

1. A or H. She should be given i.v. heparin or s.c. dalteparin. Dalteparin is a purified low molecular weight heparin which is effective when given subcutaneously once per day. It is, therefore, more convenient (but more expensive) than unfractionated heparin.

2. F or none at all! A trick question. Your answer here depends on your answer to question 1. If given i.v. heparin, then the correct answer is the APTT, which should be twice as long as a normal control. If using dalteparin, then no monitoring is generally required.

3. G and B. The drug is, of course, warfarin, monitored by the INR (the ratio of the time taken for a patient's blood to clot when exposed to standardised reagents compared with that of a normal control). The desired range is usually 2–3.

4. There are several possibilities here. *D. Aspirin* may cause a pharmacodynamic interaction: by interfering with platelet aggregation it may increase the tendency to bleed. It might also cause gastric erosions or peptic ulcer disease, leading to bleeding. There might be a possible kinetic interaction also if aspirin displaces warfarin from plasma proteins, but this is not usually very significant (see Ch. 1). *L. Cimetidine* is a liver enzyme inhibitor and might cause an enhancement of the action of warfarin. *I. Vitamin K* would decrease the effect of warfarin; warfarin acts as a competitive vitamin K antagonist.

5. I definitely and possibly J. Vitamin K is the antidote which works by increasing production of clotting factors. However, this may take hours and if an immediate effect is required (e.g. if the patient is actively bleeding) then replacing the clotting factors directly in the form of fresh frozen plasma might be necessary. In most cases of over-anticoagulation, withdrawing warfarin for a few days is adequate.

6. K. Protamine is a physiological antagonist. It is less effective against LMWH than against unfractionated heparin and the dose is determined by the extent of heparin excess activity. If too much protamine is given, it has an anticoagulant effect of its own.

Theme: Thrombolytic drugs in coronary heart disease

1. A and B both inhibit cyclo-oxygenase. Indometacin is a reversible inhibitor in contrast to aspirin and as a result, and unlike aspirin, is not useful in preventing cardiac ischaemic events.

2. D. Tirofiban is a glycoprotein IIb/IIIa inhibitor which works in this way.

3. E alteplase and J streptokinase are plasmin activators and hence thrombolytics. H, tranexamic acid, reduces activity of plasmin and may reduce bleeding.

4. There are several possible combinations, but all involve aspirin which is the best established antiplatelet drug. A and C (dipyridamole) in cerebrovascular disease, A and D (tirofiban) in severe acute coronary syndromes and A and I (clopidogrel) in less severe acute coronary syndromes are commonly used combinations. All the combinations may carry an increased risk of bleeding over aspirin alone.

5. A and J, by different mechanisms. Aspirin like other cyclo-oxygnease inhibitors, may cause a pseudo-allergy by driving substrate down alternative metabolic routes to produce leukotrienes. It can cause fatal hypersensitivity reactions. It is a pseudo-allergy because there is no antibody–antigen reaction. Streptokinase may cause a hypersensitivity reaction if the patient has previous antibodies to streptokinase, e.g. after a streptococcal infection.

6. F. Only dalteparin of the current list is used subcutaneously.

Drugs used in CNS disease

6.1 **Anxiety and insomnia**   85

6.2 **Epilepsy**   87

6.3 **Depression and hypomania**   90

6.4 **Schizophrenia**   93

6.5 **Parkinsonism**   94

6.6 **Migraine**   96

6.7 **Other disorders**   97

    Self-assessment on Chapter 6: questions   98

    Self-assessment on Chapter 6: answers   102

Overview

The observation that certain substances could alter consciousness was probably the start of primitive pharmacology, and alcohol, nicotine, caffeine and illicit recreational drugs remain in common use. Over the last 200 years, the empirical approach of isolating active molecules from naturally occurring materials has continued and doses have been formalised. It is only very recently that we have started to understand the molecular mechanisms by which drugs work in the central nervous system (CNS). Nearly all CNS drugs modify chemical synaptic transmission by changing the synthesis, storage, catabolism, release or receptor interactions of transmitter substances, or by perturbing transmitter-regulated ion conductance. One of the key factors in neurological disease is using knowledge of these processes to identify the problem area and to decide on the correct drug. This understanding of molecular mechanisms is also likely to see advances both in our understanding of disease mechanisms and in new drug design.

6.1 Anxiety and insomnia

Learning objectives

At the end of this section you should be able to:
* distinguish the terms 'sedation' and 'hypnosis'
* describe the therapeutic use of sedative/ hypnotics and appreciate the risks of their prolonged use
* list some commonly used benzodiazepines
* describe the mode of action, clinical pharmacokinetics and adverse effects of the benzodiazepines.

Clinical sketch

A middle-aged man has recently been bereaved and has insomnia as a result. His GP prescribes lormetazepam for 2 weeks.

Comment: this is an appropriate use of the drug to treat an acute problem with a clearly defined cause.

Clinical sketch

A middle-aged man has always suffered from anxiety and insomnia. He has been taking benzodiazepines during the day (for anxiety) and at night (for insomnia) for many years. The doses of both drugs have gradually been increased (at the patient's request) over the years because of diminishing effectiveness.

Comment: this inappropriate long-term use of sedatives can sometimes be hard to avoid. However, the drugs have probably become part of the problem instead of offering any therapeutic benefit. The diminishing effectiveness of the drug is termed 'tolerance'.

The benzodiazepines

Gamma-aminobutyric acid (GABA) is a major inhibitory neurotransmitter that works by opening post-synaptic chloride channels. The benzodiazepines potentiate GABA and receptors for these drugs are found in close proximity to GABA receptors and chloride channels (Fig. 31). The dose–response curve (see Fig. 8) of benzodiazepines is shallow, and overdoses tend not to cause life-threatening toxicity other than in patients with respiratory impairment.

Examples and therapeutic uses

Diazepam is one of the older drugs, and less used now because of its slow elimination. Diazepam is converted (in the liver) to *active* metabolites, many of which have very long half-lives: these may accumulate in elderly patients.

Lormetazepam is a shorter-acting benzodiazepine, with fewer 'hangover' effects than diazepam. It is mainly used as a hypnotic.

Lorazepam is a short-acting drug used mainly as an anxiolytic; an i.v. preparation is available for use in epilepsy.

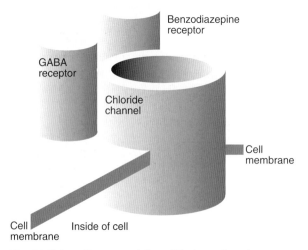

Benzodiazepine receptor

GABA receptor

Chloride channel

Cell membrane

Cell membrane   Inside of cell

Fig. 31 Schematic representation of the benzodiazepine receptors.

Clonazepam is used for the treatment of epilepsy; a parenteral form is available for i.v. use.

Midazolam is usually given i.v. and has a very short half-life. It is commonly used for medical procedures.

Adverse effects

- benzodiazepines impair intellectual function and motor skills: care is needed with machinery and patients should be advised not to drive after taking benzodiazepines
- psychological or physical dependence occurs (Ch. 18)
- natural sleep is distinguished by two patterns: non-rapid eye movement (NREM), which accounts for about 75% of sleep time, and rapid eye movement (REM), during which most recallable dreams occur. Hypnotics reduce the time spent in REM and deep NREM. Patients may complain that their sleep is not fully satisfactory
- patients with respiratory impairment may be worsened by sedative drugs
- some patients develop 'paradoxical' adverse effects including aggression and excitement.

Contraindications

- respiratory impairment
- severe liver impairment.

Drug interactions

- other sedative drugs (including alcohol, non-benzodiazepine sedatives (below), opiates, barbiturates, neuroleptics (see Section 6.4) and antihistamines): cause additive CNS depression
- cimetidine: inhibits the metabolism of midazolam
- antimicrobials: some inhibit the metabolism of midazolam
- the specific benzodiazepine antagonist *flumazenil* can be used in life-threatening overdoses.

Non-benzodiazepine sedative/hypnotics

Zopiclone, zaleplon and zolpidem are not structurally related to the benzodiazepines but all are thought to enhance the effects of GABA via the same 'benzodiazepine receptor'. All are indicated for short-term use in insomnia and can cause dependence.

6.2 Epilepsy

Definitions in epilepsy

- Epilepsy comprises recurrent episodes of abnormal cerebral neuronal discharge. The resulting seizures are usually clinically obvious and vary in pattern according to which parts of the brain are affected.
- Epilepsy can be caused by many neurological diseases, including infection, trauma, infarction and neoplasia.
- Heredity has an important role (especially in the idiopathic generalised epilepsies).

Common seizure types

The clinical manifestations of seizures are related to the part of the brain thought to be affected; classification based on these clinical features is of practical value since the response to drugs can often be predicted.

1. Generalised seizures
   a. Absence (*petit mal*). These seizures, which are most commonly seen in children, have abrupt onset and cessation, with impaired consciousness, but with normal posture often retained. The EEG shows a typical 'spike and wave' pattern. First choice drugs: *valproate, ethosuximide*.
   b. Tonic/clonic (*grand mal*). Consciousness is impaired and the patient usually falls to the floor. A phase of muscle contraction ('tonic') is followed by irregular muscle clonus and then by sleep. Injury may occur. First choice drugs: *carbamazepine, lamotrigine or sodium valproate*.
2. Partial seizures
   a. Simple partial seizures. Features depend on the part of the brain affected, e.g. motor seizures ('Jacksonian seizures') result from discharge in the precentral gyrus. Consciousness is unimpaired. First choice drugs: *carbamazepine lamotrigine or sodium valproate*.
   b. Complex partial seizures (temporal lobe epilepsy). Consciousness is impaired with complex, often repetitive, actions. First choice drugs: *carbamazepine, lamotrigine or sodium valproate*.

Management of epilepsy

Patients require supportive care during a seizure: the airway should be protected and the patient laid in a semiprone safe position (in case of vomiting). Most seizures stop spontaneously within 5 minutes; however, major seizures occurring in sequence without remission, *status epilepticus*, require emergency management (Box 4).

Box 4 Emergency management of status epilepticus

- Status epilepticus, when seizures follow one another without recovery of consciousness, is a medical emergency and has a high mortality rate. Death is from cardiorespiratory failure.
- A dose of lorazepam should be given i.v.; this may be repeated.
- In resistant cases, phenytoin may be given as a *slow* i.v. infusion, following British National Formulary (BNF) guidelines.
- Paraldehyde (which may be given rectally) causes little respiratory depression, and can be useful in settings where facilities for resuscitation are not available.
- If the seizures are thought to be related to alcohol abuse, then intravenous thiamine (vitamin B_1) should be given.

Drugs used in epilepsy

Benzodiazepines

Lorazepam is the first choice drug in status epilepticus. Clonazepam is used in maintenance. Benzodiazepines are described in more detail in Section 6.1.

Clinical sketch

A patient with longstanding epilepsy is admitted because of recurrent tonic-clonic seizures for the preceding 12 hours. She is unconscious, stiff and is having repeated episodes of clonic limb movements. Management comprises protection of the airway, oxygen, i.v. lorazepam and perhaps i.v. phenytoin.

Comment: status epilepticus is a medical emergency. A benzodiazepine such as lorazepam is the first choice drug but if it fails, then phenytoin is often effective. If neither is effective, the patient may require sedation and ventilation in an intensive care unit.

Clinical sketch

An 18-month-old toddler is brought to the A&E department by his distraught parents. He has been unwell for 2 days with a viral illness and they have been 'wrapping him up warm'. He is having generalised clonic movements and his rectal temperature is 40°C. Treatment comprises rectal paracetamol and tepid sponging to reduce temperature, rectal paraldehyde and reassurance of the parents.

Comment: febrile convulsions are common in young children and have a good prognosis. The temperature needs to be lowered and the fit terminated.

Clinical sketch

A 30-year-old woman has had epilepsy since a head injury 10 years ago. The fits were frequent, but she now takes carbamazepine, and has been fit-free for 4 years. She now holds a driving license that is renewed every 3 years. She is pregnant and wants advice.

Comments: there are a number of issues raised here. (a) It is usually possible to control fits with only one drug, as here. (b) Doctors have a duty to advise patients to behave sensibly: this often means immediate advice 'you should not drive'. They also have the responsibility to advise patients to report seizures to the Driver and Vehicle Licensing Agency and their insurance company. Patients may be allowed to drive again if they are fit-free for 12 months. (c) The risk of fetal malformation is increased by antiepileptic drugs and the patient needs to know this. If the woman decides to have the baby, the risks of the drug (to the fetus) need to be weighed against its benefits (to both mother and fetus); in most cases the drug is continued.

Carbamazepine (for partial and tonic-clonic seizures)

Carbamazepine blocks sodium channels postsynaptically, thereby reducing the response to excitatory neurotransmitter binding. Giving carbamazepine with food slows its absorption, and this can allow patients to tolerate higher doses. Carbamazepine is mainly cleared by hepatic metabolism. One of its metabolites (oxcarbamazepine) is also used as an antiepileptic. The half-life is about 36 hours after the first dose but, because it is a potent inducer of hepatic enzymes, half-life can fall by up to 50% with long-term use: this translates clinically into a need for dose adjustment. Carbamazepine plasma concentration is routinely measured but is not often a useful guide to management.

Therapeutic uses

- drug of choice for partial seizures
- extensively used for tonic-clonic seizures but is not effective against other generalised seizure types
- chronic pain: including trigeminal neuralgia
- manic-depressive disorders.

Adverse effects

- concentration-related diplopia, ataxia and sedation
- hyponatraemia leading to water intoxication
- idiosyncratic reactions include aplastic anaemia, agranulocytosis, rashes and hepatic dysfunction
- teratogenicity: spina bifida.

Contraindications and warnings

- previous adverse drug reaction
- porphyria can be exacerbated
- women of childbearing age should be advised of the teratogenic effects.

Drug interactions

- carbamazepine is a potent inducer of liver enzymes and very prone to drug interactions. Notable examples include reduced effect of both oral contraceptive steroids and warfarin
- carbamazepine levels can rise when it is combined with sodium valproate.

Sodium valproate (for both partial and generalised seizures types)

The mode of action of sodium valproate is not completely understood, but its effects include increased CNS levels of GABA with potentiation of this transmitter and changes in both Na^+ and K^+ conductance. Giving valproate with food slows its absorption, and this may reduce symptomatic adverse effects. It is cleared by hepatic metabolism with a half-life of

10–20 hours. At high concentration, blood levels rise disproportionately to dose increment (in clinical terms, because of saturation of metabolising enzymes, so called 'zero order' processes). Plasma concentration monitoring is not a good guide to dose changes, and concentrations do not correlate well with effect (perhaps in part because of variability in protein binding).

Therapeutic uses

Valproate has useful effects in most commonly seen seizure types.

Adverse effects

- symptomatic toxicity includes gastrointestinal upset, weight gain, fine tremor (at high levels) and alopecia
- idiosyncratic effects are uncommon but can be life-threatening; these include hepatotoxicity (particularly in children) and thrombocytopenia
- teratogenicity: spina bifida and skeletal anomalies.

Contraindications and warnings

- liver disease
- women of childbearing age should be advised of the teratogenic effects.

Drug interactions

Valproate can inhibit the metabolism of other anticonvulsants including carbamazepine.

Lamotrigine (for partial and tonic-clonic seizures)

Lamotrigine inhibits the release of excitatory amino acid neurotransmitters (principally glutamate) which may be involved in the generation of seizure activity and is mainly eliminated by glucuronidation in the liver. The therapeutic range is yet to be established and concentration monitoring is not routine. Lamotrigine can be used as monotherapy but is also given in combination with other antiepileptic drugs for cases refractory to a single agent. Skin rashes are quite common (around 3%) but resolve when the drug is stopped. Rarely, lamotrigine has caused severe skin reactions, angioedema and multiorgan failure.

Therapeutic uses

Lamotrigine is used in partial and tonic-clonic seizures, as monotherapy or as an adjunct to other drugs.

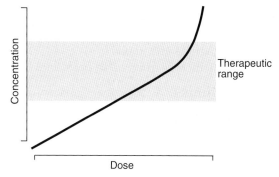

Fig. 32 Relationship between phenytoin dose and steady-state plasma concentration.

Adverse effects

- symptomatic toxicity includes gastrointestinal upset, dizziness and diplopia
- idiosyncratic effects include serious rashes (which are quite common, especially in children) and influenza-like syndromes. Blood dyscrasias have been reported; hepatotoxicity is uncommon.

Contraindications and warnings

Close monitoring is needed to detect the start of potentially serious adverse effects, like skin rash.

Phenytoin (for partial and tonic-clonic seizures)

Phenytoin is an old compound, prone to symptomatic adverse effects; it is rarely the first choice agent for newly diagnosed epilepsy. It is usually well absorbed from the gut but this is very dependent on formulation; phenytoin absorption is unpredictable when given i.m. and this route should not be used. Phenytoin is cleared by hepatic metabolism, but this can be saturated at concentrations readily reached in clinical practice. The therapeutic range is relatively narrow and therapeutic drug monitoring is considered *essential* (Fig. 32).

Therapeutic uses

- In status epilepticus i.v. phenytoin is a second choice drug after a benzodiazapine. Phenytoin i.v. is dangerous and it *must* be given slowly (*read instructions in the BNF*) while monitoring the ECG and vital signs. Phenytoin readily precipitates if diluted in i.v. fluids; it is usually given by syringe-driver.
- Phenytoin can be used for partial seizures and tonic/clonic seizures, but not for other generalised seizure types.

Adverse effects

- acute, concentration-dependent effects include diplopia, nystagmus and ataxia
- chronic effects include gingival hyperplasia.

Drug interactions

Phenytoin is an inducer of hepatic enzymes, reducing the effect of many drugs including warfarin, carbamazepine, oral contraceptive steroids and theophylline.

Phenobarbital (for partial and tonic-clonic seizures)

Phenobarbital potentiates the effects of GABA and antagonises the effects of the excitatory transmitter glutamate. It may be given orally, i.m. or by slow i.v. injection. Phenobarbital is used for partial and tonic-clonic seizures but is not the first-choice drug in industrialised nations; however, because of its low cost it is commonly used in developing countries. Adverse effects include sedation and respiratory depression (especially in overdose). Phenobarbital is contraindicated in porphyria. Like carbamazepine and phenytoin, phenobarbital is an inducer of liver enzymes and increases the clearance of many drugs; in addition the sedative effects of phenobarbital are additive with other sedative/hypnotic drugs.

Gabapentin (for adjunctive treatment of refractory partial and tonic-clonic seizures)

Gabapentin is an amino acid analogue of GABA, but its mode of action does not seem to involve binding to GABA receptors; it may perturb GABA metabolism. Gabapentin is eliminated by the kidneys as the unchanged drug; drug concentrations are not routinely measured. Gabapentin is used in addition to other drugs in the treatment of refractory partial seizures and tonic-clonic seizures. It also has a role in refractory neurogenic pain (such as the neuralgias). The most common adverse effects are sedation and ataxia.

Topiramate (as monotherapy or adjunctive therapy for tonic-clonic seizures and for partial seizures)

The mode of action of topiramate may involve effects on both sodium channels and GABA. Most of a dose is eliminated by the kidneys as the unchanged drug; there is no established concentration-therapeutic range. Topiramate is used as monotherapy or adjunctive therapy for tonic-clonic seizures and for partial seizures. Dizziness, cognitive slowing and fatigue are commonly reported. Topiramate increases the risk of nephrolithiasis (formation of kidney stones) and it is important to ensure adequate hydration.

Ethosuximide

Ethosuximide is used for generalised seizures (mainly absence) in children. The drug is well absorbed from the gut and is eliminated by metabolism (mainly hydroxylation). Gastrointestinal adverse effects are common and include pain and vomiting. Lethargy is also common. Life-threatening toxicity is rare.

Levetiracetam

This new drug is used for the adjunctive treatment of partial seizures. It should be used with caution in patients with liver impairment. The main adverse effects include drowsiness and dizziness.

Vigabatrin

Vigabatrin is used in combination with other anti-epileptic drugs as supplementary therapy for refractory seizures, particularly complex partial seizures. As many as a third of patients on this drug develop visual field defects, so counselling and careful monitoring are required. The other main adverse effects are sedation, weight gain, confusion and (uncommonly) psychosis.

6.3 Depression and hypomania

Learning objectives

At the end of this section you should:
- be able to describe bipolar affective disorder
- be able to summarise the 'amine hypothesis'
- know the clinical pharmacology of tricyclic antidepressants, selective serotonin reuptake inhibitors and monoamine oxidase inhibitors
- be aware that antidepressant drugs can take several weeks to work
- be aware of the toxicity of antidepressant drugs, especially in overdose.

Clinical sketch

A 40-year-old woman has been depressed since the death of her husband 6 months ago. She has lost about a stone in weight and is unable to work. The doctor starts her on amitriptyline but there is no improvement for 2 months.

Clinical sketch – cont'd

Comment: sadness is a normal reaction to many life events. Usually this abates with time; but the term depression is used for abnormally protracted or severe sadness. It is common and, if ignored, may result in anorexia, 'retardation' (slow mental processes), somatic symptoms and disruption of normal life. Suicide may be attempted, and suicidal ideas should be asked about when assessing such patients. Choice of antidepressant drug can be difficult and is usually empirical: trials show them to be equipotent, and improvement in mood can take several weeks with all agents. The SSRIs (e.g. fluoxetine) are safer than the tricyclic antidepressants after overdose.

Clinical sketch

A 60-year-old man has a long history of 'bipolar affective disorder'. Before he started treatment with lithium he had frequent episodes of suicidal depression. Equally problematic were episodes of hypomania, which proved to be destructive to his family life and job.

Comment: hypomania is less common than depression but is equally disruptive; it may alternate with depression in so-called 'bipolar affective disorder'.

The amine hypothesis

The amine hypothesis that depression results from a 'depletion' of monoamine neurotransmitters (5-hydroxytryptamine (or serotonin; 5-HT) and noradrenaline (norepinephrine)) is at the centre of antidepressant development. Drugs that interfere with monoamine release or storage, such as reserpine (a disused antihypertensive), can cause depression. Drugs that potentiate monoamines (such as tricyclic antidepressants and selective serotonin reuptake inhibitors (SSRIs)) can relieve it.

Drugs in depression and hypomania

Selective serotonin reuptake inhibitors (SSRIs)

SSRI drugs cause selective inhibition of 5-HT reuptake by postsynaptic nerve terminals.

Examples

Fluoxetine is well absorbed from the gut and is metabolised to an equipotent metabolite. Both parent drug and active metabolite are very slowly eliminated and may accumulate in severe liver or kidney disease. *Sertraline* in contrast, has a shorter elimination half-life and is metabolised to inactive derivatives. Other members of this group of drugs include *citalopram* and *paroxetine*.

Therapeutic uses

There is considerable delay between starting treatment and the onset of benefit. Unlike the tricyclic drugs, SSRIs do not have marked sedative, hypotensive or anticholinergic effects and have less effect on cardiac conduction. In overdose, the SSRIs are better tolerated than tricyclic antidepressants.

Adverse effects and contraindications

- suicidal behaviour is a recognised risk in people under 18 years, and the SSRIs should not be used in this group
- vasculitic rash: a rare but serious reaction to fluoxetine
- seizures: SSRIs can exacerbate seizures
- symptomatic adverse effects include anorexia and sexual dysfunction
- anorexia and weight loss
- SSRIs can cause hyponatraemia.

Drug interactions

The combination of lithium with fluoxetine may increase the risk of seizure.

Tricyclic antidepressants

Tricyclic antidepressants, which are older drugs than the SSRIs, block the reuptake into the presynaptic neurone of noradrenaline (norepinephrine) and 5-HT, thereby increasing their availability to the postsynaptic membrane (so-called uptake 1; Fig. 33). *Amitriptyline*, an example of this drug group, is completely absorbed from the gut; however, it slows gut motility and its absorption is consequently slow. There is extensive first pass metabolism. Amitriptyline's principal metabolite, nortriptyline, is active. Like all tricyclic antidepressants, amitriptyline has a large volume of distribution. The elimination half-life is slow.

Therapeutic uses

- depression: there is a delay of about 2 weeks before benefit is seen. Amitriptyline is sedative, and this can be a useful property. Other tricyclics can be chosen that lack this sedative effect
- chronic pain: tricyclic antidepressants are also used for the treatment of neuralgia.

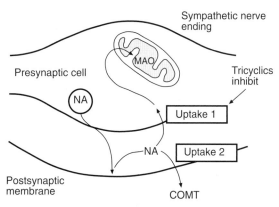

Fig. 33 Mode of action of tricyclic antidepressants. NA, noradrenaline (norepinephrine); MAO, monoamine oxidase; COMT, catechol-*O*-methyltransferase.

Adverse effects

As well as their therapeutic effect via uptake 1, tricyclic drugs are antagonists of muscarinic and histamine H_1 receptors and α_1-adrenoceptors.

- anticholinergic effects include urinary retention, constipation and tachyarrhythmias (especially problematic in overdose; see Ch. 17)
- cardiac arrhythmia may also occur because of effects on intracardiac conduction
- sedation is particularly a problem with amitriptyline
- weight gain can occur
- exacerbation of epilepsy
- idiosyncratic adverse reactions include hepatotoxicity and blood dyscrasias.

Contraindications

- glaucoma: pupil dilatation from antimuscarinic effects causes intraocular pressure to rise
- prostatic hypertrophy: acute retention of urine is a risk
- immediately after a myocardial infarction: risk of arrhythmias
- epilepsy: reduced seizure threshold.

Drug interactions

Additive sedation is seen when amitriptyline is combined with alcohol or other sedatives. Tricyclic drugs should not be combined with non-selective monoamine oxidase inhibitors (MAOIs) because of a rare, but potentially fatal, hyperthermia syndrome.

Reversible inhibitors of monoamine oxidase A (RIMA)

There are two subtypes of monoamine oxidase: MAO-A metabolises noradrenaline (norepinephrine) and 5-HT and is, therefore, relevant to depression, while MAO-B metabolises dopamine (see Section 6.5). *Moclobemide* is a reversible inhibitor of MAO-A. It is well absorbed from the gut and cleared by hepatic metabolism; its half-life is very short and it is given twice daily. Unlike older MAOIs, moclobemide does not carry a high risk of hypertensive crises with sympathomimetics, but patients should avoid heavy intake of tyramine-rich foods (such as mature cheese).

Other antidepressant drugs

Venlafaxine and mirtazapine are structurally dissimilar to all the drug groups above, and are in reasonably common use. Venlafaxine is contraindicated in the presence of severe hepatic and renal disease. Mirtazapine should be used with caution in the presence of epilepsy, and both hepatic and renal impairment. St John's wort is a popular herbal treatment for mild depression and seems to produce benefit; the amount of active ingredients vary between preparations. St John's wort is a hepatic enzyme inducer, and interacts with a wide variety of therapeutic drugs.

Lithium

The mode of action of lithium, which is used for the prophylaxis and treatment of bipolar affective disorder, is unknown. It is well absorbed orally and is excreted by the kidney. Its clearance is reduced in patients with renal impairment. There is an established therapeutic range for lithium and monitoring is *mandatory*. Exceeding the upper limit of the therapeutic range is dangerous and a serum lithium concentration, 12 hours postdose, greater than 3.5 mmol/L is life-threatening. Common adverse effects include renal damage (nephrogenic diabetes insipidus), hypothyroidism, rashes and oedema. Lithium may be teratogenic and women of childbearing age must be made aware of this and offered contraception. Lithium should be avoided in patients with renal impairment because of the risk of accumulation. Psoriasis may be worsened by lithium, making this a relative contraindication. Diuretics and non-steroidal anti-inflammatory drugs can cause accumulation of lithium.

6.4 Schizophrenia

Learning objectives

At the end of this section you should:

- be able to describe schizophrenia
- be able to outline the 'dopamine hypothesis' of schizophrenia and appreciate the limitations of this hypothesis
- know the clinical pharmacology of the 'standard' neuroleptic drugs and their main adverse effects
- understand that clozapine, an 'atypical' neuroleptic drug, is reserved for resistant cases because of its adverse effect profile.

Schizophrenia is a common, severe 'functional' mental disorder that mainly affects young adults. The disease is characterised by:

- delusions (unshakable beliefs at variance with observed reality; these are commonly 'paranoid' or 'grandiose')
- hallucinations (most commonly auditory)
- disordered thinking (the patient is oriented in person, place and time, but logical connections between ideas are perturbed)
- lack of motivation or emotion (in chronic schizophrenia, this 'negative' symptom may become more prominent).

The aetiology is not fully understood. There is a large genetic element. In addition, abnormalities of the temporal lobes are detectable, and abnormality of dopaminergic transmission may have a role.

Clinical sketch

An 18-year-old student is seen in the A&E department after a determined suicide attempt. His parents are distraught. Over the previous year, his work has been deteriorating and he has lost touch with his family. He has few friends in college. Detailed assessment by a psychiatrist reveals paranoid delusions and auditory hallucinations. A diagnosis of schizophrenia is made and he is started on depot injections of a neuroleptic drug. He improves on this treatment, but not enough to resume his studies.

Comment: schizophrenia most commonly presents in young adulthood. Disruption of social contacts and work are major features. Most people respond to neuroleptics, but complete control of symptoms is unusual.

Clinical sketch

A 30-year-old woman has been schizophrenic since she was 20. Psychiatrists have tried many different drugs without much success. Eventually, clozapine is started, and improvement is noted.

Comment: clozapine is one of several 'atypical' neuroleptic drugs that are reserved for difficult cases. Serious adverse effects are common and monitoring of white cell counts is mandatory.

Older neuroleptic drugs

Neuroleptics (otherwise known as 'major tranquilisers') are structurally heterogeneous drugs that reduce the thought disorder that characterises schizophrenia. All act by blocking dopamine D_2 receptors, primarily in the mesolimbic system. Antagonism of D_1 receptors does not contribute therapeutically but may cause dystonic adverse reactions. Neuroleptics may also block receptors to 5-HT, histamine (H_1), acetylcholine (muscarinic receptors) and noradrenaline (α_1-adrenoceptors), and these actions contribute to their adverse effect profile. Examples include *chlorpromazine*, *haloperidol* and *flupentixol*.

Therapeutic uses

- schizophrenia and related disorders
- severe organic psychosis.

Adverse effects

- exacerbation of depression
- blockade of D_1 receptors may result in parkinsonism and other extrapyramidal reactions including akathisia (severe restlessness) and acute dystonia (including torticollis). All these syndromes may respond to anticholinergic drugs. Tardive dyskinesia, the late onset of choreoathetoid movements, may occur in up to 40% of patients; it is probably caused by dopamine receptor upregulation and can be very difficult to treat
- autonomic effects include postural hypotension, premature ejaculation, visual disturbance, dry mouth, retention of urine and constipation (more common with chlorpromazine)
- jaundice, rashes and agranulocytosis are rare but serious adverse effects
- hyperprolactinaemia can result from chronic dopamine antagonism and may cause gynaecomastia
- neuroleptic malignant syndrome is a rare but serious reaction to all these drugs, comprising hyperpyrexia and muscle rigidity.

Contraindications and cautions

- hepatic and renal impairment
- hypersensitivity
- glaucoma
- Parkinson's disease
- impaired consciousness.

Drug interactions

Most of the interactions are pharmacodynamic and predictable from knowledge of the receptor groups blocked by the drugs. Additive effects are seen between neuroleptics and other antidopaminergic, antimuscarinic, antihistaminergic and antiadrenergic drugs.

'Atypical' neuroleptic drugs

The atypical neuroleptics differ chemically from any of the established (older) compounds described above. All are thought to work by their effects on D_2 receptors and all tend to cause fewer extrapyramidal adverse effects: hence their attraction. The 'atypical' drugs are gradually becoming more commonly used by psychiatrists. The atypical neuroleptics have not generally been associated with prolongation of the ECG QT interval, but should be used with care if patients are taking drugs that have this effect, or in patients with heart disease. Some examples are briefly described below.

Risperidone

The most common symptomatic adverse effects with risperidone include sleep disturbance, anxiety and rhinitis. Sudden death has occurred in a small number of patients with pre-existing cardiac disease, and this is a relative contraindication to the use of risperidone.

Olanzapine

Olanzapine was introduced in the late 1990s and its adverse effect profile is incompletely documented. Life-threatening adverse effects have included agranulocytosis and cardiac arrhythmias.

Quetiapine

Quetiapine commonly sedates, and can cause dyspepsia. QT prolongation may be exacerbated.

Clozapine

Clozapine is often effective in resistant cases of psychosis. However, because of the high prevalence of associated agranulocytosis, it was withdrawn in the 1970s. It was reintroduced in the 1990s but is reserved for resistant schizophrenia under close hospital monitoring. Other adverse effects include weight gain and convulsions.

6.5 Parkinsonism

Learning objectives

At the end of this section you should:
- be able to summarise the accepted neurotransmitter problem that underlies parkinsonism
- know the clinical features of parkinsonism
- appreciate that parkinsonism can be idiopathic (Parkinson's disease) or have identified causes
- be able to describe the clinical pharmacology of dopaminergic and anticholinergic antiparkinsonism drugs
- appreciate that the natural history of idiopathic Parkinson's disease is one of steady deterioration and that none of the existing drugs reduces mortality.

Clinical sketch

A 65-year-old man notices difficulty turning in bed and rising from a chair. This symptom worsens and is accompanied by shaking and a tendency to fall. His doctor diagnoses Parkinson's disease and starts bromocriptine.

Comment: these symptoms are typical of parkinsonism. Bromocriptine is a dopamine agonist derived from ergot. Patients need to be monitored for fibrotic reactions (described below).

Clinical sketch

A 50-year-old patient with schizophrenia has been on neuroleptic drugs for many years. The features of parkinsonism are noted, and an anticholinergic preparation is started.

Comment: neuroleptic-induced parkinsonism is common. Dopaminergic therapy would be illogical: the problem has resulted from the dopamine antagonism of the neuroleptic drug. Furthermore, dopaminergic drugs may worsen psychosis. Treatment aims to oppose the effects of cholinergic fibres, by using antimuscarinic drugs.

Parkinsonism comprises bradykinesia (or difficulty initiating movement), coarse tremor, rigidity and disordered posture. The patient shuffles ('festinating gait') and has a tendency to fall. The cause is degeneration of the substantia nigra in idiopathic disease, with marked reduction in local dopamine concentrations; this reduces the inhibition of excitatory cholinergic fibres.

Neuroleptic drugs can cause parkinsonism by blocking dopamine receptors. The aim of therapy is to restore the balance between dopamine and acetylcholine either by increasing the concentration of dopamine (dopaminergic drugs) or by blocking acetylcholine production (anticholinergic drugs).

Parkinson's disease

This is a common disease of unknown cause that mainly afflicts the elderly. The commonest symptoms are tremor and slowness of movement. The patient's writing may become small and spidery ('micrographia').

The main physical signs are:

- coarse 'pill rolling' tremor; this settles during sleep but worsens during emotion; it is often asymmetric
- rigidity
- bradykinesia: movements are slow and there is difficulty initiating movement
- postural changes: the patient is characteristically stooped, and the gait shuffles (so called 'festination')
- speech is characteristically monotonous.

The natural history is one of gradual deterioration. The rate of progress is very variable.

Dopaminergic drugs

The dopaminergic drugs act by (a) acting as dopamine agonists, or (b) providing the precursor of dopamine , or (c) reducing dopamine metabolism or (d) causing local release of dopamine.

Direct dopamine agonists

Bromocriptine, cabergoline, lisuride, pergolide and *ropinirole* are direct agonists at dopamine receptors; all but ropinirole are derived from ergot. All are subject to extensive presystemic metabolism and are cleared mainly by hepatic metabolism. These drugs may be used as monotherapy in early Parkinson's disease, especially in younger patients, and can be given with levodopa preparations in more advanced disease.

Adverse effects

The ergot derivatives (bromocriptine, cabergoline, lisuride and pergolide) may cause fibrotic reactions (in the chest, abdomen or pericardium) and patients need to be monitored with this in mind. All dopamine agonists may cause nausea, dizziness, visual disturbance, vivid dreams and postural hypotension. The non-ergot drug ropinirole may cause leg oedema.

Levodopa

Levodopa (dihydroxyphenyl-L-alanine; L-dopa) is the precursor of dopamine and, unlike the latter, can cross the blood–brain barrier. Both within the CNS, and elsewhere in the body, levodopa is metabolised (by decarboxylation) to dopamine; it is the 'peripheral' synthesis of dopamine that results in many of the adverse effects of levodopa. To offset this, levodopa is combined with a decarboxylase inhibitor (either *carbidopa* or *benserazide*) that does not cross the blood–brain barrier. Consequently, peripheral decarboxylation is reduced but the CNS is unaffected. Clinical response to levodopa is usually good initially but declines with time.

Adverse effects

- Nausea and vomiting: dopamine is the principal neurotransmitter of the vomiting centre in the brainstem, and dopamine agonists can cause nausea; this is reduced by the combination of levodopa with a decarboxylase inhibitor
- Dyskinesias (caused by overactivity in some dopaminergic pathways): seen in 80% of patients with prolonged use, including facial choreoathetosis, hemiballismus, dystonia, tics and myoclonus
- Cardiovascular: postural hypotension is common but some patients develop hypertension; tachyarrhythmias may occur
- Erratic response: marked variation in drug response occurs in a high proportion of patients after several years of treatment; in some, severe bradykinesia is seen several hours after dosing (end of dose phenomenon) while in others the fluctuation in response seems unrelated to drug doses and periods of severe bradykinesia alternate with periods of dyskinesia (on–off phenomenon). This is partly a pharmacokinetic phenomenon and may be limited by either frequent small doses or the use of a long-acting formulation.

Contraindications

- glaucoma: intraocular pressure is increased
- psychosis.

Drug interactions

Levodopa should not be given to patients taking a non-selective MAOI because of the risk of severe hypertension.

Selegiline and entacapone

Dopamine is metabolised in the CNS by MAO-B which is inhibited by *selegiline*. Levodopa is metabolised peripherally by catechol-*O*-methyltransferase (COMT), which may be inhibited by using entacapone.

Entacapone is given as an adjunct to levodopa.

Selegiline may be used in combination with levodopa either to restore the clinical response to the latter where this has been lost or in patients with 'on–off' symptoms.

Adverse effects

Both entacapone and selegiline cause gastrointestinal upset and may induce confusion.

Amantadine

Amantadine, an antiviral drug, probably increases dopamine release in the CNS. Its antiparkinsonian effects are weak, and it is not frequently used for this indication.

Anticholinergic drugs

Depletion of striatal dopamine, as in idiopathic parkinsonism, or blockade of dopamine receptors, as seen with neuroleptics, reduces inhibition of excitatory cholinergic neurones. This balance may be restored using antimuscarinic drugs. Examples include *trihexyphenidyl* and *procyclidine*. Anticholinergic drugs are most often given to patients with neuroleptic-induced parkinsonism. Their use in idiopathic Parkinson's disease is less common because the dopaminergic drugs are more effective. The adverse effects are those of systemic antimuscarinic drugs (Ch. 8), and contraindications include glaucoma and prostatic hypertrophy.

6.6 Migraine

> **Clinical sketch**
>
> A 14-year-old boy complains of periodic severe headache and facial pain. It is preceded by visual disturbance. The pain is severe, unilateral and associated with photophobia and vomiting.
>
> *Comment: this is classical migraine (it is worth noting that only a small proportion of cases are as obvious as this). An acute attack can be helped by paracetamol and aborted with 5-HT antagonists.*
>
> As the same boy approaches his GCSE examinations the frequency of the headaches increases and his parents wonder whether anything can be done to hold attacks at bay.
>
> *Comment: several classes of drug reduce migraine frequency. It is important to be sure that the benefits of the drug outweigh its risks.*

5-hydroxytryptamine (5-HT) is a vasoactive amine that is released from platelets. The main organ-specific effects of 5-HT are:

- vasoconstriction (except in skeletal muscles and heart where it is vasodilator)
- venoconstriction, causing cutaneous flush
- increased peristalsis
- platelet aggregation.

Migraine is probably caused by the abnormal release of 5-HT within intracranial blood vessels, resulting in vasoconstriction; it is this that causes the typical 'aura', which may involve visual disturbance, speech abnormalities or even temporary hemiparesis. Vasodilatation, possibly caused by 5-HT depletion, then follows and it is this that is associated with the headache, which is severe, classically unilateral and often causes prostration and nausea. Migraine is common, particularly in adolescents, is often familial and tends to decrease in frequency as age advances. Most attacks show some response to simple analgesics, which should be tried first.

Drugs for the acute attack

Simple analgesics

Paracetamol (often combined with an antiemetic) is the drug of choice for most attacks.

5-HT agonists

Sumatriptan, naratriptan and a range of newer drugs are specific 5-HT agonists that oppose the vasodilatation responsible for the headache. Sumatriptan is formulated for oral and s.c. administration, while naratriptan lacks the parenteral formulation. Sumatriptan is well absorbed but is subject to presystemic metabolism when taken orally. It is used early in an attack to abort acute migraine. Adverse effects include:

- ECG changes and chest pain (especially after s.c. injection); it is contraindicated in ischaemic heart disease and severe hypertension
- drowsiness, nausea and vomiting.

Prophylaxis of migraine

Beta-blockers and tricyclic drugs

Beta-blockers and tricyclic drugs can be used to reduce the frequency of attacks.

Pizotifen

Pizotifen is an antihistamine with anti-5-HT activity. It can reduce the frequency of migraine attacks but often causes mild sedation and weight gain.

Methysergide

Methysergide is a semi-synthetic ergot alkaloid reserved for patients with very severe symptoms. It should be used with great caution under hospital supervision because of the high risk of serious adverse effects. Treatment should be gradually withdrawn and stopped, for at least 4 weeks, every 6 months. Adverse effects include:

- fibrotic reactions: most commonly retroperitoneal fibrosis causing ureteric obstruction
- vasoconstriction: may exacerbate angina.

6.7 Other disorders

Alzheimer's disease

Alzheimer's disease is a degenerative brain disease of unknown cause that leads to dementia. It is characterised by a relative lack of the neurotransmitter acetylcholine, and by the presence of plaques of amyloid proteins. The predominant early features are memory loss and personality change. The disease is progressive, leading to global impairment of higher cerebral function. *Donepezil* is a reversible inhibitor of acetylcholinesterase. It is indicated for patients with mild to moderate Alzheimer's disease and may improve around 40% of such patients.

Multiple sclerosis

Multiple sclerosis is a common disease of unknown cause in which episodes of inflammation of white matter (of brain or cord) cause progressive disability. The disease generally starts in young people and pursues a course of relapses and remissions over many years. Acute exacerbations are generally identified by the development of new symptoms (such as optic neuropathy, cranial nerve lesions or cerebellar dysfunction). Such exacerbations are managed with short courses of *corticotropin* (adrenocorticotrophic hormone) or steroids, which shorten the duration of such episodes. Patients with relapsing-remitting multiple sclerosis can benefit from *interferon beta*; it is indicated for the reduction of frequency and severity of relapses. Interferon-beta should not be used in patients with severe depression or poorly controlled epilepsy. It is generally held that the use of interferon beta should be monitored by a neurologist.

Six

Self-assessment on Chapter 6: questions

Multiple choice questions

1. Diazepam:
   a. Causes sedation, which is abolished by the elimination of the drug
   b. Interacts adversely with amitriptyline
   c. Can prove useful in very anxious asthmatics during an attack
   d. Can be given orally, over prolonged periods, to prevent seizures
   e. Is a suitable choice for the sedation of outpatients undergoing endoscopy

2. Carbamazepine:
   a. Is an appropriate choice to treat a patient with absence seizures (*petit mal*)
   b. Can be considered to be a prodrug
   c. Induces its own metabolism
   d. May be eliminated from the body after overdose using haemodialysis
   e. Potentiates the effects of warfarin

3. Sodium valproate:
   a. Is the treatment of choice for atonic seizures
   b. Induces the metabolism of warfarin
   c. Should always be withdrawn if a woman is trying to become pregnant
   d. Is the anticonvulsant of choice in patients with cirrhosis
   e. Potentiates phenytoin

4. Amitriptyline:
   a. Enhances the uptake of catecholamines by the presynaptic neurone (uptake I)
   b. Can be expected to lift mood within a week
   c. Is contraindicated in patients with glaucoma
   d. Is free of sedative effects
   e. Is the treatment of choice for someone who has become depressed following a myocardial infarction

5. Monoamine oxidase A inhibitors:
   a. Reduce noradrenaline (norepinephrine) metabolism
   b. Reduce 5-HT metabolism
   c. Predispose to hypertensive crises
   d. Are safely combined with tricyclic antidepressants in the treatment of depression
   e. Are safely combined with levodopa

6. Chlorpromazine:
   a. Should always be combined with an anticholinergic antiparkinsonian drug
   b. Works by enhancing the effect of dopamine at D_2 receptors
   c. Often improves depressive symptoms in patients with psychosis
   d. Is the treatment of choice for confusion in the elderly
   e. Is potentiated in chronic liver disease

7. Levodopa:
   a. Has a high oral bioavailability
   b. Should be given at higher dosage in parkinsonism if facial tics develop
   c. Should be withdrawn without delay if the 'on–off' phenomenon develops
   d. May be combined with monoamine oxidase B inhibitors
   e. Is converted to dopamine by monoamine oxidase B

8. In the management of migraine:
   a. 5-HT agonists may be used to abolish headache
   b. Methysergide is an alternative to 5-HT agonists for the treatment of an attack
   c. 5-HT agonists (in case of vomiting) may be used in patients with ischaemic heart disease
   d. Beta-blockers can give effective prophylaxis
   e. Most patients can be managed with simple analgesics such as paracetamol

9. Bromocriptine:
   a. May be used as monotherapy in the treatment of idiopathic parkinsonism
   b. Must be used in combination with levodopa in the treatment of neuroleptic-induced parkinsonism
   c. Should be monitored with periodic chest X-rays and lung function tests in long-term use

d. May be used in combination with levodopa in the treatment of idiopathic parkinsonism

e. Works by inhibition of dopa decarboxylase.

Case history questions

Case history 1

An 80-year-old woman is given diazepam to help her sleep at night. After 2 weeks, neighbours discover her in a state of self-neglect. She is taken to hospital where she is found to be somnolent and confused.

1. Why was diazepam a bad choice of drug in this case?
2. How should she be treated in hospital?

Case history 2

A woman with epilepsy, taking 200 mg phenytoin per day, continues to have seizures at an unacceptable rate. The drug level is measured and found to be 30 mmol/L (therapeutic range 40–80 mmol/L), so the dose is increased to 400 mg daily. After 1 week, the patient has nystagmus and cannot walk because of ataxia.

1. What has happened?

Case history 3

A 19-year-old man has gastroenteritis and is given metoclopramide. He develops acute torticollis (involuntary spasm of the neck muscles) 2 days later, which is very painful.

1. What is the likeliest diagnosis and what should be done?

Case history 4

A 60-year-old woman with schizophrenia has been taking haloperidol for many years and has been well controlled. However, her doctor thinks that her control is 'slipping' as she has recently started to move very strangely: when doing nothing, her arms writhe continuously in a rather jerky but semi-purposeful way.

1. What is the likeliest diagnosis and what should be done?

Case history 5

A patient with longstanding idiopathic Parkinson's disease finds that she is no longer getting so much benefit from her levodopa/carbidopa combination. Specifically, she finds that she is unable to rise from a chair because of stiffness well before her next dose is due.

1. What is the problem, and what should be done?

The same patient had her dose of levodopa increased; her parkinsonism was improved marginally, but after a couple of months she complains that shortly after taking the drug she suffers an hour of uncontrollable facial grimacing.

2. What is the problem, and what should be done?

The same lady develops nausea and dizziness, from an intercurrent illness, and is started on prochlorperazine.

3. What is the principal risk?

Case history 6

A 50-year-old man who smokes cigarettes suffers from frequent migraine headaches. He takes propranolol as prophylaxis for migraine and uses sumatriptan for the treatment of acute attacks.

1. Does this seem like a sensible therapeutic strategy to you? If not, say why.
2. What risks might be caused by the sumatriptan under these circumstances?

Case history 7

A 65-year-old man is given amitriptyline because of prolonged grief following the death of his wife. He is a cigarette smoker and suffers from angina pectoris. He is admitted to hospital 2 weeks later with confusion. He is dehydrated, his pulse is irregular at 140 beats/min and he is anuric.

1. Advance some possible causes of his problems.

Short note questions

Write short notes on the following:

1. The therapeutic use of drugs for status epilepticus.

2. The clinical pharmacology of the drugs used in status epilepticus: deal with mechanisms of action, relevant pharmacokinetics, adverse effects and drug interactions.

3. The therapeutic use of drugs for complex partial seizures.

4. The clinical pharmacology of the drugs used in complex partial seizures: deal with mechanisms of action, relevant pharmacokinetics, adverse effects and drug interactions.

5. The modes of action, disposition and adverse effects of the drugs used in the treatment of depression.

6. Predicting the possible effects of chronic renal disease on response to (a) phenytoin and (b) lithium.

Extended matching items questions

Theme: The clinical pharmacology of antiparkinsonian drugs

Options

A. It stimulates dopamine receptors

B. It crosses the blood–brain barrier

C. It blocks the metabolism of dopamine

D. It inhibits conversion of dopa to dopamine in the CNS

E. It does not cross the blood–brain barrier

F. It blocks acetylcholine receptors, thereby restoring the dopamine/acetylcholine balance

G. Because drug-induced parkinsonism results from the blocking of dopamine receptors by neuroleptics (so-called 'major tranquillisers')

H. Because drug-induced parkinsonism results mainly from excess acetylcholinergic activity in the CNS

For each of the questions below, choose the most appropriate answer from the options above. Each option may be used once, more than once, or not at all.

1. Why is dopamine not used for idiopathic Parkinson's disease?

2. Carbidopa, with which levodopa is formulated, is a dopa decarboxylase inhibitor (it blocks the conversion of dopa to dopamine): so why does its use not abolish the therapeutic effect of levodopa?

3. Why is levodopa contraindicated in drug-induced parkinsonism?

4. How does selegiline work?

Theme: The clinical pharmacology of antiepileptic drugs

Options

A. Carbamazepine

B. Phenobarbital

C. Sodium valproate

D. Ethosuximide

E. Lamotrigine

F. Phenytoin

G. Phenytoin binds strongly to plasma proteins and displaces warfarin from binding sites

H. Phenytoin competes with warfarin for the active site of the drug metabolising enzymes of the CYP450 group, thereby diminishing the response to warfarin

I. Phenytoin 'induces' drug metabolising enzymes of the CYP450 group, thereby enhancing the response to warfarin

J. Phenytoin increases the renal clearance of warfarin

K. Phenytoin decreases the renal clearance of warfarin

For each of the questions below, choose the most appropriate answer from the options above. Each option may be used once, more than once, or not at all.

1. Which is the first choice drug for tonic-clonic epilepsy which starts as a simple partial seizure, but then becomes generalised?

2. Which is the first choice drug for absence seizures?

3. Which is the first choice drug for complex partial seizures?

4. How does phenytoin interact with warfarin?

Theme: The clinical pharmacology of sedative/hypnotic drugs

Options

A. Status epilepticus

B. Type I respiratory failure

C. Type II respiratory failure

D. Ventricular tachycardia

E. Bronchospasm

F. Flumazenil

G. Naloxone

H. N-acetyl cysteine

I. Activated charcoal

J. Benzodiazepines and alcohol interactions: alcohol 'induces' CYP450, thereby diminishing the clinical effect of the benzodiazepine

K. Benzodiazepines and alcohol interactions: alcohol 'inhibits' CYP450, thereby enhancing the clinical effect of the benzodiazepine

L. Benzodiazepines and alcohol interactions: alcohol and benzodiazepines interact pharmacodynamically, yielding an additive effect

M. Benzodiazepines and alcohol interactions: alcohol and benzodiazepines interact pharmacodynamically, yielding a synergistic effect

For each of the questions below, choose the most appropriate answer from the options above. Each option may be used once, more than once, or not at all.

1. In the setting of severe benzodiazepine overdose, what would be the most likely life-threatening problem?

2. In the setting of severe benzodiazepine overdose, what antagonist may be used?

3. How do benzodiazepines and alcohol interact?

Self-assessment on Chapter 6: answers

Multiple choice answers

1. a. **False.** Diazepam is converted to pharmacologically active metabolites that persist in the body after the parent drug has been eliminated.

   b. **True.** Amitriptyline has marked sedative effects; if diazepam is taken simultaneously, the two sedatives produce additive sedation.

   c. **False.** Diazepam might well kill asthmatics during an attack by causing respiratory depression. Anxiety in an asthmatic is appropriate and should be treated by tackling the asthma.

   d. **False.** Though diazepam can be used to stop a seizure, it is not used in prevention.

   e. **False.** Diazepam's effects are too long lived; a more appropriate choice would be midazolam.

2. a. **False.** Carbamazepine is indicated for partial seizures; it is useful for tonic-clonic seizures, but for no other generalised seizure types.

   b. **False.** Though carbamazepine does have a pharmacologically active metabolite, the parent drug possesses anticonvulsant activity.

   c. **True.** Carbamazepine is a potent enzyme inducer and, with chronic therapy, this enhances the elimination of the drug.

   d. **True.** Though structurally similar to the tricyclic antidepressants, carbamazepine has a small volume of distribution and can be removed by dialysis (this topic is more fully covered in Ch. 6).

   e. **False.** Carbamazepine induces the metabolism of warfarin and, therefore, reduces its effects.

3. a. **True.** Atonic seizures are not common; they are characterised by sudden loss of muscle tone causing the patient to collapse. Consciousness is often retained. Valproate is the drug of first choice.

   b. **False.** Valproate is a selective enzyme inhibitor, but it does not interact with warfarin.

   c. **False.** Standard advice for women on antiepileptic drugs is that treatment should continue during pregnancy despite the relatively small risk to the fetus.

   d. **False.** Valproate is contraindicated in patients with chronic liver disease because of the increased risk of drug-induced hepatic dysfunction.

   e. **False.** Valproate probably does not have clinically relevant effects on phenytoin.

4. a. **False.** Tricyclic antidepressants block uptake I.

   b. **False.** Usually no therapeutic response is seen within the first month.

   c. **True.** The anticholinergic effects of tricyclic drugs raise the intraocular pressure.

   d. **False.** Amitriptyline is a potent sedative and is usually given at night for this reason.

   e. **False.** Tricyclic antidepressants are contraindicated immediately after a myocardial infarction because of their effects on intracardiac conduction, and their anticholinergic effects.

5. a. **True.** MAO-A metabolises noradrenaline (norepinephrine); MAO-B metabolises dopamine.

   b. **True.** MAO-A metabolises 5-HT.

   c. **True.** Sympathomimetics, as occur naturally in some foods and are the active ingredients in some proprietary cough mixtures, can cause severe hypertension in patients taking MAO-A inhibitors.

   d. **False.** The combination of tricyclic drug plus a MAO-A inhibitor may cause 'malignant hyperthermia'.

   e. **False.** The combination of levodopa and an MAO-A inhibitor may cause severe hypertension.

6. a. **False.** Not all patients develop parkinsonism, and there is no benefit starting therapy until they do.

   b. **False.** Neuroleptics are dopamine antagonists.

   c. **False.** Neuroleptics frequently exacerbate depression.

d. **False.** Although neuroleptics may be indicated in organic psychosis, confusion in elderly patients is often worsened by sedative drugs.

e. **True.** Chlorpromazine is metabolised in the liver.

7. a. **False.** Levodopa is subject to extensive first pass metabolism.

b. **False.** Levodopa may cause dyskinesias such as tics.

c. **False.** Sudden withdrawal of antiparkinsonian drugs may cause life-threatening deterioration; drugs must be withdrawn slowly in hospital.

d. **True.** Selegiline may be combined with levodopa to restore the clinical response to the latter where this has been lost.

e. **False.** Levodopa is formed by dopa decarboxylase.

8. a. **True.** 5-HT agonists (the 'triptans') can abolish the headache of migraine. They probably work by opposing the vasodilatation that happens after 5-HT induced vasospasm. (Confusingly, 5-HT antagonists such as pizotifen are used for migraine prophylaxis. These probably work by opposing the first step of the process, namely 5-HT induced vasospasm.)

b. **False.** Methysergide is used prophylactically. This drug can have dangerous adverse effects and is best employed, as a last resort, under hospital supervision.

c. **False.** 5-HT agonists are contraindicated in patients with ischaemic heart disease because they may exacerbate angina.

d. **True.** Beta-blockers, pizotifen and the tricyclic antidepressants may be used for prophylaxis.

e. **True.** The majority of patients gain relief from paracetamol.

9. a. **True.** Bromocriptine may be used on its own, especially in newly diagnosed younger patients.

b. **False.** Neuroleptic drugs are dopamine antagonists, while bromocriptine is a dopamine agonist. The logical class of drugs here is the anticholinergics.

c. **True.** Ergot derivatives can cause fibrotic reactions.

d. **True.** Bromocriptine can be helpful in patients with advanced disease who are on levodopa preparations.

e. **False.** Bromocriptine is a dopamine agonist.

Case history answers

Case history 1

1. Diazepam itself is slowly eliminated, as are its active metabolites, and impaired hepatic or renal function slow their rate of elimination further. The elderly often have subclinical renal or hepatic impairment, and benzodiazepines accumulate, causing a so-called 'hangover effect'. With continued use confusion may develop.

2. The benzodiazepine should be stopped even though confusion may initially become worse. A specific benzodiazepine antagonist such as flumazenil is indicated in respiratory failure after overdose but not in the present circumstances. Prescription of further sedative drugs (e.g. in the event of noisy confusion at night) should be avoided.

Case history 2

The relationship between the dose of phenytoin and its plasma concentration is not linear (as it is with most drugs): relatively small dose increases frequently lead to a large rise in blood level. Doubling the dose, as here, can cause major toxicity.

Case history 3

This is an involuntary movement disorder induced by the antidopaminergic actions of the drug. Acute reactions, as in this patient, are common with some neuroleptics and antiemetics (see Ch. 11) and may come in the form of akathisia (inability to sit still) or acute dystonias such as torticollis (as here) or retrocollis. The pharmacological basis of the reaction is not clear, but anticholinergic drugs such as benzatropine or procyclidine are indicated; as the latter may be given i.v., it is probably indicated here because of the pain. After i.v. dosing, improvement should occur within about 5 minutes.

Case history 4

This patient's symptoms illustrate tardive dyskinesia. This complicates chronic neuroleptic use in about 40% of cases. Elderly women are the most common group affected, though it can occur in either sex and at any age. The movements described are typical: so-called choreoathetoid movements. Early recognition is advisable as neglected cases can be more difficult to treat. The current hypothesis is that there is increased sensitivity to dopamine, possibly receptor upregulation, resulting from the chronic use of an antagonist. Most doctors would reduce the neuroleptic dose (and stop the drug if possible), even though this may worsen the dyskinesia in the short term; diazepam is often helpful to control symptoms.

Case history 5

1. This unfortunate patient has developed a common problem in late Parkinson's disease referred to as 'end of dose akinesia'. She may be helped by increasing the frequency of her levodopa doses.

2. She has gone on to develop 'on–off' effects where the high concentration of levodopa shortly after dosing induces acute dyskinesia; such patients seesaw between akinesia and dyskinesia, with only brief spells of normal movement. This can be difficult to treat: the dose of levodopa should probably be reduced, and a supplementary drug such as bromocriptine or selegiline started. In the worst cases, the patient may need admission to hospital to allow gradual withdrawal of all drugs, a 'drug holiday'; when reintroduced, the benefit from levodopa is restored, but this is usually only temporary.

3. Prochlorperazine is a neuroleptic drug (though it is not used for schizophrenia) that works by blocking dopamine receptors: the patient's parkinsonism could be made much worse. This is very poor prescribing.

Case history 6

This does not seem like sensible therapeutics to us. A 50-year-old smoker is at quite high risk of atherosclerosis and COPD. There is the risk that the β-blocker will exacerbate COPD (and peripheral vascular disease, if he has it). While propranolol would have useful antianginal properties (if tolerated) sumatriptan is best avoided in patients with ischaemic heart disease. No features of ischaemic heart disease are given for this man in the question; and yet he is an obvious candidate for this common problem.

Case history 7

At this man's age, a degree of prostatic hypertrophy can be expected. Tricyclic antidepressants have anticholinergic effects, which tend to increase the tone of the sphincter while reducing the tone of the bladder wall: this can cause acute retention of urine. His bladder should be easily palpable. Acute retention is painful and causes tachycardia and confusion. He should be catheterised and the tricyclic drug should be stopped. However, it sounds as if this patient either has atrial fibrillation, which may have been precipitated by the anticholinergic effects of the drug, or else multiple ectopic beats. The possibilities of myocardial infarction and of tricyclic overdose should be considered.

Short note answers

1. Status epilepticus (multiple seizures without recovery of consciousness between episodes) is life-threatening because it causes hypoxia, and it may damage the brain independently of hypoxia. Diazepam (given slowly i.v.) or lorazepam are the drugs of first choice. If these fail to stop seizures, then phenytoin (given as a very slow i.v. injection) is the next choice.

2. Refer to the relevant sections above.

3. Complex partial seizures (temporal lobe seizures) respond to carbamazepine, sodium valproate and lamotrigine. Monotherapy is usually achievable. Doses of drug should start small, and dose increases should be judged by the patient's response to treatment, rather than 'drug levels'. Therapeutic drug monitoring of carbamazepine does have a role, especially in the assessment of (a) apparent lack of response to a large dose and (b) suspected drug toxicity.

4. Refer to the relevant sections above.

5. Deal with each of the following areas.

   Modes of action
   - For the tricyclic antidepressants, describe the fate of noradrenaline (norepinephrine) after release into the synaptic cleft; mention uptake 1 and uptake 2.
   - For SSRIs, the role of blockage of the reuptake of 5-HT into the neurone is not fully understood, but 5-HT may modulate noradrenaline (norepinephrine) release.
   - For MAOIs, describe the substrates of MAO-A (noradrenaline (norepinephrine)

and 5-HT) and MAO-B (dopamine). Mention that MAOIs selective for MAO-A(RIMA) are now available.

Disposition

- Tricyclic drugs are mostly well absorbed from the gut. All have large volumes of distribution (this is relevant to the overdose situation, they are not dialysable). Most are metabolised to active metabolites.
- SSRIs. Fluoxetine is well absorbed, metabolised to an equipotent metabolite and eliminated slowly.
- Most MAOIs are well absorbed and metabolised to active derivatives.

Adverse effects

- Mention the antimuscarinic properties of tricyclic antidepressants, which may, therefore, exacerbate glaucoma, retention of urine, constipation and tachyarrhythmias. Mention weight gain, sedation (especially amitriptyline) and idiosyncratic reactions.
- For SSRIs, mention vasculitis, anorexia and exacerbation of seizures.
- Mention weight gain, anticholinergic effects and gastrointestinal upset with MAOIs. Mention the risk of hypertensive crisis with sympathomimetic compounds found in cough medicines, cheese and red wine; this is not a problem with RIMAs.

6. Chronic renal diseases may alter drug response either by changing their plasma protein binding (albumin concentrations may fall and waste products may compete for binding sites) or by reducing their clearance. (This subject is dealt with more fully in Ch. 20.)

Phenytoin is extensively bound to albumin but cleared by hepatic metabolism to inactive derivatives. Hypoalbuminaemia or uraemia cause the unbound drug fraction to rise: at a given total plasma concentration the drug, therefore, seems to be more effective and more toxic. Phenytoin doses should be reduced.

Lithium is a metallic ion that is distributed in body water and is not bound to plasma proteins. It undergoes no metabolism but is cleared unchanged by the kidney. Renal impairment causes drug accumulation.

Extended matching items answers

Theme: The clinical pharmacology of antiparkinsonian drugs

1. E. Levodopa crosses the blood–brain barrier, where it is metabolised to the neurotransmitter dopamine. Dopamine itself cannot easily cross the blood–brain barrier.

2. E. Carbidopa does not cross the blood–brain barrier easily, so its effects are confined to the extracerebral metabolism of levodopa (which is responsible for many of the drug's adverse effects).

3. G. It would be illogical to give levodopa in this setting. Instead, the acetylcholinergic system is antagonised using drugs such as benzatropine and trihexyphenidyl.

4. C. Selegiline is an inhibitor of the enzyme monoamine oxidase B (MAO-B), which metabolises dopamine. MAO-A metabolises noradrenaline (norepinephrine) and 5-HT.

Theme: The clinical pharmacology of antiepileptic drugs

1. A, E, C or F. Most physicians would probably opt for carbamazepine as first choice in this situation (A). Phenytoin (F) was probably first choice some years ago, but carbamazepine is easier to use and better tolerated. Lamotrigine (E) is a relatively newer drug, and so rather less is known about its adverse effect profile than is the case for carbamazepine; and yet lamotrigine is increasingly employed as monotherapy in this setting. Valproate (C) is another commonly used drug for this type of epilepsy.

2. D and C. Ethosuximide is probably first choice, but valproate is also commonly used.

3. A, E, C or F.

4. J. Phenytoin causes increased synthesis of CYP450 by the hepatocyte (a process that takes several days, unlike the 'opposite' type of drug interaction where compounds such as erythromycin compete very rapidly for the enzyme's active site) and this increases the hepatic clearance of warfarin, reducing its clinical effects.

Theme: The clinical pharmacology of sedative-hypnotic drugs

1. C. Severe benzodiazepine overdose depresses respiration and can cause hypoxia and hypercapnia – type II respiratory failure. This is a less likely problem with the benzodiazepines than with the barbiturate sedatives, and mainly occurs in patients with pre-existing cardiorespiratory disease.

2. F. Flumazenil is the specific benzodiazepine antagonist. Naloxone antagonises the opiates (and of course some patients may need both drugs if they have taken both opiate and benzodiazepine). Activated charcoal may have a role in severe overdose, to reduce drug absorption, but it is not an antagonist.

3. L. Both benzodiazepines and alcohol are sedative, and they interact pharmacodynamically by simple addition.

Analgesics

7.1	**Pain**	**107**
7.2	**Analgesic drugs**	**108**
	Self-assessment on Chapter 7: questions	**111**
	Self-assessment on Chapter 7: answers	**113**

Overview

Pain can arise from damage to somatic areas (e.g. skin, bone), the viscera (e.g. heart, gut) or the central nervous system (CNS; neurogenic pain). Analgesics are classified by their mode of action and include opioids, non-opioids and non-steroidal anti-inflammatory drugs. Analgesics vary widely in their potency and the right drug should be chosen for the type and level of pain.

7.1 Pain

Learning objectives

At the end of this section you should:
- be aware of the different sources of pain and the occurrence of referred pain
- be able to assess likely levels of pain and the therapeutic response needed.

Somatic pain can arise from damage of any kind, to skin, bone, fascia, meninges, peritoneum, pleura and teeth. Somatic pain is usually well localised; the sensory modality is conducted to the CNS along small myelinated *delta* fibres and non-myelinated *C-fibres*.

Visceral pain can arise from damage to heart, gut and bladder, but not brain, liver, lung and spleen. Visceral pain is often poorly localised and may be *referred* to a distant site. It is not transmitted to the CNS by specific fibres but rather by changes in the rate of discharge of afferent autonomic fibres.

Neurogenic pain can result from damage to the CNS itself: such neurogenic pain is felt in the periphery. Neuralgia is a classical example. Such pain tends not to respond to the drugs described below and it can be difficult to treat (see Ch. 6); tricyclic antidepressants or antiepileptic drugs may be useful.

Endorphins

The endorphins are endogenous compounds released in the CNS in response to pain. Many endorphins have been identified; they vary widely in structure but are all small peptides. The endorphins act by binding to opioid receptors in the CNS, of which there are three main subtypes: μ, κ and σ.

- μ-receptors cause analgesia at a supraspinal level and are also responsible for drug-induced euphoria, respiratory depression and drug dependence
- κ-receptors cause analgesia at a spinal level and also induce miosis and sedation
- σ-receptors seem to have no clinically useful properties but cause dysphoria and hallucination.

The morphine-like (opiate) drugs are the only class known to act by mimicking these peptides. Development work in new pain relief drugs is also looking at potential inhibitors of endorphin breakdown and other molecules that might interfere with nociception (sense of pain).

7.2 Analgesic drugs

Learning objectives

At the end of this section you should:
* know the mode of action of the opiates and their major actions in the intact individual
* appreciate that opiates are mainly eliminated by hepatic metabolism
* be able to list the major adverse effects of opiates and know how naloxone reverses their effects
* be able to describe the appropriate clinical use of opiates and appreciate that they can be addictive
* be aware that strict law governs the storage of many opiates, and the records that must be kept by medical staff
* appreciate that the antipyretic effects of paracetamol are useful in lowering fever
* appreciate that paracetamol is useless against inflammatory diseases such as arthritis
* appreciate that some NSAIDs are also used as analgesics (at a lower dose than that used for anti-inflammatory effects)
* appreciate that compound analgesics, although in common use, rarely have much benefit over the use of paracetamol or low-dose NSAID.

Analgesics are classified according to their mode of action, into opiates, non-opiates, and non-steroidal anti-inflammatory drugs (NSAIDs). As suggested by their name, this last group has the additional therapeutic property of reducing inflammation (Ch. 9). Analgesics vary in their potency and are used for a wide variety of pains ranging from mild, such as 'tension headache', to severe, such as terminal malignancy.

Opiate analgesics

Clinical sketch

A young man is involved in major trauma and sustains both pelvic and head injuries. He is given diamorphine for the pain from his fractures, but his level of consciousness gradually worsens in the next hour; arterial gases reveal carbon dioxide retention. A computed tomographic (CT) scan shows brain swelling.

Comment: opiate analgesics are contraindicated in patients with head injury. Respiratory depression causes retention of carbon dioxide and may worsen brain swelling.

Clinical sketch

A man with severe alcoholic liver disease is admitted with an exacerbation of chronic liver failure, brought on by pneumonia. He is given dihydrocodeine for headache, and becomes comatose.

Comment: all opiates are contraindicated in patients with decompensated liver disease, because they are not metabolised at the usual rate. Even drugs of relatively low potency, such as codeine, can worsen the level of consciousness.

Clinical sketch

A woman with ischaemic heart disease presents with a myocardial infarction. She is in great pain, clammy and breathless. She is given i.v. diamorphine as a slow injection. This relieves the pain and dyspnoea but makes her vomit.

Comment: this is appropriate use of diamorphine, but the nausea could have been anticipated as it is a common type-A adverse effect of the drug. It is usual to co-prescribe an antiemetic under such circumstances. The breathlessness may have been caused by pulmonary congestion, and the vasodilator effects of diamorphine are useful. Her blood pressure would be very likely to fall, and this is also a common adverse consequence.

Clinical sketch

A 30-year-old man has been using opiates (mainly heroin) illegally for many years. He takes them intravenously but has run out of usable veins in his arms and now uses his femoral veins. After several deep vein thromboses and groin abscesses, and a major pulmonary embolism, he decides to quit and seeks help. The Drug Dependency Clinic uses methadone as part of his management.

Comment: this is a frequently encountered clinical problem in cities. IVDUs are at risk of serious infections including endocarditis, HIV and hepatitis. Methadone is a slowly-eliminated opiate and is given by mouth (usually in very dilute liquid formulations). Although it can be abused, if part of a management strategy, methadone has a role in helping to stabilise such patients.

Mode of action of opiates

Opiate analgesics, which are structurally quite different from the endorphins, are agonists at endorphin receptors. The effects of opiates on specific organs are as follows:

* CNS
  — analgesia: the perception of both somatic and visceral pain is impaired, and the response

to pain is altered; the patient may feel 'at ease' even though pain is still perceived
— euphoria: a sensation of wellbeing; this is the main sensation sought by addicts
— sedation: a dose-dependent effect that may lead to respiratory depression
— other effects: cough suppression, nausea and miosis (small pupils)
- gastrointestinal tract
— reduced gut motility leading to constipation
— tone of biliary tree may be increased
— sphincter of Oddi may contract.
- cardiovascular system
— peripheral arteriodilatation and venodilatation, possibly as a result of effects on the vasomotor centre in the CNS
— blood pressure may fall in subjects with reduced blood volume.

Examples and clinical pharmacokinetics

The examples have certain features in common. All are well absorbed from i.m. and s.c. sites but are subject to extensive first pass metabolism in the liver if given orally. All are widely distributed and cross the blood–brain barrier readily. All are metabolised in the liver.

Morphine is a potent analgesic with a duration of analgesia of about 4–6 hours.

Diamorphine (heroin) is more potent than morphine, possibly because it crosses the blood–brain barrier more readily. The duration of analgesic action is 4–6 hours.

Pethidine is a synthetic opiate with a shorter duration of action (2–4 hours) than morphine or diamorphine and a lower potency.

Codeine has a higher bioavailability than morphine but is less potent.

Buprenorphine is a synthetic opiate with both agonist and antagonist effect at opioid receptors. It may precipitate a withdrawal reaction in opiate addicts. Its oral bioavailability is low, and buprenorphine is given either sublingually or parenterally. Buprenorphine has a long duration of action (4–8 hours) but is less potent than morphine.

Fentanyl is a potent synthetic opiate mainly used in anaesthesia.

Tramadol is a synthetic compound that, like buprenorphine, has mixed agonist and antagonist activity. It also has effects on other, non-opiate, receptors. There is probably no major advantage over opiates.

Methadone is a slowly eliminated opiate and forms part of management strategies in opiate addicts, since it helps prevent the symptoms of withdrawal. Patients can be helped to break the habit of intravenous drug abuse. This is an example of harm reduction.

Therapeutic uses

Somatic and visceral pain. Opiates are useful for both types of pain. They are, however, contraindicated in biliary colic (see above) and are useless against neurogenic pain. The severe visceral pain of myocardial infarction is treated with morphine or diamorphine, usually by slow i.v. injection accompanied by an antiemetic. In terminal disseminated cancer, s.c. infusions (often at a rate controlled by the patient) can be very useful, and oral slow-release preparations are also available.

Pulmonary oedema. Morphine and diamorphine are commonly used to treat pulmonary oedema, in combination with loop diuretics. The opiate acts partly by relieving respiratory distress and partly by reducing venous return. Caution is needed because of their effects on the blood pressure.

Diarrhoea. Oral opiates can be useful against diarrhoea, though the priority is maintenance of hydration, especially in children.

Cough suppression. This effect may be particularly useful in terminal illness.

Adverse effects

- addiction is a risk if opiates are used regularly for long periods: withdrawal then causes an unpleasant, but not clinically serious, reaction (Ch. 18). With continuous exposure larger doses are required to produce the same effects: this is called tolerance. These problems should not be used to deny patients necessary analgesia (but careful judgment is often called for)
- respiratory depression is a problem after overdose and in patients with chronic respiratory disease
- nausea
- constipation.

Contraindications

- acute or chronic respiratory disease: patients with chronic retention of carbon dioxide caused by type 2 respiratory failure are particularly at risk
- hepatic failure (see the clinical sketches on p. 108)
- head injury (see the clinical sketches on p. 108).

Drug interactions

Opiates produce additive sedation when given with other sedative drugs or alcohol.

Opiate antagonists

Naloxone is the main antagonist in widespread use for opiate overdose. Opiate effects, such as respiratory depression and coma, are dramatically reversed within 2 minutes of giving i.v. naloxone. However, naloxone has a short half-life and must sometimes be given repeatedly to those who have taken large overdoses.

Paracetamol (acetaminophen)

Mode of action

Paracetamol probably works by inhibiting the enzyme prostaglandin synthetase within the CNS. Furthermore, inhibition of prostaglandin E_2 synthesis in the hypothalamus accounts for the drug's antipyretic effects. (NB: paracetamol does not lower a normal body temperature.) Little inhibition of prostaglandin synthesis is seen peripherally and paracetamol has little or no anti-inflammatory properties.

Clinical pharmacokinetics

The clearance of paracetamol is described in Ch. 17, where the effect of overdosage is covered.

Therapeutic uses

- analgesia: paracetamol is effective, safe and causes little gastric irritation. In standard doses it is virtually free of adverse effects
- to correct fever: this can prevent febrile convulsions in young children (in this setting the drug may be given as rectal suppositories).

There is now an intravenous formulation of paracetamol for use in moderately severe pain.

Non-steroidal anti-inflammatory drugs as analgesics

NSAIDs inhibit cyclo-oxygenase and block production of prostaglandin E_2 both centrally and peripherally. They are effective both as anti-inflammatories and as analgesics.

Aspirin and *ibuprofen* are available as simple analgesics without prescription in the UK.

Most other NSAIDs require a prescription. They are intended for use in inflammatory conditions (see also Ch. 9) but are often used, sometimes inappropriately, as simple analgesics.

Therapeutic uses

- analgesia in common pain: aspirin and ibuprofen are widely used for common pain, such as headache and dysmenorrhoea
- analgesia in bone metastases: NSAIDs can be a useful adjunct to opioids in the terminal care of patients with bone metastases
- antipyretic: aspirin used to be a common remedy for childhood fevers, but fears about its role in Reye's syndrome have caused a switch to paracetamol for paediatric use.

Adverse effects

- gastrointestinal upset (Ch. 9)
- peptic ulcer disease
- allergy
- renal impairment.

Compound analgesics

Many analgesic drug combinations are marketed: they are often expensive, are rarely more potent than use of a single drug and can be dangerous in overdosage. Examples include *co-codamol:* paracetamol plus codeine.

Neuropathic pain

Neuralgia, and other syndromes caused by damage to the CNS, can cause severe morbidity and may be unresponsive to analgesics, including the opiates. This can present major clinical difficulty and require specialist help. Pain clinics are now common. A diverse range of drugs can have benefit including the tricyclic antidepressants, and some antiepileptic drugs (including carbamazepine, pregabalin and gabapentin).

Self-assessment on Chapter 7: questions

Multiple choice questions

1. The following are appropriate choices of drug:
   a. Diamorphine for pulmonary oedema
   b. Pethidine for biliary colic
   c. Paracetamol for arthritis
   d. Aspirin for dyspepsia
   e. Morphine for joint pain in haemophiliacs

2. Paracetamol plus dihydrocodeine (co-dydramol):
   a. Is safe in patients with severe renal failure
   b. Is safe in patients with liver impairment
   c. Is as potent an analgesic as morphine
   d. Can induce addiction
   e. If taken in overdose, may cause both CNS and hepatic dysfunction

3. In patients with painful bony metastases:
   a. Oral morphine may be used
   b. The combination of an opiate with a non-steroidal anti-inflammatory drug (NSAID) is beneficial
   c. Opiates do not produce important adverse effects in such patients
   d. When using parenteral morphine (via an infusion pump) it is important that the rate of infusion is not controlled by the patient
   e. Carbamazepine or tricyclic antidepressants may have better analgesic effects than opioids

Case history questions

Case history 1

A registered i.v. drug abuser is admitted with a deep vein thrombosis and pleuritic chest pain. Ventilation-perfusion scanning reveals a pulmonary infarct. Blood cultures grow *Staphylococcus aureus*. He is treated with dalteparin and antibiotics. He claims to be on methadone, but it is the weekend and you cannot check with the drug dependency centre. His pleuritic pain is severe, and he wants painkillers.

1. What should you do?
2. What are the risks of stopping methadone abruptly?

Case history 2

A man is admitted with severe abdominal pain: you suspect acute appendicitis. The surgeon is scrubbed and will not be available for about half an hour.

1. What should you do?

Short note question

Contrast the modes of action, disposition, clinical use and adverse effects of aspirin and paracetamol.

Extended matching items questions

Theme: Prescribing the best drug

Options
A. Paracetamol
B. Dihydrocodeine
C. Aspirin
D. Ibuprofen
E. Methysergide
F. Indometacin
G. Diamorphine
H. Diamorphine *and* a NSAID
I. Paracetamol-codeine compound tablet
J. Carbimazole
K. Carbamazepine

For each of the cases below prescribe the best drug for the patient from the options above. Each option may be used once, more than once, or not at all.

1. A 30-year-old man with unilateral headache, which was preceded by visual disturbance and is accompanied by nausea and prostration.
2. A 65-year-old woman with osteoarthrosis and reflux oesophagitis.

3. A young woman with tendonitis.

4. A patient with advanced metastatic cancer.

5. A man with severe facial neuralgia.

Theme: Predicting adverse effects of analgesics

Options

A. Liver damage

B. Kidney damage

C. Gastro-intestinal bleeding

D. Coma

E. Worsened pain

F. Angioedema

G. Shock

H. Rash

I. Respiratory arrest

For each of the cases below predict the most likely adverse reaction to the named drug from the list of options above. Each option may be used once, more than once, or not at all.

1. A 50-year-old man with alcoholic cirrhosis is admitted with mild confusion. He complains bitterly of severe back pain, and the doctor prescribes dihydrocodeine.

2. A woman with a past history of peptic ulcer disease is given diflunisal for dysmenorrhoea.

3. An 80-year-old man with severe chronic bronchitis suffers a nasty fall and is admitted 24 hours afterwards with pneumonia. The partial pressure of oxygen in his arterial blood is found to be very low, while that of carbon dioxide is markedly elevated. He is in a great deal of pain from two broken ribs, and this is making physiotherapy very difficult. The doctor gives him an injection of diamorphine.

4. A mildly jaundiced man with cholelithiasis takes codeine for biliary colic.

5. A patient involved in major head and neck trauma is given diamorphine.

Self-assessment on Chapter 7: answers

Multiple choice answers

1. a. **True.** Diamorphine reduces anxiety and breathlessness and is vasodilator, thereby reducing venous return.

   b. **False.** Pethidine can cause smooth muscle contraction and may exacerbate biliary colic.

   c. **False.** Paracetamol has no anti-inflammatory properties.

   d. **False.** Aspirin may exacerbate peptic ulcers and, because of its effects on clotting, may cause gastrointestinal bleeding.

   e. **False.** Haemophilia is a lifelong problem that causes repeated painful intra-articular bleeds. Frequent use of opioids may lead to addiction.

2. a. **False.** The effects of dihydrocodeine are enhanced in renal failure; paracetamol, however, is safe.

   b. **False.** Opiates undergo extensive liver metabolism and, in the presence of hepatic failure, may induce fatal coma. The role of paracetamol in severe liver disease is more contentious; in theory the patient may be more prone to toxicity, but in practice many physicians are forced to use the drug because alternatives are usually less safe.

   c. **False.** Dihydrocodeine is less potent than morphine.

   d. **True.** Full agonist opiates can induce dependence.

   e. **True.** Co-dydramol is particularly dangerous when taken in large doses: the opioid effects are clinically obvious (depression of consciousness and respiration) but those of the paracetamol may be missed unless drug levels are assayed. Co-proxamol (a combination of paracetamol and the opiate dextropropoxyphene) was withdrawn from the market for this reason. It also had a tendency to cause serious cardiac arrhythmias in overdose.

3. a. **True.** Although morphine has a low bioavailability, it is given in a slow-release formulation, which can easily be used in the community.

   b. **True.** The NSAID is often a very effective addition to the opiate.

   c. **False.** Constipation is the main problem encountered, and this is often very distressing to the dying patient. It needs to be tackled vigorously.

   d. **False.** Current practice is to give limited control of infusion rates to the patient: doses of drug are often found to be lower, and many patients find analgesia improved.

   e. **False.** Terminally ill patients may need antidepressants, but these drugs have 'analgesic' properties only in neurogenic pain.

Case history answers

Case history 1

1. It is reasonable to give him *oral* methadone, in a moderate dose, until you can check with his usual doctor. Such patients are manipulative and will often request that the dose be increased. This should be resisted: it is not in the patient's best interests.

2. Stopping opiates abruptly does cause a somatic illness, 'cold turkey': sweating, shivering, goose bumps and drug-craving. However, this is not life threatening. A NSAID would be the best choice for relief of the pleuritic chest pain: parenteral opiates should be avoided.

Case history 2

There is the concern about 'masking' important abdominal signs that may influence a surgical opinion and delay a decision to operate. Ideally the surgeon will want to assess an alert patient and examine the abdomen in the absence of strong analgesia. This needs to be weighed against a patient's need for analgesia. This is a clinical judgement that has to be made carefully in each individual circumstance. This dilemma should also be sympathetically explained to patient and family.

Short note answer

Modes of action. Both inhibit prostaglandin synthetase, paracetamol weakly and aspirin relatively more strongly. Aspirin has anti-inflammatory, analgesic and antipyretic effects; paracetamol is analgesic and antipyretic but has no significant anti-inflammatory properties.

Disposition. Both drugs are well absorbed from the gut. Aspirin is hydrolysed, by tissue esterases, into salicylic acid and acetate. Both drugs are extensively bound to plasma proteins. Paracetamol is eliminated by hepatic metabolism (conjugation reactions at therapeutic doses; in overdose, paracetamol is oxidised to a reactive, and toxic, metabolite; Ch. 17). Salicylate is mainly eliminated by conjugation in the liver, but a clinically relevant fraction is excreted unchanged by the kidney: renal clearance of salicylate is increased by alkalinisation of the urine.

Clinical use. Both drugs are available without prescription in the UK. Paracetamol is used to treat mild pain (including headache and dysmenorrhoea) and to lower temperature, especially in young children at risk of febrile seizures. Aspirin should not be given to children because of the possible association with Reye's syndrome; otherwise, aspirin is used for mild pain. Few patients can tolerate the doses of aspirin required for anti-inflammatory effects, and alternative NSAIDs are usually employed. Aspirin is also standard therapy for primary and secondary prevention in cardiovascular disease including myocardial infarction and non-haemorrhagic stroke.

Adverse effects. At therapeutic doses, it is unusual for paracetamol to cause adverse effects, but aspirin causes gastrointestinal bleeding even at therapeutic doses. Aspirin may exacerbate peptic ulcer. In patients with haemophilia or von Willebrand's disease, aspirin should be avoided because of its antiplatelet effects. In overdose, paracetamol causes concentration-dependent liver damage, which can develop into fulminant hepatic failure; aspirin overdose is characterised by a metabolic acidosis.

Extended matching items answers

Theme: Prescribing the best drug

1. A. The brief description is typical of migraine, which is usually relieved by simple analgesics such as paracetamol. Methysergide (Ch. 6) is used for the *prevention* of migraine as a drug of final resort (because of the frequency of severe adverse effects). Indometacin (Ch. 9) can cause headache and is not indicated in migraine. Dihydrocodeine may exacerbate nausea, as may aspirin and (to a lesser extent) ibuprofen.

2. A or B. This is a difficult, but common, problem. The pain of osteoarthritis can be very disabling, but the various NSAIDs exacerbate

oesophageal reflux or peptic ulcer. Some doctors might give NSAIDs while also giving either a histamine H_2 antagonist (e.g. ranitidine) or a proton pump inhibitor (e.g. omeprazole). However, paracetamol and dihydrocodeine, either separately or in combination, may give adequate pain relief.

3. D. Ibuprofen will be better tolerated than aspirin by most patients. Indometacin may be used for severe cases, but adverse effects are much more common.

4. H. Although diamorphine is very valuable in this setting, NSAIDs may give added benefit.

5. K. Carbamazepine, although an antiepileptic drug, can be beneficial in neurogenic pain like this. (Carbimazole was used as an option to make the point that drug names can be similar; this anti-thyroid drug has no utility in this situation, of course). Alternatives might have been gabapentin, amitriptyline and phenytoin.

Theme: Predicting adverse effects of analgesics

1. D. Opiates, even mild ones, are absolutely contraindicated in patients with liver failure.

2. C. Diflunisal (which you may have needed to look up in BNF) is one of the many commonly used NSAIDs. Gastrointestinal bleeding is a common adverse effect.

3. I. This man has type 2 respiratory failure (Ch. 10) in that he has carbon dioxide retention. All sedative drugs, including opiates, which can cause marked sedation are contraindicated.

4. E. Opiates (with the possible exception of pethidine) increase the tone of the sphincter of Oddi. Cholelithiasis confined to the gallbladder (cholecystolithiasis) will not usually be complicated by jaundice so this suggests a bile duct stone (choledocholithiasis). Thus the codeine might actually worsen his pain.

5. D. In general, opiates are best avoided after serious head injury. Hypoventilation (a consequence of the opiate) will tend to increase arterial CO_2, and this risks worsening cerebral oedema.

Drugs used in anaesthesia

Chapter 8

8.1 Pain prevention	**115**
8.2 Local anaesthetic agents	**115**
8.3 General anaesthetic agents	**117**
8.4 Relaxation of skeletal muscle and its reversal	**119**
Self-assessment on Chapter 8: questions	121
Self-assessment on Chapter 8: answers	122

Overview

Anaesthetics are used to prevent pain for a limited period during surgery or other procedures whereas analgesics are used to control pain. In this chapter, the use of local and general anaesthetics is described as is the use of skeletal muscle relaxants, which facilitate surgery by reducing muscle tone.

8.1 Pain prevention

Learning objectives

At the end of this section you should:
- be aware of the indications for use of local or general anaesthetics
- understand the principles upon which drug use in surgery is based.

Broadly, surgery may cause two types of pain: *somatic* pain, which is produced by cutting the skin, peritoneum or other ectodermal structures, and *visceral* pain, which is produced by traction on organs or omentum. While analgesics are used to *control* pain, anaesthetics are used to *prevent* it, for a limited period, during surgery. This has long been attempted with drugs, probably since prehistory: alcohol or opioids were the (unsatisfactory) mainstay until the discovery of ether, other inhaled drugs and cocaine.

Local anaesthetic agents are extensively used for both minor and major procedures: instilled locally they prevent somatic pain and abolish much tactile sensation; instilled epidurally, they allow abdominal surgery, though visceral pain may not be entirely prevented.

The state of general anaesthesia is complex but includes loss of consciousness, amnesia, analgesia and impairment of sensory and autonomic function. Depending on the drug, general anaesthetics may be given i.v., most frequently for *induction*, or by inhalation often for *maintenance* of anaesthesia.

Even with general anaesthetics, much surgery would be technically difficult because of the high tone of abdominal and other muscles. Skeletal muscle relaxants are widely used to facilitate major surgery and during mechanical ventilation; consequently, these drugs will also be dealt with in this chapter.

8.2 Local anaesthetic agents

Learning objectives

At the end of this section you should:
- be able to describe the mode of action of local anaesthetics at both the molecular and whole neurone levels
- appreciate that drug absorption, from injection site into the circulation, usually *terminates* the effects of local anaesthetics
- be aware of the relevance and dangers of formulation of local anaesthetic with adrenaline (epinephrine)
- appreciate that local anaesthetics are eliminated by hepatic metabolism
- be able to list the main adverse effects of local anaesthetics.

Mode of action

At the molecular level. When a neurone is stimulated, sodium channels open and Na⁺ rapidly diffuses into the cell from the higher extracellular concentration; this depolarises the cell membrane and transmits the nerve impulse. Local anaesthetics reversibly block activated sodium channels (Fig. 34) by binding to receptors situated 'within' the channel. They have low affinity for the receptor when the channel is resting (Fig. 34A) and bind mainly to activated and inactivated channels (Fig. 34B, C). Local anaesthetics are mainly ionised at physiological pH, but only the unionised (lipid-soluble) fraction is capable of crossing the cell membrane and gaining access to the receptor.

At the neurone level. Local anaesthetics block the conduction of action potentials along axons (and other excitable membranes such as cardiac muscle; see Ch. 3). Their effects are more marked in rapidly firing neurones than in resting fibres because of the higher affinity of the drug for the receptor in the active state. Furthermore, the effects of local anaesthetics vary between differing neurones: Small diameter fibres (e.g. those carrying pain modalities) with little or no myelination are more susceptible than the larger, more extensively myelinated fibres (e.g. motor neurones). See the clinical sketch below.

Examples and clinical pharmacokinetics

Lidocaine. This is one of the most commonly used local anaesthetics. The drug achieves local anaesthesia when applied to conjunctiva and mucous membranes. It is most often used as a local injection. Lidocaine is extensively metabolised to inactive derivatives (see also Ch. 3). It can be formulated with adrenaline (epinephrine), which causes local vasoconstriction and slows its absorption (this usually terminates local anaesthetic action). Gangrene can result if this preparation is used to 'ring block' a digit (see the following clinical sketches).

Cocaine. Cocaine is mainly used topically in ear, nose and throat (ENT) surgery. Indeed, it is rarely used outside this speciality, now it has been largely replaced by less toxic alternatives. It need not be formulated with adrenaline (epinephrine) because it prevents the uptake of catecholamines and, therefore, produces vasoconstriction. It is extensively metabolised.

Clinical sketch

A dentist chooses lidocaine plus adrenaline (epinephrine) for anaesthesia during routine work.

Comment: by causing vasoconstriction, adrenaline (epinephrine) slows lidocaine absorption and, therefore, prolongs its activity.

Clinical sketch

After dental anaesthesia, a patient is apprehensive because he can still feel the dentist's touch.

Comment: this is expected, and the patient should be reassured. Neurones for light touch are myelinated and hence less susceptible than those carrying pain awareness. The level of anaesthesia is likely to be acceptable.

Clinical sketch

Lidocaine plus adrenaline (epinephrine) is drawn up by an A&E doctor for 'ring block' anaesthesia, to allow him to suture the finger of a young child. Just before injection, he checks the label on the ampoule and discovers his error.

Comment: the vasoconstriction can cause gangrene. You should always double-check the content of a syringe before it is injected.

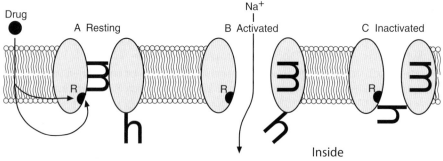

Fig. 34 Effect of local anaesthetic agents on sodium channels. **A.** When resting, the 'm' gate is shut and Na⁺ cannot diffuse. **B.** On activation, the 'm' gate opens and the 'h' gate begins to shut. **C.** When inactivated, the 'h' gate has interrupted the influx of Na⁺ and energy must be expended to return the channel to its resting configuration. Local anaesthetics must access their receptors (R) from within the cell or from within the membrane; they have no direct access from outside the cell. They have greater affinity for activated and inactivated channels than for resting channels.

Bupivacaine. This drug, which is more lipophilic than lidocaine, has a longer duration of action than other local anaesthetics. This is its principal advantage in local anaesthesia, often being used in lumbar epidural blockade. It is thus particularly suitable as continuous analgesia during labour, often mixed with an opioid analgesic.

Adverse effects

- CNS: in the doses used for minor local procedures, serious CNS toxicity is very rare; high plasma drug concentrations, resulting from incautious or accidental i.v. use, may result in seizures or perturbations in conscious level
- cardiovascular system: the antiarrhythmic and proarrhythmic effects of local anaesthetics have been described in Chapter 3. The membrane stabilising activity of anaesthesia can also be of use in cardiac arrhythmias. Like all antiarrhythmics, however, they can also be proarrhythmic
- hypersensitivity.

8.3 General anaesthetic agents

Learning objectives

At the end of this section you should:
- understand the clinical use of injected general anaesthetic drugs such as thiopental and propofol as induction agents
- appreciate the clinically important aspects of the pharmacokinetics of thiopental and propofol
- be able to describe the clinical use of ketamine
- appreciate the diverse nature of the inhaled general anaesthetic drugs and our poor understanding of their modes of action
- know the role of inhaled agents in the maintenance of anaesthesia and appreciate why they are used less often for induction
- be able to describe the pharmacokinetic principles underpinning the use of anaesthetic gases and their use clinically in combination
- know the main adverse effects of the main inhaled anaesthesic agents.

Injected general anaesthetics

Intravenous anaesthetics act much more rapidly than inhaled agents, producing unconsciousness in about 30 seconds, and are less intimidating for the patient. Hence they are preferred for induction of anaesthesia, although they can be used for the maintenance of anaesthesia throughout surgery. They can produce apnoea and hypotension. The airway must therefore be adequately maintained alongside ventilatory support; intravenous fluids may also need to be given.

Thiopental sodium

Thiopental sodium is a barbiturate that enhances the effect of the inhibitory transmitter gamma-aminobutyric acid (GABA). It readily crosses the blood–brain barrier, and, at standard doses, surgical anaesthesia is achieved after the lapse of one arm–brain circulation time. Thiopental diffuses out of the brain rapidly (being distributed to other tissues): this distribution phase has a half-life of about 3 minutes and terminates the anaesthetic effect. The elimination half-life is about 9 hours, but this has little bearing on the clinical effects. Elimination is mainly by hepatic metabolism. Thiopental is used for induction of anaesthesia. It is a potent respiratory depressant, but in the setting of controlled ventilation this is not usually an issue. Thiopental does not increase intracranial pressure.

Propofol

Propofol is very widely used, being associated with a rapid recovery and very little of a hangover effect. The mode of action of propofol is unknown. Propofol rapidly crosses the blood–brain barrier and, like thiopental, its CNS effects are terminated by distribution (out of the brain) rather than elimination. It may cause pain on injection and may cause tremors. Like most intravenous anaesthetics, propofol causes vasodilatation and hence may cause hypotension.

Ketamine

Ketamine is rarely used now and is not used as an induction agent. Instead, it tends to be used to induce 'dissociative anaesthesia' in which the eyes remain open and spontaneous respiration is maintained, but pain is not appreciated and the patient is amnesic. This state can be maintained for around 15 minutes after a slow i.v. injection, which is sufficient to allow re-dressing of burns or similar short-duration procedures. Ketamine is not used much in adult medicine because there is a high incidence of hallucinations and transient psychotic events during emergence from anaesthesia; this seems to be less of a problem with young children. The drug induces salivation, and the airway must be carefully protected. Heart rate, blood pressure and intracranial pressure are all increased.

Etomidate

Etomidate is used as an induction agent in a similar way to propofol, but appears to cause less hypotension than other drugs so may be preferred in the presence of other illness such as cardiac disease.

Inhaled anaesthetics

Pharmacokinetics

Rapid induction and recovery are important in inhaled anaesthesia allowing flexible control of the depth of anaesthesia. The main factors that determine the speed of these processes are the physical properties of the gas – its solubility in blood and lipid (cell membranes) – and physiological factors (lung and heart).

To achieve their effects, inhaled anaesthetics must pass from the alveolar air into the blood and thence into the CNS. This needs to happen rapidly but the extent and rate at which these happen depend upon:

- the partial pressure of the agent in the inspired air
- the solubility of the agent in blood: very blood-soluble drugs take longer to achieve high partial pressure in the blood and vice versa
- pulmonary physiology: the arterial tension of highly soluble drugs, such as halothane, is very dependent on ventilation; similarly, pulmonary blood flow changes the arterial tension of very soluble inhaled anaesthetics (e.g. in patients with low cardiac output, the reduced blood volume exposed to the drug steepens the rise in arterial tensions).

Elimination of the agent from the body is mainly by transfer from tissues to blood and from blood to alveolar air. Some hepatic metabolism also occurs (but this varies between the different drugs).

The rate at which consciousness returns after ceasing drug administration depends mainly on the relative solubility of the drug in the CNS and blood. For example, nitrous oxide, which is relatively insoluble, is 'washed out' rapidly, whereas halothane is more soluble and recovery takes longer.

The *duration* of the anaesthetic procedure is important for very soluble agents since, after long exposure, drug may accumulate in diverse tissues and clear from them slowly.

Mode of action

At the molecular level. The lack of structural similarity in the general anaesthetics has given rise to the concept that no specific receptor is involved in their mode of action. Rather, it is thought that these lipophilic drugs interact with the lipid of the cell membrane and thereby 'distort' membrane ion channels.

At the clinical level. If anaesthesia is *induced* using older inhalational agents, patients pass through four stages:

I. **Analgesia.** The patient has not lost consciousness but pain is reduced. This is exploited in the use of a mixture of nitrous oxide, N_2O, with air to achieve analgesia during the second stage of labour.
II. **Excitement.** The patient appears to be delirious, and there is amnesia thereafter.
III. **Surgical anaesthesia.** There is no blepharospasm upon brushing the eyelashes. Breathing is regular.
IV. **Respiratory depression.** This develops as stage III deepens, and eventually respiration ceases in stage IV. Mechanical ventilation is therefore, of course, needed.

Nowadays anaesthesia is almost always induced with i.v. drugs and these stages are not recognisable. However, they do indicate an important point about the action of inhaled general anaesthetics, which is that different neurones manifest different sensitivity: the dorsal horn cells of the spinal cord are particularly sensitive to inhaled agents, whereas brainstem neurones are fairly resistant.

Examples and clinical pharmacokinetics

Nitrous oxide. This drug, which is a gas at room temperature, has a rapid onset of action and recovery because of its low solubility (see above). It is not metabolised. It is not particularly good as a sole agent, but when mixed with oxygen is used to produce analgesia without loss of consciousness, hence its valuable role in obstetric analgesia.

Halothane. This is a volatile liquid at room temperature, is more soluble than nitrous oxide and, therefore, has slower onset and recovery rates; it is more potent than nitrous oxide. The drug is mainly eliminated via the lungs. However, the fraction metabolised in the liver may be important to the adverse effect profile – the processes involved are complicated, but involve production of free radicals within the liver. Halothane causes cardiorespiratory depression.

Isoflurane and enflurane. These drugs are volatile liquids at room temperature; their solubility and potency is somewhere between those of nitrous oxide and halothane. Enflurane undergoes a degree of hepatic metabolism, but that of isoflurane is negligible.

Therapeutic use

Inhaled general anaesthetics are often used in combination to minimise the disadvantages of any one drug (e.g. the relatively low potency of nitrous oxide) while taking full advantage of their 'strengths'.

Adverse effects

- *Cardiovascular.* Halothane, enflurane and isoflurane all reduce the blood pressure, mainly by lowering cardiac output, though isoflurane also reduces systemic vascular resistance. Nitrous oxide has little effect on blood pressure.
- *CNS.* All inhaled general anaesthetics, with the exception of nitrous oxide, reduce tidal volume and depress responses to carbon dioxide. This is not usually a practical problem as ventilation is under careful control during general anaesthesia. More of a problem is the increase in intracranial pressure induced by all these agents (nitrous oxide the least), especially in the setting of head injury.
- *Liver.* Halothane frequently causes asymptomatic elevation of transaminases and may infrequently cause severe hepatitis. This appears to occur more frequently after repeated exposure.
- *Uterus.* Halothane, isoflurane and enflurane relax uterine muscle. This is a problem if vaginal delivery is in progress but can be used therapeutically if uterine contraction needs to be inhibited.
- *Malignant hyperthermia.* This is a rare, but potentially fatal adverse reaction to halothane, resulting from violent muscle fasciculation.

8.4 Relaxation of skeletal muscle and its reversal

Learning objectives

At the end of this section you should:
- appreciate that skeletal muscle relaxants allow adequate muscle relaxation to avoid potentially hazardous levels of general anaesthetic
- appreciate that, under the influence of muscle relaxants, breathing ceases and secure artificial ventilation is immediately essential
- be able to describe the basic physiology of the motor end-plate and the modes of action of depolarising and non-depolarising agents
- be able to describe the mode of action of the anticholinesterases and their clinical use to reverse depolarising muscle relaxants
- be able to describe the use of anticholinesterases in myasthenia gravis
- know how the 'edrophonium test' is used in myasthenia gravis
- be able to list the major adverse effects of the different drug groups.

Skeletal muscle relaxants

The motor end-plate

Somatic motor neurones terminate at specialised parts of the cell membrane of striated muscle fibres termed *motor end-plates*. When the transmitter acetylcholine is released into the synaptic cleft, it binds to *nicotinic acetylcholine receptors* on the motor end-plate. This causes the opening of cation channels in the cell membrane and depolarisation; if sufficient acetylcholine is released, then a wave of depolarisation spreads through the fibre, which goes on to contract.

Acetylcholine is removed from the motor end-plate partly by acetylcholinesterase, an enzyme present in the cleft, and partly by diffusion.

Contraction of skeletal muscle can be prevented by *antagonists* of acetylcholine at the nicotinic receptor (*non-depolarising drugs*) and also, paradoxically, by *agonists* at the same receptor (*depolarising drugs*).

Non-depolarising drugs (acetylcholine antagonists)

These non-depolarising agents structurally resemble acetylcholine and are competitive antagonists at nicotinic acetylcholine receptors. All examples are given i.v. after the induction of anaesthesia but usually before endotracheal intubation. They have no sedative or analgesic effects (and hence are always employed with other agents). The effects of all examples may be reversed by anticholinesterases such as neostigmine.

Examples

Tubocurarine. This is the prototype non-depolarising muscle relaxant, replaced by more modern drugs. Tubocurarine is eliminated unchanged via the kidneys and has a long terminal half-life; its gross effects last between 30 and 60 minutes.

Pancuronium. This is mainly excreted unchanged. This has a long duration of action and is often used in patients on mechanical ventilation in intensive care.

Eight

119

Vecuronium and atracurium. These are shorter acting drugs preferred for brief procedures.

Rocuronium. This has a very rapid action, exerting an effect within 2 minutes.

Adverse effects

Hypotension: many non-depolarising drugs cause histamine release with consequent vasodilatation; at higher doses they may block autonomic nicotinic receptors.

Contraindications

Non-depolarising drugs have more potent effects in patients with myasthenia gravis (Ch. 20).

Drug interactions

- general anaesthetics cause a degree of muscle relaxation and therefore the effects of muscle relaxants are superimposed on existing relaxation
- aminoglycosides have nicotinic antagonist properties and may enhance non-depolarising drugs.

Depolarising drugs

Like the non-depolarising drugs, these compounds also resemble acetylcholine structurally. Having bound to the nicotinic receptor, they stimulate it (i.e. they are *agonists*) and sodium channels open; this causes transient muscle contraction. Thereafter, though the end-plate remains depolarised, the muscle fibre membrane is refractory, and the muscle becomes flaccid.

Suxamethonium

Suxamethonium (succinylcholine) is the only example of a depolarising drug in common use. It has an extremely short duration of action because it rapidly diffuses away from the end-plate and is then metabolised by a plasma enzyme *butyrylcholinesterase* (also called pseudocholinesterase). It is given i.v. and has a half-life of about 5 minutes. Because its duration of action is short, it can be useful for brief procedures; it can be given in repeated doses for longer procedures.

Adverse effects

- atypical butyrylcholinesterase: about 1 in 2800 patients inherits a butyrylcholinesterase with markedly reduced activity; the drug should be avoided in such patients because of its markedly prolonged duration of action
- arrhythmias: suxamethonium can produce life-threatening bradyarrhythmias

- malignant hyperthermia: this is a rare, but potentially fatal, adverse reaction resulting from muscle fasciculation
- hyperkalaemia: can be a problem, particularly during the anaesthesia of trauma victims.

Anticholinesterases

The anticholinesterases act by inhibiting acetylcholinesterase in the synaptic cleft, thereby prolonging the duration of acetylcholine. They may therefore be used: (a) to 'compensate' for autoimmune destruction of acetylcholine receptors (as in myasthenia gravis); or (b) to 'overcome' the presence of an antagonist (such as a non-depolarising muscle relaxant).

Examples

Neostigmine forms a complex with acetylcholinesterase. Its duration of action is mainly determined by the turnover of this drug–enzyme complex, rather than by pharmacokinetic processes. In myasthenia gravis, doses are needed every 2–4 hours. Neostigmine does not readily cross the blood–brain barrier.

Pyridostigmine is similar to neostigmine but longer lasting.

Physostigmine crosses the blood–brain barrier well. This gives it utility in anticholinergic poisoning (e.g. deadly nightshade consumption by children).

Edrophonium is a very short-acting anticholinesterase used in diagnostic tests: i.v. injection rapidly produces short-lived improvement of muscle weakness in myasthenia gravis (which can be a difficult diagnosis in its early stages).

Adverse effects

- *heart*: the effects of both sympathetic and parasympathetic systems are potentiated, but the parasympathetic predominates and the heart rate and stroke volume fall
- *muscular weakness* can occur at high dosage (excessive acetylcholine causing depolarisation).

Antimuscarinic drugs

Antimuscarinic drugs such as atropine and glycopyrronium (glycopyrolate) are used before or with neostigmine to prevent the bradycardia and excessive salivation that can be seen with neostigmine use. They also have a role in preventing the bradycardia and consequent hypotension that can occur with using drugs such as propofol, halothane and suxamethonium.

Self-assessment on Chapter 8: questions

Multiple choice questions

1. Anticholinesterases:
   a. Markedly reduce peripheral vascular resistance
   b. Are negatively chronotropic
   c. Can cause muscle weakness in myasthenia gravis
   d. All cross the blood–brain barrier well
   e. Have their effects reversed by edrophonium

2. Local anaesthetic drugs:
   a. Diffuse across the cell membrane in their unionised (uncharged) form
   b. Bind to receptors on the external surface of the cell membrane
   c. Block sodium channels
   d. May be potentiated locally by combination with vasoconstrictor drugs
   e. Cause seizures at high plasma concentration

3. Nitrous oxide:
   a. Is very soluble in blood compared with other inhaled anaesthetics
   b. Is very soluble in brain tissue compared with other inhaled anaesthetics
   c. Works by binding to specific receptors on neurones
   d. Has potent analgesic properties
   e. Depresses respiration

4. Halothane:
   a. Is a liquid at room temperature
   b. Is eliminated from the body mainly by hepatic metabolism
   c. Lowers the cardiac output
   d. Increases the intracranial pressure
   e. Crosses the placenta

5. Suxamethonium:
   a. Is mainly metabolised in the liver
   b. Has a long duration of action
   c. Causes depolarisation of motor end-plates
   d. Causes histamine release
   e. Is reversed by neostigmine

Short note questions

Write short notes covering the uses, mode of action and adverse effects of the following in general anaesthesia:

1. Thiopental
2. Nitrous oxide
3. Halothane
4. Pancuronium
5. Neostigmine.

Extended matching items questions

Theme: Drug selection in anaesthesia

A. Bupivacaine
B. Cocaine
C. Isoflurane
D. Ketamine
E. Lidocaine
F. Lidocaine plus adrenaline (epinephrine)
G. Neostigmine
H. Pancuronium
I. Propofol
J. Suxamethonium

For each of the drugs described below, select the drug listed above which comes closest to the description.

1. A local anaesthetic useful in epidural anaesthesia
2. A local anaesthetic useful during minor suturing procedures to an injured finger
3. An intravenous anaesthetic agent with a rapid onset of action used at induction of anaesthesia
4. A depolarising muscle relaxant
5. A non-depolarising muscle relaxant

Self-assessment on Chapter 8: answers

Multiple choice answers

1. a. **False.** Modest vasodilatation may occur.
   b. **True.** By opposing the breakdown of acetylcholine, these drugs increase the effects of the vagus at the sinoatrial (SA) node.
   c. **True.** Paradoxically, if too much anticholinesterase is used, patients develop weakness.
   d. **False.** Only physostigmine crosses extensively into the brain.
   e. **False.** Edrophonium is a short-acting anticholinesterase used in myasthenia gravis to distinguish weakness caused by excessive anticholinesterase dosage from that caused by the disease.

2. a. **True.** In common with all drugs, the unionised fraction is lipid soluble.
   b. **False.** The receptors are internal.
   c. **True.**
   d. **True.** Cocaine needs no vasoconstrictor, since it stimulates release of catecholamines.
   e. **True.** Especially when used i.v. (e.g. to treat arrhythmias, see Ch. 4).

3. a. **False.** Nitrous oxide is relatively insoluble.
   b. **False.** Because nitrous oxide is relatively insoluble, it has a rapid onset of action and recovery.
   c. **False.** The inhaled anaesthetics are thought to act by induction of changes to neuronal membranes.
   d. **True.**
   e. **True.** In common with all general anaesthetics.

4. a. **True.**
   b. **False.** Although halothane is partly eliminated by hepatic metabolism, this is a minor pathway; most is exhaled.
   c. **True.** It therefore lowers blood pressure.
   d. **True.** A particular problem after head injury, where intracranial pressure is already raised.
   e. **True.** May cause apnoea in the neonate.

5. a. **False.** Suxamethonium (succinylcholine) is metabolised by a plasma enzyme.
   b. **False.** It acts for about half an hour in normal subjects.
   c. **True.**
   d. **False.** This is an adverse effect of the non-depolarising drugs.
   e. **False.**

Short note answers

1. Thiopental is an i.v. general anaesthetic agent with a very rapid onset of action and a short duration of activity; it is used for the induction of anaesthesia.
   - Thiopental is a barbiturate.
   - Mention its effects on the GABA receptor, its steep dose–response curve and its depressant effect on respiration.
   - Mention that its effects are terminated by distribution rather than elimination.

2. Nitrous oxide is an inhaled anaesthetic, used for the maintenance of general anaesthesia.
   - Describe the solubility of inhaled agents such as nitrous oxide in lipid membrane, and mention the current hypothesis that it is this property which explains their activity.
   - Nitrous oxide has a rapid onset of action (though not enough for its pleasant use as an induction agent) and recovery.
   - It has relatively few adverse effects and is widely used with other anaesthetic gases; however, nitrous oxide is not very potent when used alone.

3. Halothane is a volatile liquid at room temperature.
   - Halothane has a slower onset of action and recovery than nitrous oxide but is more potent.
   - It reduces blood pressure.
   - Halothane is metabolised in the liver and can be hepatotoxic if used repeatedly for the same patient.
   - It can cause a rare but potentially fatal syndrome known as malignant hyperthermia.

4. Pancuronium is a muscle relaxant, an essential class of drug for abdominal surgery.

- Describe the mode of action of non-depolarising agents like pancuronium.
- Pancuronium is excreted more rapidly than tubocurarine but even so is usually reversed using an anticholinesterase.

5. Neostigmine is used to terminate the effects of pancuronium.

- Describe the metabolism of acetylcholine by acetylcholinesterase in the cleft between the motor end-plate and the motor neurone.
- Explain that this is not confined to nicotinic receptors on striated muscle but extends to nicotinic receptors of the autonomic nervous system too (parasympathetic effects predominate and the heart rate and stroke volume fall).

Extended matching items answers

1. A. Because of its long duration of action, this property of bupivacaine can be exploited in continuous epidural analgesia during labour.

2. E. In this case the vasoconstriction brought about by the addition of adrenaline (epinephrine) to lidocaine could lead to a dangerous distortion of blood supply and hence lidocaine is employed on its own.

3. I. Propofol is an induction agent.

4. J. Suxamethonium has the most rapid onset of action of any of the muscle relaxants, ideal if a fast onset and brief duration of action is required. Unlike the non-depolarising muscle relaxants its action cannot be reversed and recovery is spontaneous.

5. H. Pancuronium is one of the non-depolarising muscle relaxants, all differing subtly in their properties and potential clinical uses.

Drugs for arthritis

9.1	**Causes of arthritis**	**125**
9.2	**Non-steroidal anti-inflammatory drugs (NSAIDs)**	**126**
9.3	**Disease-modifying antirheumatic drugs**	**128**
9.4	**Drugs used in gout**	**129**
	Self-assessment on Chapter 9: questions	**131**
	Self-assessment on Chapter 9: answers	**133**

Overview

Arthritis means joint *inflammation* (redness, local heat and loss of function) and not simply joint pain (which is termed arthralgia). The most common causes of non-suppurative arthritis are rheumatoid disease (a result of disordered immune function), osteoarthritis (a result of 'wear and tear'), and gout (caused by deposition of uric acid crystals in joints). The treatment of each differs, but the non-steroidal anti-inflammatory drugs (NSAIDs) are used in the management of all three.

9.1 Causes of arthritis

Learning objectives

At the end of this section you should:
- be aware of the causes of joint inflammation
- understand that treatment differs with the underlying mechanism by which inflammation is provoked.

Osteoarthritis is very common, especially in the elderly. It often involves large, weight-bearing joints (vertebral column, hips and knees). It is caused by the failure of normal repair of joint cartilage following minor injuries. Fractures that involve an articular surface and damage caused by other joint diseases predispose towards osteoarthritis. In some patients it is a familial trait. Treatment usually involves non-steroidal anti-inflammatory drugs (NSAIDs) and may require local steroid injections; joint replacement may also become necessary.

Rheumatoid arthritis is the result of disordered immune function. It is a chronic inflammatory condition principally involving the joints but it is a multi-system disease often also involving lung, heart, eye, blood vessels and spleen. It causes a symmetrical polyarthritis, usually of small peripheral joints (hands, wrists and feet) although any joint may be involved. The disease has a very long course of relapses and remissions and may cause gross deformity. Treatment of rheumatoid arthritis usually involves NSAIDs and may require disease-modifying drugs (*penicillamine* or *gold*), *corticosteroids* (locally as injections, and systemically) and/or other immunosuppressant agents.

Gout results from excess tissue levels of uric acid, which is the end product of purine metabolism. While the cause of hyperuricaemia is usually unidentifiable, it may result from metabolic diseases or occur during treatment of malignancy (where sudden necrosis of the malignant clone during chemotherapy increases purine turnover). Acute attacks of gout typically present as a monoarthritis. The first metatarsophalangeal joints are commonly involved, but any joint (apart from the axial skeleton) may be affected.

9.2 Non-steroidal anti-inflammatory drugs (NSAIDs)

Learning objectives

At the end of this section you should:
- be able to describe the therapeutic uses of NSAIDs for inflammatory conditions and, in the case of some, for pain
- be able to list the main adverse effects, contraindications and drug interactions of NSAIDs
- know how NSAIDs work and be able to distinguish cyclo-oxygenase 2 (COX-2) inhibitors from other NSAIDs in terms of adverse effects and cost
- be aware of current concerns around the safety of COX-2 inhibitors (and all NSAIDs)
- be aware that aspirin is commonly used at low dose for its beneficial effects on platelet adhesion in the setting of cardiovascular disease.

At the whole animal level, NSAIDs are anti-inflammatory, analgesic and antipyretic (although they have no effect on temperature in the absence of fever). At a cellular level, the inflammatory response involves the release of mediator substances that attract further inflammatory cells to the locality and increase vascular permeability. Many of the mediator substances are synthesised from phospholipid in membranes of the endoplasmic reticulum, through the intermediate substance *arachidonic acid* (Fig. 35). NSAIDs inhibit *prostaglandin synthetase* enzyme, *cyclo-oxygenase (COX)*, which has two isoenzymes:

- COX-1 has housekeeping functions, including gastric cytoprotection: inhibition can have harmful effects including mucosal damage
- COX-2 is a gene product of inflammatory cells: inhibition has anti-inflammatory effects.

Fig. 35 The site of action of non-steroidal anti-inflammatory drugs (NSAIDs).

Most NSAIDs are non-selective (e.g. aspirin, ibuprofen, naproxen, indometacin), but specific COX-2 inhibitors have been developed. Rofecoxib, a COX-2 inhibitor, was withdrawn from the market when a long-term study showed an increased risk of serious cardiovascular events. The other COX-2 inhibitors (and other NSAIDs) are currently being studied with such safety concerns in mind.

Examples

Aspirin (acetylsalicylic acid). Aspirin is converted to salicylate, its active metabolite, in the tissues. Salicylate is partly excreted unchanged and is partly conjugated; its half-life is about 4 hours. Aspirin overdose is covered in Chapter 17.

Ibuprofen is extensively metabolised in the liver. Its half-life is about 2 hours.

Naproxen has a longer half-life (about 12 hours) and is excreted as an inactive glucuronide.

Indometacin is partly excreted unchanged and partly as inactive metabolites.

Therapeutic uses

Anti-inflammatory. Although aspirin and ibuprofen are NSAIDs at high dose, at usual doses their effects are confined to analgesic and antipyretic actions; anti-inflammatory doses of aspirin are often poorly tolerated because of gastrointestinal effects. Naproxen is used as a NSAID in the treatment of rheumatoid arthritis, osteoarthritis, gout and other inflammatory conditions. Indometacin is the most potent NSAID generally available, though it is also prone to common adverse effects. Many other structurally heterogeneous NSAIDs are available. Selective inhibitors of COX-2 (such as celecoxib and valdecoxib) can be expected to have fewer serious gastrointestinal adverse effects than non-specific agents. However, their cardiovascular safety profiles are currently a matter for concern (see above) and these drugs are contraindicated in patients with ischaemic heart disease and cerebrovascular disease; they are also much more expensive than the older drugs.

Antipyretic effects. All NSAIDs are antipyretic, but their use for this indication is limited by their toxicity relative to paracetamol. In children, fever can be complicated by febrile convulsions, and thus antipyretics are commonly used. Ibuprofen syrup is available over the counter for this purpose; paracetamol is also more commonly used.

Analgesia. See Chapter 7.
Antiplatelet. See Chapter 5.

Clinical sketch

A 50-year-old woman has metastatic breast cancer with bone pain. Her doctor has prescribed morphine, and subsequently added naproxen.

Comment: NSAIDs are very useful additions in pain relief from bony secondaries.

Clinical sketch

A 75-year-old woman with heart failure has painful, swollen knees. She takes ramipril and big doses of furosemide for her heart failure. The doctor gives her indometacin for her knees. She is admitted to hospital with severe pulmonary oedema and renal failure 2 weeks later.

Comment: indometacin is a very potent NSAID. It causes salt and water retention, hence the worsening of this lady's heart failure. The combination of ACE inhibitor (ramipril), loop diuretic (furosemide) and NSAID may have contributed to the renal failure.

Clinical sketch

A 60-year-old man is taking warfarin for atrial fibrillation; he has not read the 'drug interaction booklet' that the hospital gave him when the warfarin was started. Reading about the benefits of aspirin in heart disease, he starts himself on a regular dose of aspirin. He is admitted with life-threatening gastrointestinal bleeding.

Comment: NSAIDs can cause gastric erosions. Furthermore, aspirin predisposes to bleeding (see text for the mechanism). Warfarin and aspirin have very different effects on the blood clotting process: warfarin is anticoagulant whilst aspirin is antiplatelet. While some physicians may choose to use both in the same patient, the risks of bleeding (particularly gastrointestinal bleeding) are increased.

Clinical sketch

A 50-year-old man develops an acutely painful big toe; his foot is red and swollen and he cannot put on his shoe or walk. The doctor diagnoses gout and starts naproxen: the inflammation begins to settle within the next 48 hours.

Comment: gout can be extremely disabling. NSAIDs are the drug of choice for acute attacks, and steroids may also sometimes be needed.

Clinical sketch

A 70-year-old man is taking aspirin because he has angina and a history of two myocardial infarctions. The aspirin has never caused indigestion. Because of worsening osteoarthritis in his knees, his GP starts diclofenac. He develops dyspepsia, which he fails to report to the doctor, and is admitted to hospital with lifethreatening gastrointestinal bleeding.

Comment: probably the commonest regular use of aspirin is for its effects in coronary heart disease. NSAIDs are often prescribed in addition to 'low dose aspirin' and the combined risk of GI bleeding is greater. Antidepressant drugs also seem to increase the risk of GI bleeding, especially when prescribed with NSAIDs.

Adverse effects

- *gastrointestinal effects:* all NSAIDs can cause dyspepsia and also peptic ulceration and bleeding. Peptic ulceration may be asymptomatic or may manifest as dyspepsia, iron-deficiency anaemia, haematemesis and melaena or ulcer perforation; the COX-2 inhibitors are less prone to this adverse effect, although the risk is not completely eliminated
- *sodium and water retention:* a particular problem in heart failure and hypertension
- *renal impairment:* chronic exposure to large doses of NSAIDs may cause papillary necrosis; acutely, all NSAIDs may reduce the glomerular filtration rate, particularly when combined with certain other drugs (see drug interactions below)
- *asthma:* attacks may be precipitated by NSAIDs
- *indometacin:* rarely causes hepatitis and blood dyscrasias.

Contraindications

- peptic ulcer
- renal failure
- haemophilia: aspirin worsens the bleeding diathesis, but ibuprofen and indometacin are usually safe
- asthma (only in those sensitive to NSAIDs).

Drug interactions

Aspirin

- warfarin is potentiated: the interaction is mainly pharmacodynamic – through inhibition of platelet aggregation – and partly pharmacokinetic because of displacement of warfarin from protein binding
- probenecid and sulfinpyrazone: at low dose, aspirin opposes their uricosuric effects.

All NSAIDs, including aspirin

- diuretics: NSAIDs cause salt retention and reduce the potency of diuretics. This may result in deterioration in blood pressure or heart

Nine

failure control. Less commonly the combination of potent diuretic (e.g. furosemide) and a NSAID may precipitate or worsen renal impairment
- lithium: clearance of lithium is reduced
- aminoglycosides, semisynthetic penicillins and cephalosporins: acute renal failure may occasionally be precipitated (especially when multiple 'nephrotoxic drugs' are combined).

9.3 Disease-modifying antirheumatic drugs

Learning objectives

At the end of this section you should:
- understand the role of 'disease-modifying drugs' in the management of rheumatoid disease
- be aware that the decision to start such drugs is usually made with specialist advice
- be able to list the main adverse effects of the commonly used drugs
- be aware that these drugs can take a very long time to produce appreciable benefit.

Clinical sketch

A 30-year-old woman presented to her GP a year ago with severe arthritis: this required a hospital admission. She was started on a regular NSAID. However, her rheumatologist is unhappy with her progress: in particular, radiographs show inexorable worsening of joint erosions. Oral penicillamine is started. After several months her clinical progress is improved, but she has many adverse effects from the drug.

Comment: penicillamine takes months for its therapeutic benefit to become evident, and adverse effects are common (and often serious).

Although NSAIDs are the mainstay of treatment in rheumatoid arthritis, they do not alter the natural history of this crippling disease. The disease-modifying antirheumatoid drugs (DMARDs) improve symptoms (as do NSAIDs) but they also slow disease progression. They include sulfasalazine, methotrexate, gold, penicillamine, some antimalarial drugs and immunosuppressive agents. Their effects take months to become apparent, and their use (which should be supervised by rheumatologists) is often limited by toxicity. Although formerly used as 'reserve' drugs, they are often now used early in the course of the disease.

Sulfasalazine

Sulfasalazine is mainly unabsorbed until it reaches the colon: microorganisms then split the molecule to produce 5-aminosalicylic acid (5-ASA) and sulfapyridine, both of which are absorbed. In rheumatoid arthritis, it is the sulfonamide component, not the 5-ASA, that has disease-modifying activity (see also Ch. 11). Adverse effects are common (see Ch. 11) and include severe skin reactions and blood dyscrasias.

Methotrexate

This is a folate antagonist which can also be used as an antineoplastic drug. In the setting of rheumatoid disease methotrexate is often employed in a twice weekly or thrice weekly regimen, to avoid toxicity. The main toxic effects of methotrexate are on the bone marrow, and megaloblastic anaemia is the main outcome. The effects of methotrexate may be reversed using folinic acid.

Gold (sodium aurothiomalate)

Sodium aurothiomalate is given as intramuscular injections; an oral dosage form is available but this is incompletely absorbed. Gold is reserved for patients with active and progressive disease. About one-third of patients develop adverse reactions including serious skin reactions, nephritis and blood dyscrasias.

Penicillamine

The mode of action of penicillamine is unknown. It induces changes in white cells and alters immune function. Little is known about the drug's disposition because of difficulties in assay. The drug is given orally for prolonged periods. Severe adverse effects occur in about 40% of patients, and include nephropathy, blood dyscrasias, skin reactions and autoimmune disorders.

Antimalarial drugs

Chloroquine and hydroxychloroquine have 'disease-modifying activity'. Both can cause retinopathy when given for many years.

Other drugs

Glucocorticoids. This group of drugs (see Ch. 12) is used for its anti-inflammatory properties in many diseases, including rheumatoid arthritis and gout (see below).

Azathioprine. This is a derivative of the anticancer drug 6-mercaptopurine. Azathioprine is used in severe rheumatoid arthritis and other inflammatory diseases (such as systemic lupus erythematosus). The chief toxicity, which is dose dependent, is bone marrow suppression. The toxicity of azathioprine correlates to the activity of thiopurine S-methyltransferase (TPMT), whose interindividual variation is a consequence of genetic polymorphisms: clinical tests for TPMT genotype are becoming available.

Ciclosporin. This drug is the mainstay of treatment to prevent graft rejection. Its use in rheumatoid disease is restricted to severe and unresponsive disease. Its adverse effects include hair growth, liver dysfunction and nephrotoxicity. In common with all drugs that suppress immunity over long periods of time, ciclosporin increases the risk of malignancy (particularly lymphoma). Ciclosporin has little bone marrow suppressing effect.

Infliximab. This is a monoclonal antibody against tumour necrosis factor. It is used in both rheumatoid disease and Crohn's disease. In rheumatoid disease, it is used when disease-modifying drugs have failed, and it is generally given in combination with methotrexate.

9.4 Drugs used in gout

Learning objectives

At the end of this section you should:
* know the therapeutic options in the management of acute gout
* be aware that allopurinol and uricosuric drugs may make acute gout worse, and know their therapeutic use
* be able to list the main adverse effects of colchicine, allopurinol and uricosuric drugs.

Acute attacks of gout are typically treated with high doses of NSAIDs such as diclofenac or indometacin (see above). Colchicine is an alternative, particularly in those patients who may be at risk from NSAIDs, including those who have experienced gastrointestinal complications from such drugs. Allopurinol and uricosurics are used as drugs to prevent further attacks.

Clinical sketch

A 50-year-old man develops agonising inflammation of his first metatarsophalangeal joints on both feet. He is unable to walk and has a low-grade fever. The joints are red, exquisitely tender and the surface skin shows signs of desquamation. His plasma urate level is extremely high. His doctor starts the NSAID naproxen and gives a short course of prednisolone.

Comment: this treatment will probably improve the symptoms within a week, at which point the steroid would be stopped. Drugs such as allopurinol or uricosuric agents are contraindicated at this stage: they will precipitate a further attack. Such prophylactic drugs should be delayed for several weeks and then started under 'cover' from a NSAID.

Clinical sketch

A 60-year-old man, who still suffers acute attacks of gout periodically, has tissue deposits of urate crystals (*tophi*). His doctor gives him sulfinpyrazone to lower his plasma urate levels. During an episode of severe viral gastroenteritis, when he is very dehydrated, he develops agonising loin pain which radiates to his left testicle.

Comment: this is likely to be a ureteric uric acid stone. By raising the urine concentration of urate, drugs like sulfinpyrazone can cause stone formation, especially during dehydration.

Clinical sketch

A 12-year-old boy has acute leukaemia. His doctors start allopurinol before the first dose of chemotherapy.

Comment: the destruction of the malignant clone will release a great deal of purine, which will be metabolised into urate in the absence of allopurinol. This urinary urate load may threaten renal function.

Colchicine

Colchicine is as effective as NSAIDs in the treatment of an acute attack of gout: its major use is in those patients who cannot take NSAIDs, mainly those on anticoagulants or those with heart failure at risk of fluid retention. The major problem with colchicine is the toxicity experienced with high doses. Gastrointestinal disturbance is common – profuse diarrhoea can limit treatment.

Allopurinol

Allopurinol inhibits the enzyme xanthine oxidase (Fig. 36), thereby interrupting purine metabolism

Fig. 36 The mode of action of allopurinol.

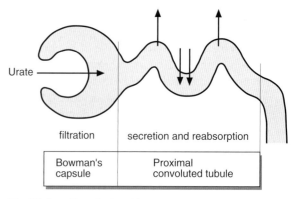

Fig. 37 Excretion of uric acid.

to produce hypoxanthine, a much more soluble compound than uric acid. Hypoxanthine does not cause arthritis and is readily excreted. Allopurinol is given orally but is incompletely absorbed. It is used for the prophylaxis of gout; it is also used during the chemotherapy of haematological malignancy (e.g. leukaemia) to prevent renal dysfunction from the massive uric acid excretion that results from the death of the malignant clone.

Adverse effects

- gout may be precipitated or exacerbated because of the early rise in uric acid concentration and the drug should not be used until about 3 weeks after an acute attack; many physicians start allopurinol under 'cover' from a NSAID to minimise the chances of a new acute attack
- gastrointestinal effects are common
- allergic rashes.

Drug interactions

- 6-mercaptopurine and azathioprine are both potentiated. They are structurally similar to allopurinol and are metabolised by xanthine oxidase
- warfarin is potentiated.

Uricosuric agents

Uric acid is filtered by the glomerulus but, in common with other relatively strong acids and bases, it is subject to both reabsorption and secretion in the proximal tubule (Fig. 37). Uricosuric drugs inhibit reabsorption, increasing uric acid clearance. Examples include *probenecid* and *sulfinpyrazone*, which are used for the prophylaxis of acute gout and the treatment of patients with large accumulations of uric acid in their tissues ('chronic tophaceous gout'). Urinary levels of this relatively insoluble acid are increased, and precipitation may occur – especially when urine volumes are small and at low pH.

Adverse effects

- exacerbation of acute attacks: when first given, uricosurics inhibit urate secretion rather than its reabsorption; this increases urate levels and may worsen gout and, consequently, uricosuric drugs are generally started about 3 weeks after an acute attack, and many physicians routinely start treatment under the 'cover' of a NSAID or colchicine
- gastrointestinal upset
- uric acid stones can form in the urinary tract
- allergic rashes.

Contraindications

- previous urinary tract stones
- impaired renal function
- recent acute gout.

Self-assessment on Chapter 9: questions

Multiple choice questions

1. Aspirin:
   a. Should be avoided in patients taking warfarin
   b. Commonly causes gastrointestinal bleeding
   c. Is the drug of first choice for rheumatoid arthritis
   d. Should be avoided in all asthmatics
   e. Is excreted unchanged

2. Indometacin:
   a. May be used to treat headache
   b. Causes few gastrointestinal adverse effects
   c. Is less likely than aspirin to interact adversely with warfarin
   d. Reduces the clearance of lithium
   e. Is relatively contraindicated in heart failure

3. Penicillamine
   a. Is indicated for gout
   b. Is the first choice drug for rheumatoid arthritis
   c. Should not be combined with NSAIDs
   d. Can only be given by injection
   e. Is usually well tolerated

Case history questions

Case history 1

An 84-year-old woman takes a NSAID for osteoarthritis; she is also taking furosemide and enalapril for heart failure. Following a fall, she breaks her hip and receives emergency surgery during which a prosthetic joint is implanted. The surgeons start her on cefuroxime as prophylaxis against infection. Postoperatively her renal function declines alarmingly.

1. What may account for her renal failure, and what should be done?

Case history 2

A 60-year-old man with mild hypertension presents with arthritis, which is diagnosed as acute gout. He takes bendroflumethiazide for his blood pressure.

1. Which of the following treatments would it be correct to start:
   a. Indometacin and allopurinol
   b. Indometacin and probenecid
   c. Indometacin alone, and allopurinol in due course
   d. Aspirin alone
   e. Allopurinol alone

The man gets better from the acute attack and remains on the thiazide for his hypertension, and allopurinol for gout prophylaxis. Over the next year he has six further bad attacks of gout.

2. What do you think about his drug treatment?

Short note questions

Write short notes on:
1. Drug treatment of acute and chronic gout.
2. Drug treatment of severe, progressive rheumatoid disease.

Extended matching items questions

Theme: The clinical pharmacology of NSAIDs

Options
A. Bleeding from the large bowel
B. Perforated peptic ulcer

C. Upper GI haemorrhage

D. Deterioration in renal function

E. Pulmonary oedema

F. Acute asthma

G. Megaloblastic anaemia

H. Myocardial infarction

For each of the clinical scenarios below, choose the most appropriate answer from options A–H, above. Each option may be used once, more than once, or not at all.

1. An 86-year-old woman has had systemic hypertension as long as she can remember. An ex-smoker with diabetes, she also suffers from heart failure and renal impairment. Her regular medications are: lisinopril, furosemide and spironolactone. She is started on diclofenac by her GP because of severe osteoarthritis in her hips and worsening mobility. She is admitted to hospital 2 weeks later with breathlessness. What two adverse events are the most likely to explain her symptom?

2. An elderly man has been depressed for a considerable period and takes an antidepressant drug and a NSAID. What adverse effect is the most likely to occur?

Self-assessment on Chapter 9: answers

Multiple choice answers

1. a. **True.** Aspirin increases the bleeding time by its effects on platelet function; furthermore, by causing gastrointestinal bleeding diatheses, all NSAIDs may induce life-threatening bleeds in patients with prolonged prothrombin times.

   b. **True.**

   c. **False.** Aspirin needs to be given at high dose to induce an anti-inflammatory effect. Many patients cannot tolerate these high doses.

   d. **False.** Aspirin may precipitate asthma in some patients who are sensitive; this is thought to occur through its inhibition of prostaglandin synthetase.

   e. **False.** Aspirin (acetylsalicylic acid) is hydrolysed to salicylate (phase I metabolism) and thereafter conjugates (phase II).

2. a. **False.** Indometacin is a potent NSAID that is not used as a simple analgesic but for its anti-inflammatory properties; indometacin may cause headache.

   b. **False.** It is very prone to cause gastrointestinal effects.

   c. **True.** Although warfarin is displaced from plasma protein binding, this is not clinically important; indometacin has less potent antiplatelet effects and interacts little with warfarin.

   d. **True.** See Chapter 6.

   e. **True.** Indometacin may cause pronounced salt and water retention.

3. a. **False.** Penicillamine is not used for gout. It is used as a disease-modifying drug in rheumatoid arthritis.

   b. **False.** NSAIDs are usually first choice agents. Penicillamine is used for aggressive disease (often for extra-articular manifestations, such as vasculitis). It is started and monitored by specialists.

   c. **False.** Penicillamine is often used with NSAIDs.

   d. **False.** It is given orally.

   e. **False.** It frequently causes adverse events.

Case history answers

Case history 1

It is possible that her blood pressure may have fallen as a result of the fracture or the anaesthetic causing acute tubular necrosis, but her drugs are probably responsible. NSAIDs, furosemide, enalapril and cefuroxime are all nephrotoxic, and their effects are additive. The necessity for antibiotic prophylaxis needs to be reconsidered, the enalapril should probably be stopped and the NSAID should certainly be stopped. The patient's state of hydration and the risk of withdrawal of furosemide (acute pulmonary oedema) need to be carefully considered. Specialist advice would certainly be required.

Case history 2

1. It would only be correct to start (c): indometacin alone with allopurinol in due course. Most physicians would start a NSAID alone for immediate therapy: this should begin to control symptoms within 2 days, but failure to improve may necessitate addition of a more potent corticosteroid. Aspirin would not be a good choice because it causes retention of urate when first started. Any NSAID may worsen control of hypertension, but this can be compensated for by increasing antihypertensive dosage. When symptoms have resolved, a prophylactic drug may be started (under NSAID cover to begin with). Starting either allopurinol or a uricosuric alone immediately would worsen the gout.

2. Thiazide diuretics elevate plasma urate and should be changed to an alternative drug.

Short note answers

1. The urgent priority in *acute gout* is relief of symptoms using an anti-inflammatory drug:

   • the usual choices are indometacin, naproxen or ibuprofen, although any NSAID may be used

- in the presence of peptic ulcer disease, or recent upper gastrointestinal haemorrhage, treatment becomes more difficult; colchicine may be used but generally causes severe diarrhoea
- patients with severe gout may require systemic steroids as well as NSAID treatment.

The NSAID should be continued until the arthritis has subsided; most physicians would continue to give a NSAID during the introduction of allopurinol or uricosuric therapy.

The treatment of *chronic gout* aims to reduce the risk of further acute arthritis, to preserve renal function and to avoid formation of gouty tophi. Patients who have had more than one clinical attack of gout should probably be offered treatment with either:

- uricosuric drugs (probenecid or sulfinpyrazone) which increase the renal clearance of uric acid; they are contraindicated in patients with renal failure because there is the risk of uric acid stone formation, which may further worsen renal function, and the uricosurics work less well in the presence of renal impairment

  or

- allopurinol (more commonly used) which inhibits the enzyme xanthine oxidase and reduces the formation of uric acid; it is preferable in patients with renal failure (although doses should be reduced, as the risk of adverse effects increases in renal failure).

A summary of the main adverse effects of NSAIDs, colchicine, uricosurics and allopurinol should be given.

2. The usefulness and limitations of NSAIDs should be covered:

- NSAIDs reduce inflammation and help symptoms but do not change the rate of disease progression
- the principal adverse effects of NSAIDs should be discussed: gastrointestinal bleeding, gastrointestinal ulceration, dyspepsia, antiplatelet effects, salt retention and exacerbation of heart failure, exacerbation of renal impairment.

The use of gold, penicillamine and sulfasalazine should be covered:

- indications
- route of administration
- course of therapy
- adverse effects.

Extended matching items answers

Theme: The clinical pharmacology of NSAIDs

1. D, E or F. Salt and water retention can worsen congestive cardiac failure and precipitate pulmonary oedema, and this seems the most likely explanation. However, patients with pre-existing renal impairment can have this worsened by NSAIDs, especially if they already take 'nephrotoxic' medicines – and she is on an ACE-inhibitor. Finally, NSAIDs can precipitate asthma.

2. C. The combination of antidepressant tricylics or selective serotonin reuptake inhibitors (SSRIs) with NSAIDs increases the risk of GI bleeding.

Respiratory disorders and hypersensitivity

10.1 Drugs for asthma and chronic obstructive pulmonary disease   **136**

10.2 Respiratory failure: oxygen therapy and respiratory stimulants   **139**

10.3 Cough suppressants and expectorants   **140**

10.4 Hypersensitivity   **140**

Self assessment on Chapter 10: questions   **143**

Self-assessment on Chapter 10: answers   **146**

Overview

This chapter covers the use of drugs and oxygen in the treatment of asthma, chronic obstructive pulmonary disease (COPD) and respiratory failure. Asthma is caused by inflammation of the small bronchi. Most attacks are mild. Acute severe attacks of asthma are potentially life-threatening. Drugs are used both in acute asthma and to control chronic asthma. COPD results from damage to respiratory cilia as well as inflammation, and requires antibiotics for acute attacks as well as drugs to dilate airways as in asthma. Respiratory failure can complicate a number of conditions (including both asthma and COPD) and requires oxygen therapy, drugs or mechanical ventilation, depending on the circumstances. Because the immune system plays a role in asthma, it is convenient to cover hypersensitivity in this chapter, but some parts of this section are more relevant to adverse drug reactions and should be read in conjunction with Chapter 21.

Learning objectives

At the end of this section you should be able to:

- describe the basic pathophysiology of asthma and COPD
- understand what is meant by 'acute severe asthma', and appreciate the severity of this condition
- outline a management plan for a patient with acute severe asthma and discuss the indications for mechanical ventilation in this condition
- outline a management plan for patients with stable asthma and COPD, both to prevent attacks and treat acute episodes
- list the main classes of drug used for asthma and COPD, their main adverse effects and the interactions of these drugs
- describe the use of controlled oxygen therapy in respiratory failure.

Clinical sketch

A 60-year-old cigarette smoker developed asthma aged around 40. He is now on regular doses of inhaled salbutamol (he has a nebuliser at home) and cannot drop his dose of oral prednisolone below 7.5 mg daily (the doctor has tried him on inhaled high-dose beclometasone, but systemic steroids have always been found essential to avoid hospital admissions). He suddenly develops severe back pain. Radiographs confirm a collapsed thoracic vertebra and osteopenia.

Comment: some patients do need long-term systemic steroids. As always the risks of such treatment need to be weighed against the benefits. Osteoporosis is a common hazard, which might be reduced by specific therapies.

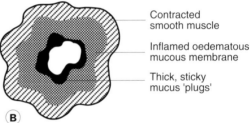

Fig. 38 Airways obstruction in asthma. **A**. Normal airway. **B**. Airway during an asthmatic attack.

10.1 Drugs for asthma and COPD

Asthma is caused by inflammation of small bronchi – usually resulting from type I hypersensitivity (see Section 10.4 below) – resulting in recurrent, reversible episodes of airways obstruction. This causes three main features: dyspnoea, wheeze and cough. The antigen (commonly the excreta of the house dust mite or pollen) is usually inhaled. However, asthmatics also have attacks in response to non-allergic stimuli including exercise, emotion and viral respiratory infection; in many cases (often where symptoms have come on later in life), no allergy can be demonstrated. Obstruction results from (a) mucous membrane oedema secondary to inflammation; (b) contraction of bronchial smooth muscle, under the influence of the autonomic nervous system and inflammatory mediators; and (c) thick mucus plugs, which may obstruct the lumen altogether in the most severe cases (Fig. 38). The principal clinical features are paroxysmal cough, wheeze and shortness of breath. Most attacks are mild, but asthma still kills around 2000 people in the UK annually, despite available drugs.

Chronic obstructive pulmonary disease (COPD) is a very common complication of cigarette smoking and results from damage to respiratory cilia, which causes chronic colonisation of the lower airways by *Haemophilus influenzae* and *Streptococcus pneumoniae*. It includes emphysema and chronic bronchitis: most patients have elements of both. Chronic bronchitis is clinically defined as 'a cough productive of sputum for more than 3 months in 2 consecutive years' but, in addition, there is usually associated small airways obstruction, and so patients are often wheezy and breathless. The airway obstruction in COPD is often fixed rather than reversible, and inflammation is not such a prominent feature. The drugs used to treat COPD are the same as those used for asthma, but patients with COPD usually require antibiotics for exacerbations.

Anti-inflammatory drugs

Glucocorticoids

The preferred route of administration for glucocorticoids is by inhalation: high local concentrations of steroid can then be achieved with small doses, which minimises systemic adverse effects (Box 5). *Beclometasone* and *budesonide* are formulated for inhalation via several different devices. The mode of action, pharmacokinetics and adverse effects of steroids are dealt with in Chapter 21. Inhaled glucocorticoids are useful for the *prevention* of attacks by the reduction of bronchial inflammation. Inhaled steroids are not used on their own for acute attacks. Systemic steroids (particularly hydrocortisone) are life-saving drugs under such circumstances.

Box 5 Topical use of drugs in asthma

In acute severe asthma (see text below), which is a medical emergency, drugs are often used systemically: steroids may be given by injection or by mouth and beta-agonists may be given by i.v. infusion.

For the maintenance of patients with asthma, it is logical to use drugs topically when possible:

- if the drug is delivered directly to its site of action, high concentrations can be rapidly achieved
- total doses can be kept low, thereby reducing adverse effects; this is particularly important with the use of topical steroids.

Drugs can be delivered topically in three main ways (although there is a wide range of commercially available delivery systems).

1. Nebulisation of drug solution: this is usually done in hospital (using a stream of oxygen or air) but can be achieved at home using electric pumps.
2. Hand-held metered-dose inhalers, using pressurised canisters: essentially the same technology as furniture polish!
3. Hand-held dry-powder devices: these usually rely on puncturing a plastic capsule, which contains the drug, followed by dispersal of the drug by a 'turbine', which is powered by the patient's inspiration through the mouthpiece.

Sodium cromoglicate and nedocromil

It is not entirely clear how cromoglicate and nedocromil work. Neither is absorbed when given orally, but both are formulated as aerosols. They are used to *prevent* asthma attacks (i.e. prophylaxis), and are *useless* in the treatment of an attack. Cromoglicate and nedocromil reduce bronchial response to inhaled antigens and to nonspecific triggers such as exercise. They are of most use in atopic asthmatics, though non-topic patients may also benefit. Used regularly, they seem to reduce inflammation and may abolish bronchial hyperreactivity. Different formulations of cromoglicate are also used for seasonal rhinitis (hay fever). Cromoglicate is useless in COPD. Adverse effects are confined to laryngeal irritation.

Leukotriene pathway inhibitors

The leukotrienes (see below under type I hypersensitivity) are inflammatory mediators and potent bronchoconstrictors. Leukotriene receptor antagonists (such as montelukast and zafirlukast) may be taken orally for the prophylaxis of asthma attacks.

Bronchodilators

Beta-agonists

Selective β_2-adrenoceptor agonists are used as bronchodilators in asthma. (See Ch. 2 for details of adrenoceptor classification and function.)

Salbutamol is well absorbed when given orally but is subjected to extensive first pass metabolism. More usually, the drug is given as an inhaled aerosol either for treatment of acute attacks or for maintenance. If salbutamol is given as a nebulised solution (driven either by pressurised oxygen or by electronic pump) then high concentrations can be achieved in the lungs. Salbutamol may be given i.v. in an emergency.

Terbutaline is also given topically as a metered-dose inhaler or as nebulised solution. It has a longer duration of action than salbutamol.

Salmeterol and *formoterol* are longer-acting β_2-agonists, used for maintenance treatment by inhalation only, in patients not adequately controlled by inhaled steroids.

Therapeutic uses

- acute severe asthma: nebulised β_2-agonists, usually salbutamol, usually give rapid symptomatic improvement
- maintenance of symptomatic asthma: most asthmatics take inhaled β_2-agonists as required for symptomatic relief; some patients need regular doses. Salmeterol or formoterol can be useful for patients with bad asthma and are added to inhaled steroids
- COPD: bronchodilators are used both in acute exacerbations of COPD and as maintenance treatment.

Adverse effects

- tachycardia: sinus tachycardia is a common adverse effect but does not usually necessitate a change in therapy; a reduction in dose is sometimes required
- fine tremor is a frequent finding but is rarely severe enough to warrant changing therapy.

Anticholinergics

Stimulation of the bronchi by the parasympathetic fibres of the vagus nerves causes bronchoconstriction and secretion of mucus. Muscarinic antagonists, such as ipratropium and tiotropium, oppose these effects. Ipratropium is used topically by inhalation and can be given by nebuliser in severe bronchospasm. Tiotropium is also used by inhaler but differs from ipratropium in that (a) it is longer acting and (b) it is unsuitable for relief of acute symptoms. Because neither is extensively absorbed, systemic effects are few. Local absorption in the mouth may result in diminished salivary flow. Rarely, ipratropium may exacerbate glaucoma.

Aminophylline

Aminophylline is a soluble derivative of theophylline that is widely used, especially for maintenance treatment of COPD. The mode of action is unknown (aminophylline blocks the metabolism of cyclic AMP, but it is doubtful whether this is the basis of the therapeutic benefit). Aminophylline may be given orally, rectally or i.v. Aminophylline is mainly cleared by hepatic metabolism (to inactive derivatives); the elimination half-life is short but sustained-release formulations allow less frequent dosing (once or twice daily). The drug has a narrow therapeutic range (5–20 mg/L) and therapeutic drug monitoring is recommended, given the drug's adverse effects at high concentration.

Therapeutic uses

- acute severe asthma. Aminophylline is *not* a first choice agent but may usefully be combined with β_2-agonists. Aminophylline is usually given as a *slow* i.v. loading dose followed by constant rate infusion until improvement is seen. *Caution* is needed if the patient takes oral theophylline preparations, as toxicity is more likely
- control of asthma and COPD. Regular doses of oral aminophylline may be needed in addition to other bronchodilators.

Adverse effects

- seizures occur at high aminophylline concentrations and are most common when the drug is given rapidly i.v.
- tachyarrhythmias may be life-threatening; like seizures, they are concentration related and common if the drug is given rapidly i.v.
- tremor
- nausea
- insomnia.

Drug interactions

Because aminophylline is mainly cleared by biotransformation, its effects are enhanced by enzyme inhibitors and opposed by enzyme inducers (see Ch. 21).

Acute severe asthma and its management

Severe asthma is a medical emergency, and patients need careful observation even though they may respond rapidly to initial treatment. An attack of asthma in an adult should be considered severe if any of the following are present:

- the patient is unable to complete sentences in one breath
- respiratory rate is greater than 25 breaths/min
- the heart rate is greater than 110 per minute
- the peak expiratory flow rate is less than 50% the value predicted.

An attack should be considered to be *life-threatening* if any of the following features develop:

- PEFR is less than 33% of predicted value
- the chest is silent on auscultation
- cyanosis
- feeble respiratory effort
- bradycardia
- hypotension
- exhaustion, confusion or coma
- Pao_2 less than 8.0 kPa; $Paco_2$ in the normal range.

Management

1. The patient must be admitted to hospital, and given a high concentration of oxygen.
2. Inhaled nebulised β_2-agonist and ipratropium should be given; intravenous therapy is reserved for patients in whom inhaled drugs cannot be given reliably.
3. High doses of systemic steroid should start at once.
4. A single i.v. dose of magnesium sulphate has been shown to be effective in cases that fail to respond to initial therapy.
5. Clinical monitoring (including charting of PEFR, and repetition of arterial gases) should be intensive.
6. Patients who need mechanical ventilation (see below) or those who fail to respond to initial treatment should be managed in either an intensive care unit or a respiratory high dependency unit.

Clinical sketch

A 20-year-old woman is admitted with severe asthma and mild left-sided 'sharp' chest pain. She is hypoxic. Initial treatment is with inhaled 40% oxygen, regular nebulised salbutamol and regular i.v. hydrocortisone. She fails to improve and becomes exhausted. The doctor is asked to give a night sedative 'to settle her down': this is declined. Auscultation reveals reduced breath sounds on the left and a chest radiograph shows a pneumothorax. She is moved to the intensive care unit; a chest drain is inserted and she is ventilated.

Comment: this sort of case is not unusual. You should remember that (a) not all asthmatics respond satisfactorily to first line treatment, (b) pneumothorax must always be excluded and (c) sedative drugs are contraindicated.

Chronic asthma and its management

Many patients with chronic asthma can be managed with occasional use of a bronchodilator such as a β_2-agonist. If this is required more than once daily, regular inhaled anti-inflammatory drugs are needed:

- in adults, inhaled steroids are most commonly used

- in children, *sodium cromoglicate* may be preferred (mainly because of the possible adverse effects of regular steroid exposure); its effectiveness is uncertain

- some patients need high doses of inhaled steroids and regular use of bronchodilators

- a very small minority of patients need regular oral steroid.

Patients need to understand:

- which of their drugs are indicated for acute attack

- which of their drugs are indicated mainly for prevention of attacks

- how to take their drugs (particularly in the case of complicated inhaler devices) (see Box 5)

- when to seek urgent medical help.

10.2 Respiratory failure: oxygen therapy and respiratory stimulants

Learning objectives

At the end of this section you should be:

- conversant with the classification of respiratory failure into types I and II

- able to contrast the use of oxygen in type I and type II failure

- able to describe the role of mechanical ventilation.

Respiratory failure is defined as an arterial partial pressure of oxygen (Po_2) less than 8.0 kPa (when breathing atmospheric air at sea level). It may complicate asthma, COPD, pneumonia, pulmonary embolism and pulmonary fibrosis, pulmonary oedema and CNS 'depression' (including the effects of respiratory depressant drugs, such as opiates). 'Controlled oxygen therapy', respiratory stimulant drugs and mechanical ventilation may be needed, depending on the circumstances.

Clinical sketch

A young woman on oral contraceptive steroids suddenly collapses with vague chest pain and severe dyspnoea. She is centrally cyanosed, has a pulse rate of 140 beats/min, a blood pressure of 60/20 mmHg, and marked jugular venous engorgement. Her arterial gases are Po_2 6.0 kPa, Pco_2 1.2 kPa and pH 7.52. The chest radiograph is normal, but spiral computed tomographic scans show massive pulmonary emboli in both main pulmonary arteries.

Comment: this patient probably needs urgent thrombolysis, or perhaps surgery. The inspired oxygen concentration should be as high as is needed to normalise the arterial partial pressure. Oxygen masks deliver up to 80%, depending on flow rate, while nasal cannulae will deliver up to 35%. In some cases even 80% oxygen will often be inadequate, in which case positive-pressure ventilation may be needed.

Clinical sketch

A 70-year-old cigarette smoker with severe COPD is admitted with an infective exacerbation. Her arterial gases are Po_2 5.0 kPa, Pco_2 9.2 kPa and pH 7.10. She is started on 35% oxygen, on which her gases are: Po_2 6.5 kPa, Pco_2 10.2 kPa and pH 6.98. She is changed to 28% oxygen and given bronchodilator nebulisers, steroids, aminophylline, antibiotics and physiotherapy. Her gases improve to Po_2 6.9 kPa, Pco_2 8.8 kPa and pH 7.22.

Comment: in chronic type II failure, high inspired oxygen concentrations may worsen carbon dioxide retention, may cause acidosis and may lead to death. In this circumstance, 24–28% inspired oxygen is usually recommended with cautious monitoring of the arterial blood gases. In this case, non-invasive ventilation (NIV) may be considered because of the extent of the abnormalities.

Ten

Classification of respiratory failure

Type I

Type I respiratory failure is caused by ventilation–perfusion mismatching; Po_2 is low and Pco_2 is normal or low. Common causes include:

- pulmonary embolism
- pneumonia
- asthma
- adult respiratory distress syndrome (ARDS).

  Management involves:

- inhaled oxygen concentrations high enough to normalise arterial gases
- mechanical ventilation if arterial oxygen cannot be maintained otherwise
- treatment of the underlying cause.

Type II

Type II respiratory failure is caused by hypoventilation and the Pco_2 is high. Common causes include:

- sedative drug overdose (acute and self-limiting if supportive therapy is adequate)
- other causes of severe CNS 'depression' (e.g. massive cerebrovascular accident)
- COPD.

It is crucially important to remember that, whereas normal respiration is mainly driven by changes in pH, in patients with chronic type II failure, respiration is driven by hypoxia. Too great a correction of hypoxia can be life-threatening.

Management involves:

- carefully monitoring of inhaled oxygen concentrations
- respiratory stimulants may be useful
- mechanical ventilation is indicated for acute cases (such as drug overdose) and non-invasive ventilation with bi-level positive airways pressure (BiPAP) has a role in the setting of acute exacerbations of chronic cases complicated by respiratory acidosis.

10.3 Cough suppressants and expectorants

In general, coughing serves the useful function of expelling bronchial secretions, and its suppression is often unwise. However, in the setting of terminal care, cough can be a distressing symptom (especially at night). Diverse drugs including mild opiates (commonly codeine) and sedating antihistamines are used, and may give benefit; both classes are dealt with elsewhere.

Expectorants are claimed to promote expulsion of bronchial secretions and are often used in COPD. There is little evidence of benefit over that of a placebo function. Proprietary examples are too numerous to list.

10.4 Hypersensitivity

Learning objectives

At the end of this section you should:

- be able to describe briefly the mechanisms of the four types of hypersensitivity
- be able to describe the clinical syndromes of anaphylaxis and angioedema, and outline the emergency management of these syndromes
- appreciate that 'type B' adverse drug reactions are often caused by hypersensitivity.

The immune system, there for our protection against microorganisms, can cause disease when inappropriate responses lead to tissue damage: this is termed *hypersensitivity*. Hypersensitivity responses can be 'triggered' by environmental agents (as is often the case in asthma), but also by drugs. It causes diverse clinical syndromes including asthma, anaphylaxis, vasculitis, glomerulonephritis and arthritis. Hypersensitivity can be classified into four groups, I–IV, based on the immune response.

Type I (immediate)

Environmental materials such as pollen and avian proteins can be antigenic. In contrast, drugs are too small to function as antigens, but they may be capable of binding to a protein to form an antigen: the drug is then termed a hapten. Exposure stimulates production of antigen-specific IgE antibodies by plasma cells and these become attached to the membrane of mast cells and basophils (Fig. 39). Repeat exposure results in recognition of the antigenic drug–protein complex by IgE, and the release by the mast cells and basophils of preformed mediator substances (histamine, kinins and 5-HT) and the rapid synthesis of others (leukotrienes and prostaglandins). The net effects of the mediators are mucosal inflammation, increased capillary leakiness, secretion of mucus and contraction of smooth muscle. Drugs commonly producing type I reactions are *penicillins* and *cephalosporins*. Common syndromes are asthma (above), rhinitis/conjunctivitis/eczema, angioedema and anaphylaxis.

Clinical sketch

A 40-year-old woman has had penicillin in the past without incident. During a hospital admission she is given high-dose benzylpenicillin i.v. for cellulitis of the leg. While the infusion is running, she becomes breathless and wheezy: the nurses stop the infusion and summon the doctor. Five minutes later, when the doctor arrives, the patient is cold and clammy and stridor is audible from the end of the bed. Her blood pressure is unrecordable. She is given adrenaline (epinephrine) i.m.; i.v. access is obtained and chlorphenamine, hydrocortisone and fluids are given i.v.

Comment: this woman has developed anaphylaxis and angioedema in response to benzylpenicillin. The life-saving actions were immediate interruption of the suspect drug and i.m. adrenaline (epinephrine). The steroid and antihistamine may be helpful, but the former can take many hours to produce clinical benefit.

Seasonal rhinitis

People prone to seasonal rhinitis/conjunctivitis, asthma and eczema are termed 'atopic'. Seasonal rhinitis is common and, although not life-threaten-

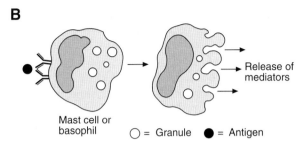

Fig. 39 Type I hypersensitivity. **A**. First exposure. **B**. Re-exposure.

ing, is a frequent cause of time off school and work. The classical pathogenesis is illustrated in Figure 39. Symptoms are maximal in the summer months when pollen counts are high and comprise rhinorrhoea, sneezing and sore eyes.

Treatment

Treatment is with systemic antihistamines and topical sodium cromoglicate and topical steroids. Histamine type I receptor antagonists (of which there are many, some available without prescription) 'block' those histamine receptors found on mucus-secreting cells and capillaries in the mucous membranes of the upper airways. Older examples are usually short-acting and have major sedative effects: if a sedative effect is required (e.g. in the management of a child with sleep disturbance because of urticaria), then a drug like chlorphenamine is preferred. More usually, sedation is an undesirable effect, because it impairs skills such as driving and the use of machinery. Under these circumstances a drug like loratadine or cetirizine is indicated. Both these drugs are long-acting, and can be taken once daily. Although loratadine and cetirizine are labelled 'non-sedating', patients should be warned that sedation can occur, and that skilled tasks and excess alcohol should be avoided.

Anaphylaxis/angioedema

Mediator-induced venodilatation may be marked enough to lower cardiac output, causing life-threatening shock: this is termed anaphylaxis. Capillary leakiness in the larynx can cause life-threatening upper airways obstruction, termed angioedema. Anaphylaxis and angioedema may be present simultaneously.

Management

The suspected drug should be stopped (mainly relevant to i.v. infusions), and the airway maintained. Intramuscular (or subcutaneous) adrenaline (epinephrine) is life-saving and may need to be repeated every 5 minutes (judged by response of blood pressure). Histamine H₁ antagonists (see above) should be given parenterally. A glucocorticoid should be given but is of secondary importance because of the delay in its onset of action. If the blood pressure is low, then the foot of the bed should be elevated to increase venous return. Intravenous fluid may also be necessary.

Type II (autoimmunity)

Drugs may induce immune responses to 'self'. The mechanisms are incompletely understood but include: (a) covalent binding of the drug to a cell surface so that the cell becomes haptenated; (b) binding to a circulating protein, producing a hapten that resembles a cell antigen; and (c) alteration of cell metabolism so that cellular antigens change and become recognised by the immune system as foreign. In all cases the immune system is activated, and cell damage occurs. Clinical features can include systemic lupus erythematosus (SLE)-like syndromes and blood dyscrasias. SLE is a common autoimmune disease with features that include arthritis, vasculitis, nephritis and rashes. *Hydralazine* (Ch. 3) and *isoniazid* (Ch. 13) can induce an SLE-like syndrome; this is usually reversible when the drug is stopped. *Methyldopa* can induce autoantibodies towards erythrocytes, causing haemolytic anaemia. Some drugs may induce autoimmunity towards bone marrow precursor cells, causing pancytopenia (in which all cell series are affected) or agranulocytosis (in which the granulocyte series is affected): these syndromes may prove irreversible when the drug is stopped and can be fatal.

Clinical sketch

A young man is found to be hyperthyroid and is started on carbimazole. One month later he presents with a febrile illness, conjunctivitis and a sore throat. His granulocyte count is extremely low.

Comment: this is agranulocytosis, a rare but potentially fatal adverse reaction to carbimazole.

Type III (immune-complex)

Type III hypersensitivity is characterised by circulating antigen–antibody complexes (immune complexes), and their subsequent deposition on basement membranes. Attraction of cells of the immune system and local activation of complement cause tissue damage. Drugs commonly producing the type of reaction are *penicillins* and *sulphonamides*.

Serum sickness. Commonly seen with incompatible blood transfusions, this comprises urticaria (hives), fever and arthralgia.

Clinical sketch

An HIV positive woman is given sulfamethoxazole-trimethoprim for the treatment of *Pneumocystis carinii* pneumonia. Within 24 hours she is extremely ill with fever, severe rash and ulcerating mouth lesions.

Comment: this is Stevens–Johnson syndrome resulting from a type III hypersensitivity to the sulphonamide.

Type IV (delayed)

Whereas type I responses are seen within minutes of exposure, and those of type II and III usually within hours, type IV responses can take longer to evolve. Antigens are phagocytosed by macrophages, transported to local lymph nodes and presented to lymphocytes. The lymphocyte clone then proliferates and travels to the site of antigen delivery. The classical example of a class IV reaction is that towards tuberculin injected into the skin as a Mantoux test, where inflammation takes 72 hours to develop. Contact dermatitis is the only common adverse drug reaction of this class; it may result from many skin preparations and from nickel salts.

Self-assessment on Chapter 10: questions

Multiple choice questions

1. Salbutamol:
   a. Takes about 1 hour to produce bronchodilatation
   b. Is a selective agonist at β_1-adrenoceptors
   c. Should be stopped if it causes tremor
   d. Must be taken regularly
   e. May be valuable for acute left ventricular failure

2. Ipratropium:
   a. Is a nicotinic antagonist
   b. May cause intraocular pressure to rise
   c. Is of no value in the treatment of acute severe asthma
   d. Causes a dry mouth
   e. Encourages oral candidiasis

3. The following statements are true:
   a. Cough suppressant drugs, such as codeine, are valuable in the management of asthma
   b. In acute severe asthma, the inhaled oxygen concentration should be low (24–28%)
   c. Ciprofloxacin has no effect on the disposition of theophylline
   d. Glucocorticoids potentiate the effects of salbutamol
   e. Antihistamines have no place in the treatment of acute severe asthma

4. Inhaled sodium cromoglicate:
   a. Is beneficial in chronic bronchitis
   b. Is beneficial in acute severe asthma
   c. May cause hoarseness
   d. Is beneficial in allergic conjunctivitis
   e. Is anti-inflammatory

5. Drug hypersensitivity reactions:
   a. May involve more than one hypersensitivity mechanism
   b. May cause renal failure
   c. Should always be treated with systemic steroids
   d. May cause joint pain
   e. Usually occur upon first drug exposure

6. Histamine H_1 antagonists:
   a. Have a major role in the treatment of asthma
   b. Have a major role in the prevention of asthma
   c. Should not be combined with alcohol
   d. Have a major role in the treatment of anaphylaxis
   e. May cause dyskinesia

Case history questions

Case history 1

A 20-year-old non-smoker with severe asthma presents as an emergency. She is given nebulised salbutamol, i.v. hydrocortisone and i.v. ampicillin. Later that night her breathing is no better and she is exhausted and sweaty but cannot sleep because of breathlessness. The doctor gives her temazepam because of her obvious agitation and insomnia.

1. What is likely to happen next and what comments do you have on her management?

Case history 2

A 50-year-old smoker with chronic obstructive pulmonary disease takes salbutamol, ipratropium and aminophylline. He presents to his doctor with an infective exacerbation of his bronchitis; as he is allergic to penicillin the doctor starts erythromycin.

1. What is the potential risk?

Case history 3

A woman takes co-amoxiclav (amoxicillin plus clavulanic acid) for a urinary tract infection. On the third day she feels unwell and shivery and complains of joint pains; subsequently she loses consciousness briefly. In hospital she is found to have a temperature of 38°C and lymph node enlargement. A diagnosis of bacteraemia is made and the co-amoxiclav is continued.

1. What alternative diagnosis should have been considered?

> During the night after admission, she is very unwell and develops a generalised rash plus ulceration of her buccal mucosa.

2. What should be done?

Short note questions

Write short notes on:

1. The modes of action, adverse effects and clinical use of drugs employed in the management of chronic asthma.
2. The emergency management of anaphylaxis and angioedema.

Extended matching items questions

Theme: The management of life-threatening acute asthma

> **Case history part 1.** A 17-year-old non-smoker with asthma presents as an emergency to the A&E department. He is given 35% O_2, nebulised salbutamol and i.v. hydrocortisone. There is initial improvement, but his breathing deteriorates again within the next few hours, and arterial blood is drawn to estimate gases. The salbutamol is repeated.

Options

A. Peak expiratory flow rate of 55% of the expected value

B. Heart rate of 40 beats per minute

C. Arterial partial pressure of CO_2 below the lower end of the reference range

D. Absence of wheeze upon auscultation of the chest

E. Salbutamol can be given continuously during a severe attack

F. It is unwise to give salbutamol more frequently than once every 4 hours in this context

G. It may be necessary to give salbutamol boluses every 15–30 minutes in this context

H. The steroid was given by injection because very breathless patients may have difficulty swallowing oral medication

J. The steroid was given by injection because *pharmacokinetic* factors determine the rate of onset of steroids, and intravenous steroid achieves high drug levels sooner than oral steroid

K. The steroid was given by injection because *pharmacodynamic* factors determine the rate of onset of steroids, and intravenous steroid can be expected to work sooner than oral drug

L. The steroid was given by injection because there is a risk that vomiting might expel the steroid, and this drug can prove to be life-saving

For each of the questions below choose the most appropriate answer or answers from the options above. There may be more than one correct answer. Each option may be used once, more than once, or not at all.

1. List the features which, if present, identify this as a life-threatening episode.
2. How often is it acceptable to use salbutamol by nebuliser?
3. Why do you think he was given steroids as an injection instead of by mouth?

> **Case history part 2.** Despite the repeated doses of salbutamol, the 17-year-old patient continues to worsen and is transferred to the ITU. On arrival in ITU, his gases are: pH 7.01 (normal range 7.35–7.45), PO_2 6.0 kPa (normal range 10–13.3) PCO_2 7.2 kPa ((normal range 4.8–6.1).

Options

A. Intravenous ipratropium

B. Intravenous adrenaline (epinephrine)

C. Intravenous salbutamol

D. Intravenous magnesium sulphate

E. Inhaled magnesium sulphate

F. Nebulised ipratropium

G. Intravenous chorphenamine

H. Intravenous infusion of doxapram

J. Mechanical ventilation

K. Increase inhaled O_2 from 35% to 40%

L. Intravenous aminophylline

For each of the questions below choose the most appropriate answer or answers from the options above. There may be more than one correct answer. Each answer may be used once, more than once, or not at all.

4. What should now be started to try to relieve his bronchospasm?

5. What should be done to try to improve his arterial blood gases?

Self-assessment on Chapter 10: answers

Multiple choice answers

1. a. **False.** The effect is almost immediate.
   b. **True.** Although salbutamol has greater affinity for β_2-adrenoceptors, β_1-adrenoceptors are stimulated, especially at high drug concentration. This may lead to tachycardia.
   c. **False.** Tremor is common but rarely bad enough for drug withdrawal.
   d. **False.** Salbutamol is usually taken when needed for wheeze and dyspnoea.
   e. **True.** Given i.v., salbutamol induces marked vasodilatation (β_2) as well as bronchodilatation. It is not a first choice drug for left ventricular failure but can be useful.

2. a. **False.** It is a muscarinic antagonist.
   b. **True.** This may result from systemically absorbed drug, but it is more likely that part of the aerosol reaches the conjunctiva and is absorbed locally. Antimuscarinics cause the pupil to dilate (mydriasis) and this may occlude entry to the canal of Schlemm; this is only relevant if the patient has closed-angle glaucoma.
   c. **False.** See the management of acute severe asthma at the start of this chapter.
   d. **True.** Like atropine.
   e. **False.** Inhaled steroids do this.

3. a. **False.** Cough is a frequent symptom of asthma and bespeaks the underlying airways inflammation and obstruction. Codeine and the sedating antihistamines could be expected to be harmful in the setting of severe asthma, where sedation can worsen respiratory failure.
   b. **False.** Oxygen concentrations should be high (40%) to try to correct hypoxia; caution is only needed in patients with chronic type II respiratory failure. Blood gases should be measured in all cases of severe respiratory distress to help to resolve this issue.
   c. **False.** Ciprofloxacin (Ch. 13) is an enzyme inhibitor and reduces the clearance of theophylline.
   d. **True.** Glucocorticoids interact with β_2-agonists pharmacodynamically, by upregulating the expression of receptors.
   e. **True.** Their use confers no additional benefit.

4. a. **False.** Chronic bronchitis is secondary to mucosal damage, usually from smoking, and exacerbations are caused by infection.
   b. **False.** Cromoglicate is only of prophylactic value.
   c. **True.**
   d. **True.**
   e. **True.** Though the exact mode of action is unclear.

5. a. **True.** The division into types I, II, III and IV hypersensitivity is convenient, but adverse reactions can involve more than one mechanism.
   b. **True.** Drug allergy may cause renal damage by inducing vasculitis or 'interstitial nephritis'.
   c. **False.** Systemic steroids may be needed for life-threatening disease, but most drug reactions settle quickly upon withdrawal of the drug.
   d. **True.** Arthralgia and arthritis may both be a consequence of types II or III hypersensitivity.
   e. **False.** Previous exposure is usually required.

6. a. **False.**
   b. **False.** Antihistamines are of little use in either setting.
   c. **True.** Antihistamines are sedative.
   d. **True.** After adrenaline (epinephrine) has been given subcutaneously, an antihistamine, such as chlorphenamine, should be given i.v.
   e. **True.** This is not a common adverse reaction but is well documented.

Case history answers

Case history 1

This patient has been badly managed and may die because of the sedative. She was correctly given a β_2-agonist and early systemic steroid. She needs to be closely observed. Antibiotics were not required. Exhaustion and sweating are features of life-threatening disease, and sedatives are absolutely contraindicated.

Case history 2

Erythromycin is an inhibitor of drug-metabolising enzymes and potentiates theophylline: drug levels will rise. Commonly this induces nausea, headache and insomnia; arrhythmias and seizures are less common but more serious.

Case history 3

1. Although this woman did not initially have a rash, hypersensitivity should have been considered – particularly in view of the arthralgia. Her loss of consciousness was probably simple syncope. Continuation of the drug worsened her condition, and it sounds as if she developed a severe skin reaction (like erythema multiforme) during the night.

2. Co-amoxiclav should be stopped, systemic steroids are indicated and specialist help is needed from a dermatologist.

Short note answers

1. a. In very mild asthma, occasional doses of inhaled β_2-agonist may be sufficient.

   b. If this is needed more than once daily, then an anti-inflammatory drug should be given regularly. In adults, inhaled steroid is probably the drug of first choice, but sodium cromoglicate is preferred as the drug of first choice in children.

   c. If asthma is not adequately controlled by low-dose inhaled steroid, then doses should be increased (high-dose aerosols and other delivery systems are available).

   d. Regular oral steroids are reserved for the most severely compromised patient: they will contribute to osteoporosis and other medical problems if they are needed for many years.

   e. Aminophylline (oral) and ipratropium bromide (inhaler) may be needed in addition by some patients to control symptoms.

This question, therefore, calls for the above overview, plus a summary of the clinical pharmacology of inhaled β_2-agonists, ipratropium, inhaled and oral steroids and aminophylline.

2. Describe what you mean by the terms anaphylaxis and angioedema:

   a. the main problem with anaphylaxis is shock (caused by vasodilatation)

   b. angioedema causes acute laryngeal narrowing

   c. the two often co-exist

   d. they are both medical emergencies.

Once you have clarified what you are treating, list the management steps:

   a. if a drug infusion (or blood transfusion) is in progress it should be stopped (it may be the cause of the problem)

   b. adrenaline (epinephrine) should be given i.m. and may be repeated at intervals: this drug may be life-saving

   c. high concentrations of inhaled oxygen are required

   d. the feet should be raised: this may raise the blood pressure by increasing venous return; use your judgement though as this may be difficult to achieve outside hospital and, if the patient arrests, the posture may make CPR difficult

   e. severe cases of laryngeal oedema may call for a tracheostomy.

Extended matching items answers

Theme: The management of life-threatening acute asthma

Case history part 1

1. B and D. Consult the list of features set out on page 138.

2. E and G. The British Thoracic Society guidelines on severe asthma countenance both continuous use of nebulised beta-agonist or repeat bolus doses up to every 15-minutes. It is very likely that both tremor and sinus tachycardia would result. In some patients there is a risk that significant tachyarrhythmias may occur, but the benefits outweigh the risks.

3. H and L. Very breathless patients can struggle to swallow tablets, which may remain in the oesophagus for prolonged periods (especially if inadequate water is taken with the dose) and which may be vomited. Steroids are potentially life-saving, and so the doctor wants to see that they are safely 'in the body' at an early stage. Neither J nor K is correct. Steroids do take many hours to achieve clinical benefit. This is not for pharmacokinetic reasons: the absorption phase after oral dosing is not long, and oral steroids are standard in cases of severe asthma where the patient is well enough to swallow. The slow response is for pharmacodynamic reasons (see Ch. 1), but it is illogical to suppose that the route of drug administration could affect this.

Case history part 2

4. D and F. Nebulised ipratropium is a helpful addition to salbutamol and a single intravenous dose of magnesium sulphate has been shown to have benefit. It is unlikely that intravenous salbutamol would add anything to the frequent use of this drug as nebulised boluses, and adrenaline (epinephrine) is not indicated. The sedating antihistamine chorphenamine is contraindicated: it will worsen his respiratory failure.

5. J. This man needs to be ventilated, and, once stable, his chest radiograph needs repetition to search for pneumothorax or consolidation (a possible feature of bronchial plugging by mucus). The suggested increase in inspired oxygen would be inadequate and respiratory stimulants are not indicated.

Drugs and the gastrointestinal system

11.1	Gastric acid-related conditions	149
11.2	Nausea and vomiting	153
11.3	Disorders of the bowel	155
11.4	Gallstones	156
	Self-assessment on Chapter 11: questions	158
	Self-assessment on Chapter 11: answers	161

Overview

Conditions related to excessive secretion of gastric acid are extremely common, and include peptic ulcer disease, gastro-oesophageal reflux and nonspecific dyspepsia. Acid-suppressing drugs are very important and widely used in treating these conditions. *Helicobacter pylori* is associated with peptic ulcer disease but to only a very limited extent with simple dyspepsia and not at all with reflux oesophagitis. Eradication of *H. pylori* drastically reduces the relapse rate in peptic ulcer disease.

The causes and treatment of nausea and vomiting are considered. Constipation and diarrhoea are very common symptoms and some causes and symptomatic treatment are considered. Irritable bowel syndrome is a cause of both, and antispasmodics are available for treatment. Inflammatory bowel disease is commonly treated with anti-inflammatory drugs, either locally or systemically.

11.1 Gastric acid-related conditions

Learning objectives

At the end of this section you should:
- be able to explain the control of acid secretion in the stomach
- be able to explain how drugs can affect acid secretion and the types of drug used, giving examples
- know the role of *Helicobacter pylori* in acid-related diseases
- be able to describe the regimens used for *H. pylori* eradication.

Clinical sketch

A 28-year-old man goes to his GP complaining of pain in his epigastrium. The pain occurs whenever he eats spicy foods, but also at other times and, in particular, wakes him up at night.

Comment: as many as one in ten of all GP consultations are for dyspepsia; this is a condition of epigastric pain and it is often difficult to work out from the history what the exact cause is. Causes include peptic ulcer disease, simple dyspepsia, irritable bowel syndrome or more serious pathologies such as gastric cancer. Reflux oesophagitis tends to have a more characteristic history. In at least half of all cases of dyspepsia there is no clear pathological cause. Treatment policies include early endoscopy for all patients, Helicobacter pylori *screening to identify patients for endoscopy or specific treatment, or simple empirical treatment. In a young man presenting for the first time like this, simple empirical treatment is probably reasonable management in the first instance.*

Control of gastric acid secretion

Gastric acid serves many purposes, including providing an optimal environment of proteolytic enzymes to work and enhancing the sterility of stomach contents. It is controlled by CNS and local endocrine effects.

Acid secretion is increased by:

- the vagus nerve secreting acetylcholine
- local nerve endings secreting histamine, which acts on histamine type II receptors
- gastrin secreted by the antrum of the stomach.

Acid secretion is decreased by:

- prostaglandin receptors on the luminal surface of the cell.

All of these mechanisms act ultimately via the 'proton pump' (Fig. 40). Gastrin provides a negative feedback system: an acid environment in the stomach decreases gastrin output, shutting down acid

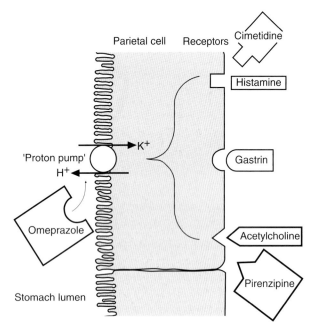

Fig. 40 The pharmacology of acid secretion.

secretion, while an alkaline environment (e.g. after eating) stimulates acid secretion.

Drugs and gastric acid

Drugs may:

* buffer acid secretion: antacids
* decrease acid secretion by
  — blocking acetylcholine receptors
  — blocking histamine H_2 receptors
  — stimulating prostaglandin receptors
  — blocking the final common pathway of all of these mechanisms, i.e. the proton pump.

The principal pathological conditions in which it is useful to reduce acid secretion are:

* simple dyspepsia
* peptic ulcers
* gastro-oesophageal reflux
* Zollinger–Ellison syndrome (a rare gastrin secreting tumour causing very high acid secretion and severe ulceration).

Peptic ulcers

In peptic ulcers, the balance between protective elements (mucus secretion, gastric blood flow) and harmful elements (acid, exotoxins, drugs) is deranged.

Duodenal ulcers

These are associated with:

* high acid output
* usually (95%+) *Helicobacter pylori* infection
* no risk of malignancy.

Duodenal ulcers can be cured by acid suppressant therapy alone but have a very high relapse rate (90% at 12 months); this can be reduced by eradication of *H. pylori* (see below).

Gastric ulcers

These:

* often have low–normal acid output
* are related to *H. pylori* infection in 60–70% of cases
* carry a risk of malignancy
* can be related in some cases to use of non-steroidal anti-inflammatory drugs (NSAIDs; see Ch. 9).

Complications of peptic ulcers

* pain
* anaemia
* severe bleeding
* perforation
* pyloric stenosis (caused by the fibrosis that follows the acute inflammatory process).

Helicobacter pylori and peptic ulcer

H. pylori is spread by the faeco-oral route. It is highly prevalent and is associated with 95%+ of duodenal ulcers and 70% of gastric ulcers. It is less clearly associated with nonspecific dyspepsia and not with gastro-oesophageal reflux disease.

H. pylori colonises the antrum of the stomach, where it protects itself by secreting urease. This breaks down urea to ammonia and creates an alkaline microenvironment. Because it interferes with the normal control of acid secretion, acid output increases (Fig. 41). *H. pylori* also secretes exotoxins, directly damaging the mucosa.

Successful eradication of *H. pylori* heals duodenal ulcers and is associated with a very low relapse rate.

Regimens for *H. pylori* eradication

The usual treatment is with a proton pump inhibitor and two antibiotics. Bismuth-based regimens are possibly slightly superior in effectiveness but they are less convenient and less well tolerated; consequently they usually form second line use only.

Proton pump inhibitor regimen. This usually comprises high-dose omeprazole and two antibiotics (any two of clarithromycin, amoxicillin and metronidazole) for 1 week. Clarithromycin regimens are probably slightly more effective.

Bismuth-based regimen. This is usually *chelated bismuth* and two antibiotics (*metronidazole* or *tinidazole*, and either *amoxicillin* or *tetracycline*, all in high doses), usually for 2 weeks.

Normal

HCl↑ − ve
Gastrin

Rise in gastrin stimulates HCl secretion, which in turn shuts down gastrin production

---

Clinical sketch

A 45-year-old woman had peptic ulcer disease diagnosed 2 years ago. She was treated with ranitidine for 12 months, which settled her symptoms, but now they have recurred.

Comment: peptic ulcer disease is most commonly caused by Helicobacter pylori. *Simple acid suppression will allow the ulcer to heal but does not remove the underlying cause and relapse is likely, as in this patient.*

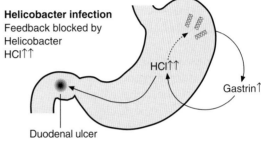

Helicobacter infection
Feedback blocked by Helicobacter
HCl↑↑

HCl↑↑
Gastrin↑

Duodenal ulcer

Fig. 41 *Helicobacter pylori* in peptic ulcer disease.

Clinical sketch

A 50-year-old man has peptic ulcer disease diagnosed as related to *Helicobacter pylori*. He is given an eradication course of treatment and his symptoms settle. However, a year later his symptoms recur and retesting shows the presence of *H. pylori*.

Comment: re-infection with H. pylori *occurs at the rate of about 1% per year. The alternative explanation in this patient is that eradication therapy was unsuccessful, either because the patient had resistant* H. pylori *or (as is frequently the case) the patient was not compliant with the full course of therapy to eradicate the infection.*

NSAIDs and peptic ulcers

NSAIDs (see Ch. 9) may cause peptic ulcer (especially gastric) by decreasing local prostaglandin secretion in the gastric mucosa and hence reducing mucosal blood flow, mucus secretion and other protective factors. This may occur regardless of the route of administration of the NSAID. Many NSAIDs may also have a direct irritant effect on the gastric mucosa. NSAIDs are a relatively common cause of gastrointestinal bleeding because of these effects.

Appropriate treatment is withdrawal of the NSAID if possible; if necessary, antisecretory drugs (see below) or the prostaglandin analogue *misoprostol* may be used.

Clinical sketch

A 72-year-old woman taking diclofenac for her arthritis presents to hospital with haematemesis (vomiting blood).

Comment: irritant drugs such as non-steroidal anti-inflammatory drugs (NSAIDs) can also cause peptic ulcer disease or can cause a flare up in existing peptic ulcer disease. These gastrointestinal complications are among the most serious for NSAIDs. They may occur without any prior warning of dyspepsia and present with a serious complication, as in this case. This patient needs to have her NSAID withdrawn and needs an urgent endoscopy. She may also require blood transfusion or even surgery if the bleeding fails to stop spontaneously. She should avoid NSAIDs in the future, probably including Cox-2 selective drugs. Many patients receive acid-suppressant drugs such as proton pump inhibitors with their NSAIDs because they are considered to be at risk of such complications. A better approach, however, would be careful selection of those patients who receive NSAIDs, which are commonly overused.

Gastro-oesophageal reflux

Gastric contents regurgitate into the oesophagus in some patients with an incompetent gastro-oesophageal sphincter, causing heartburn or severe pain. In severe cases, complications such as erosions, bleeding and stricture may occur. Management involves general measures (weight loss if obese, avoiding tight clothes around the waist, avoiding stooping, elevating the head of the bed to reduce nocturnal reflux) and, often, drug therapy.

Therapy includes:

- antacids: particularly antacids combined with alginate, which coats the oesophagus and reduces the contact with acid
- antisecretory drugs: proton pump inhibitors are usually highly effective in severe cases. Long-term use may be necessary in some patients. Histamine H_2 blockers are effective in less severe cases
- prokinetic drugs. *Metoclopramide* and *domperidone* are discussed under antiemetics (see below) but both increase lower oesophageal sphincter pressure and increase gastric clearance, in addition to their central effects.

Acid-modifying drugs

Antacids

Antacids are weak alkalis used for symptomatic relief. They:

- neutralise the acid secreted by the parietal cells
- are generally not absorbed and so cause no systemic effects
- may also reduce the absorption of other drugs, e.g. tetracyclines or digoxin.

Examples

Aluminium hydroxide (tends to cause constipation) *or magnesium trisilicate* (diarrhoea). *Sodium bicarbonate* is sometimes taken as a popular home remedy for dyspepsia. It is not recommended because it is absorbed and if used in large amounts can cause systemic alkalosis.

Histamine receptor antagonists

These drugs act by antagonising histamine at H_2 receptors. They:

- decrease acid secretion, especially at night and during fasting
- heal almost all duodenal ulcers after 4–8 weeks: gastric ulcers heal more slowly and may require higher doses for longer. There is a high relapse rate unless *H. pylori* is treated also
- are also effective in reflux oesophagitis, but here high-dose long-term therapy is often necessary
- relieve symptoms in many patients who have dyspepsia without any clear organic lesion.

Many patients take H_2 receptor antagonists indefinitely, or in repeated courses.

Clinical sketch

A 47-year-old woman has severe reflux oesophagitis confirmed on endoscopy. Initial treatment with ranitidine is partly successful, but she continues to have a lot of pain.

Comment: in severe cases of reflux oesophagitis, proton pump inhibitors are more effective. In general, proton pump inhibitors decrease acid secretion to a greater extent than histamine H_2-blockers, even in a high dose. Such intense acid suppression is not always necessary in acid-related conditions.

Examples

Cimetidine and *ranitidine* are both well absorbed after oral administration, but both can also be given i.v. They are excreted unchanged by the kidney.

Adverse effects

Cimetidine has weak antiandrogen effects and occasionally causes gynaecomastia in long-term use. This is less common with ranitidine. Either may cause confusion and drowsiness in the elderly.

Interactions

Cimetidine inhibits drug-metabolising enzymes in the liver and may increase the effects and toxicity of many drugs (see Ch. 21).

Proton pump inhibitors

The H^+/K^+-ATPase enzyme ('proton pump') is irreversibly inhibited by these drugs, and so acid production ceases. Acid secretion can only resume when new enzyme has been formed. They:

- are the most effective acid suppressants: heal acid-related diseases faster and to a greater extent than other drugs
- have a high relapse rate in peptic ulcers unless *H. pylori* is eradicated
- form long-term therapy in reflux oesophagitis commonly
- are used, in high doses, to treat Zollinger–Ellison syndrome.

Examples

Omeprazole is metabolised by the liver. Because of the irreversible inhibition of the proton pump, its duration of action is considerably longer than its half-life and omeprazole is usually administered once per day. *Lansoprazole* is similar. *Esomeprazole* is a stereo-isomer of omeprazole and is used for intermittent treatment of gastro-oesophagal reflux disease.

Adverse effects

- headache
- nausea, vomiting and diarrhoea.

Interactions

Omeprazole can inhibit some hepatic drug-metabolising enzymes.

Prostaglandin E$_1$ analogues: misoprostol

Prostaglandin E$_1$ decreases acid secretion by an action on a receptor on the surface of the parietal cell. It may have an effect in protecting the mucosa of the stomach, perhaps by increasing mucosal blood flow and mucus and duodenal bicarbonate secretion.

Example

Misoprostol is an analogue of prostaglandin E$_1$ with a half-life of 2 hours. It is well absorbed and is metabolised to active metabolites. While misoprostol can heal peptic ulcers, H$_2$-blockers or proton pump inhibitors are better and easier to take. Misoprostol is also used in the induction of abortion as it causes uterine contractions.

Contraindication

In pregnant women, it may cause miscarriages.

Adverse effects

- crampy abdominal pains
- diarrhoea.

Prophylaxis in patients taking NSAIDs (see Ch. 9)

Prophylactic therapy may be advisable in patients at high risk (e.g. those who require a NSAID despite a previous history of peptic ulcer disease); its routine use in all patients taking NSAIDs is not justified. Misoprostol may have a role in the treatment and prophylaxis of ulcers caused by NSAIDs. However, proton pump inhibitors are more pleasant to take and more widely used as prophylaxis than misoprostol.

Drugs with no effect on acid secretion

These drugs are believed to enhance the protective elements by forming a protective coating over the ulcer crater and allowing healing to occur under-neath. They may also have a separate action in stimulating local prostaglandin release. They are not used often today.

Chelated bismuth

This has some activity against *H. pylori* infection and also protects the ulcer crater and allows healing.

It is given orally and a small quantity is absorbed; this is later excreted through the kidney.

Adverse effects

- metallic taste
- blackening of faeces
- encephalopathy, if used in high doses for prolonged periods; bismuth should not be used repeatedly or for more than 2 months at a time.

Sucralfate

Sucralfate is an aluminum salt of sucrose. It heals peptic ulcers as effectively as histamine H$_2$-blockers but is less convenient.

It causes constipation.

Carbenoxolone

Carbenoxolone is a derivative of licorice. It stimulates gastric mucus secretion as well as protecting the ulcer. It is also used in treatment for reflux oesophagitis.

Adverse effects

Carbenoxolone has mineralocorticoid effects and may cause sodium retention and hypokalaemia; this could be serious in patients with cardiac failure.

11.2 Nausea and vomiting

Learning objectives

At the end of this section you should:
- understand the mechanisms that may case nausea and vomiting
- be able to describe the drugs that can be used to prevent or treat nausea and vomiting.

Clinical sketch

A patient with migraine is unable to take simple analgesics because of the associated nausea and vomiting from the migraine.

Comment: combined use of analgesic and a simple antiemetic such as metoclopramide is appropriate. This also has effects overcoming the gastric stasis common in migraine treated with an analgesic.

Nausea and vomiting are common nonspecific features of disease or drug toxicity and the cause should be diagnosed and treated where possible. Drugs to treat nausea and vomiting may be given orally or parenterally (i.m. or i.v.).

Vomiting is caused by activation of the vomiting centre in the brainstem, mainly via the vagus nerve. The vomiting centre is also influenced by the vestibular apparatus, by the cerebral cortex, by afferents from the gastrointestinal tract and by the chemoreceptor trigger zone, through muscarinic and histamine (H_1) receptors. The chemoreceptor trigger zone is another region of the brainstem and is activated by afferents (often D_2 dopaminergic) similar to those of the vomiting centre. In addition it is activated by toxins, including drugs.

Antiemetics

Antiemetics may act in several different ways (Fig. 42).

Anticholinergic drugs. These act on the vomiting centre especially but also affect the gastrointestinal tract directly, for example *hyoscine*. Adverse effects are typical of anticholinergic drugs and include dry mouth, occasionally confusion and agitation.

Antihistamines. These act on H_1 receptors in the vomiting centre and also have weak anticholinergic and sedating effects. Newer non-sedating antihistamines are not effective. The antihistamines are frequently used to treat motion sickness or vestibular disease (often inappropriately in the elderly). Example: *promethazine*.

Phenothiazines. In addition to anticholinergic, sedative and H_1-blocking effects, the phenothiazines also block dopamine receptors in the chemoreceptor trigger zone. Example: *prochlorperazine*.

Adverse effects include parkinsonism (see Ch. 6 for fuller description).

Dopamine receptor antagonists. Metoclopramide acts in the chemoreceptor trigger zone and has direct effects on the gastrointestinal tract (see above). It is given orally or parenterally for most causes of vomiting, although it is not effective for motion sickness.

Adverse effects include acute extrapyramidal reactions, such as oculogyric crisis, especially in children or young women (treat with parenteral anticholinergic such as benzatropine). Increased prolactin concentrations and gynaecomastia can occur in prolonged use.

Domperidone is similar to metoclopramide but is less likely to cause extrapyramidal reactions; it can, however, cause cardiac arrhythmias when given parenterally in high dose.

5-Hydroxytryptamine (5-HT) antagonists. Ondansetron is one of several 5-HT$_3$ antagonists, which are very effective in treating severe nausea and vomiting, particularly after anticancer chemotherapy but also postoperatively. They are often reserved for cases where other drugs are ineffective.

Adverse effects include constipation and headache.

Other drugs

Aprepitant is a neurokinin receptor antagonist and *nabilone* is a cannabinoid, both used orally to treat nausea and vomiting associated with chemotherapy which does not respond to other drugs.

Choice of drug

- Postoperatively: phenothiazines, metoclopramide or a 5-HT antagonist are used.
- Pregnancy: drugs should be avoided in pregnancy as much as possible. Simple rehydration (perhaps intravenously) is enough in many cases. If drugs are necessary, the antihistamine promethazine is usually recommended.
- After chemotherapy: in regimens which are highly likely to cause vomiting, 5-HT antagonists are usually recommended. In regimens less prone to cause vomiting, metoclopramide or domperidone may be used. Consider dexamethasone and lorazepam which are also used to treat nausea with some chemotherapeutic regimens.

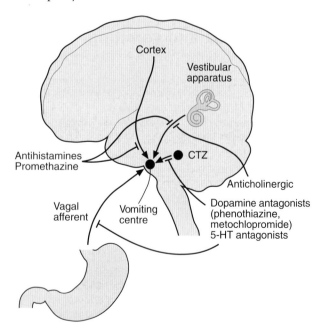

Fig. 42 Central actions of antiemetics.

- After opiates: a phenothiazine may be used.
- Motion sickness: hyoscine is best but phenothiazines or antihistamines (with some anticholinergic action) are also useful.

11.3 Disorders of the bowel

Learning objectives

At the end of this section you should:
- be aware that disorders of the bowel are common, often resolve without treatment and can be secondary to drug therapy and inflammatory conditions as well as infections
- know the main treatment possibilities and when to use them.

Disturbances of bowel habit are common and often resolve spontaneously without treatment. The cause should be identified if possible and treated as necessary. Bowel disturbance may be an adverse effect of many drugs (e.g. opiates and tricyclics can cause constipation, antibiotics can cause diarrhoea).

Treatment of constipation

Constipation can often be treated effectively with dietary modification, with increased fibre and fluids; and with careful education of the patient. Only if this fails should laxatives be used, adjusting the dose to achieve the desired effect (Fig. 43). In order of preference:

1. the bulking agents
2. osmotic laxatives
3. stimulant drugs (reserved for intermittent use)
4. the faecal softeners (used less often).

Bulking agents

Bulking agents absorb water, swell and increase the bulk of the stool. This increased bulk stimulates normal peristalsis and hence defaecation. They may take a few days to act fully and may cause flatulence and crampy abdominal pain at first. They are given orally.
Examples: *bran, ispaghula.*

Osmotic laxatives

The osmotic laxatives reduce absorption of water from the bowel. This softens the stool and increases its bulk, stimulating peristalsis.
Lactulose is a disaccharide that is broken down by colonic bacteria to acetic and lactic acid, which cause

Fig. 43 Laxatives.

the osmotic effects. Polyethylene glycols are non-absorbed inert compounds. Both are taken orally. Adverse effects include abdominal pain and flatulence. *Phosphate* or *magnesium* salts are used as enemas.

Stimulants

Stimulants are drugs used to stimulate peristalsis and are indicated for severe chronic constipation or where a more rapid effect (within 6–8 hours) is required. They may cause atony of the bowel if used chronically, creating a vicious cycle of laxative use/constipation/laxative use for the patient. Stimulants are usually given orally.
Examples: *senna, bisacodyl, castor oil.*

Faecal softeners

The faecal softeners lubricate and soften the stool and are usually given orally.
Examples: *liquid paraffin.* (There is a risk of aspiration lipoid pneumonia with liquid paraffin.)

Treatment of diarrhoea

Clinical sketch

A 22-month-old child develops profuse diarrhoea. The GP tells the mother that this is infective gastroenteritis. The mother asks the GP for an antidiarrhoeal agent and an antibiotic.

Comment: the priority in treating a child with diarrhoea is maintaining hydration of the child; oral rehydration therapy (dilute solutions of essential salts) is the correct therapy, but intravenous fluid administration in hospital may be necessary. Children die from dehydration in infective gastroenteritis. The use of antibiotics or antidiarrhoeal agents is entirely inappropriate in this setting.

Eleven

In treating diarrhoea, especially in children, it is vitally important to replace fluid and electrolyte losses. Since most cases of diarrhoea are self-limiting, this is often all that is necessary, and the use of specific antidiarrhoeal drugs is often inappropriate.

Antimotility drugs

Antimotility drugs reduce peristalsis by stimulating opioid receptors in the bowel. An adverse effect is constipation.

Examples: *loperamide, diphenoxylate* are pethidine derivatives that act only in the bowel. Diphenoxylate is often combined with atropine. *Codeine phosphate* and *morphine* (Ch. 7) are also occasionally used.

Adsorbents

Some drugs absorb water without increasing stool bulk, so making the stool firmer and smaller, for example *kaolin*.

Irritable bowel syndrome

Irritable bowel syndrome is common (30% of women, 15% of men) and is caused by dysmotility of the bowel. It overlaps in some cases with simple dyspepsia. Many new drugs are currently in development for this potentially large market.

Symptoms include intermittent diarrhoea and constipation, and abdominal pain.

Drug treatment is currently symptomatic, i.e. treat pain, constipation or diarrhoea as required.

Antispasmodics

Anticholinergic drugs decrease bowel motility by reducing peristalsis and are used orally to treat painful spasm of the large bowel.

Examples: *mebeverine*, which has little systemic anticholinergic effect; *propantheline*, which has more systemic effects and which is also used parenterally to relieve severe pain associated with spasm, e.g. in biliary colic.

Inflammatory bowel diseases

The cause of the chronic inflammatory diseases is not known. Ulcerative colitis affects the large bowel; Crohn's disease affects mainly the small bowel but also the large bowel and other parts of the gastrointestinal tract. Both diseases typically undergo exacerbations and remissions.

The aim of treatment is to resolve the acute episodes and prolong remissions. In addition to drug therapy, treatment involves correction of any nutritional deficiencies (enteral feeding may be effective in Crohn's) and sometimes surgery for complications or severe uncontrolled disease.

Anti-inflammatory drugs

Drug treatment is with anti-inflammatory drugs, especially the corticosteroids, which are used systemically in severe acute attacks (e.g. *prednisolone* or *hydrocortisone*) (see Ch. 12). They may also be given locally by means of enemas for less severe acute attacks involving the large bowel, or as maintenance therapy. Other anti-inflammatories such as *azathioprine* or *ciclosporin* (see Ch. 9) are also occasionally used.

Infliximab is a monoclonal antibody which inhibits the actions of the inflammatory cytokine tumour necrosis factor (TNF) α. It is used in refractory Crohn's disease. It is also used in rheumatoid arthritis.

Aminosalicylates

5-Aminosalicylate (5-ASA) is the active drug, effective in treatment and maintenance of colonic disease in ulcerative colitis or Crohn's disease.

Sulfasalazine is a complex of a sulphonamide, *sulfapyridine*, and 5-ASA. The complex is taken orally or rectally and is broken down by bacteria in the large bowel to release the 5-ASA. It is also used as a disease-modifying drug in rheumatoid arthritis (see Ch. 9).

Mesalazine is another name for 5-ASA and can be given orally or rectally as an enema.

Olsalazine is two molecules of 5-ASA combined, given orally.

Adverse effects

Adverse effects are mainly because of the sulfapyridine content: headache, nausea and vomiting, rashes and occasionally blood dyscrasias and renal dysfunction. Infertility in males can occur because of decreased sperm count.

Adverse effects of 5-ASA: diarrhoea, occasionally blood disorders (patients should be advised to report any purpura, unexplained bruising or sore throat or fever and a full blood count should then be done).

11.4 Gallstones

In the developed world, gallstones are usually made of cholesterol.

Bile acids

Bile acids may be used to gradually dissolve cholesterol gallstones. This is only suitable for small stones, as 3–6 months of treatment is required. Recurrence is common. Bile acid treatment for gallstones is generally reserved for patients who are unfit for surgery. Diarrhoea is an adverse effect.

Examples: *chenodeoxycholic acid, ursodeoxycholic acid*.

Self-assessment on Chapter 11: questions

Multiple choice questions

1. In duodenal ulcers:
   a. *H. pylori* is present in almost all cases
   b. Relapse after treatment with omeprazole is rare
   c. *H. pylori* secretes a urease enzyme
   d. Basal acid secretion is increased
   e. Attempts to eradicate *H. pylori* are rarely successful

2. In conditions where gastric acid secretion causes symptoms:
   a. Antacids are mainly used for symptomatic relief
   b. H_2 receptor antagonists block all acid secretion
   c. Ranitidine may commonly cause drug interactions
   d. The final common pathway of all stimuli to acid secretion is the proton pump
   e. Omeprazole is very effective in reflux oesophagitis

3. In treating peptic ulcer disease:
   a. Misoprostol is used to treat the gastrointestinal adverse effects of NSAIDs
   b. All patients taking NSAIDs should also take misoprostol
   c. Chelated bismuth can be used
   d. Long-term bismuth is used to maintain remission in peptic ulcer disease
   e. Sucralfate may cause diarrhoea

4. In the treatment of gastric motility disorders:
   a. Metoclopramide may enhance drug absorption
   b. Metoclopramide may cause severe dystonic reactions
   c. Hyperprolactinaemia may be a result of taking antidopaminergic drugs
   d. Domperidone increases large bowel motility
   e. Bisacodyl inhibits peristalsis.

5. Drugs used to treat nausea include:
   a. Ondansetron
   b. Prochlorperazine
   c. Bromocriptine
   d. Atropine
   e. Dexamethasone

6. Bowel disturbance may arise as a result of treatment with:
   a. Disopyramide
   b. Omeprazole
   c. Erythromycin
   d. Iron salts
   e. Morphine

7. In treating disturbances of bowel motility:
   a. Rehydration is more important than using antidiarrhoeal drugs
   b. Sulfasalazine is used to treat irritable bowel syndrome
   c. Lactulose is most effective for treating morphine-induced constipation
   d. In treating constipation, improving diet is often more important than drug therapy
   e. Overdose of diphenoxylate may be treated with naloxone

8. In treating inflammatory bowel disease:
   a. Corticosteroids are the main anti-inflammatory drugs used to treat acute ulcerative colitis
   b. Steroids are always used topically in inflammatory bowel disease
   c. 5-ASA may cause male infertility
   d. Patients may need to have their full blood count monitored
   e. Infliximab is given orally or rectally

Case history questions

Case history 1

A 30 year old patient complains of upper abdominal pain and is treated by his GP with omeprazole for a month. The pain recurs after the omeprazole is stopped and the patient is sent for a gastroscopy. This shows a duodenal ulcer. Antral biopsies show *Helicobacter pylori*.

1. Should this patient have received treatment to eradicate *H. pylori* on first presentation?

2. What treatment should be given to eradicate *H. pylori*?

3. What treatment might be given to heal the peptic ulcer?

4. If therapy to eradicate *H. pylori* is not given, what are the risks of recurrence?

5. Does the patient need a further endoscopy to check if the ulcer has in fact healed?

6. The patient later develops osteoarthritis of the knee; should he be given a non-steroidal anti-inflammatory drug (NSAID)?

Case history 2

A patient has gastro-oesophageal reflux proven on endoscopy.

1. Apart from non-pharmacological treatments, what drugs might be considered?

2. How might metoclopramide be helpful?

3. What drugs might aggravate this condition?

4. How should severe cases be treated?

5. What are the adverse effects of omeprazole?

Case history 3

An elderly patient resident in a nursing home is constipated, i.e. no bowel motion passed for 5 days.

1. What drugs might cause constipation?

2. What other causative factors should be considered in this patient's constipation?

3. If dietary treatment is unsuccessful in this patient, what drug treatment should be considered?

4. What are the harmful effects of long-term use of senna or other stimulant laxatives?

5. What drug therapies might be useful in acute severe constipation?

Short note questions

Write short notes on:

1. Treatment of *Helicobacter pylori* infection

2. Acid-suppressant drugs

3. Drugs in the treatment of reflux oesophagitis.

Extended matching items questions

Theme: Upper gastrointestinal disorders

Options

A. Omeprazole

B. Cimetidine

C. Clarithromycin

D. Ranitidine

E. Metronidazole

F. Lansoprazole

G. Metoclopramide

H. Erythromycin

I. Loratadine

For each of 1–6 below, choose the most appropriate option from the list above. Each option may be used once, more than once, or not at all.

1. Select three drugs that might be used together in the eradication of *Helicobacter pylori*.

2. Select a drug to treat postoperative vomiting.

3. Select a drug that binds to histamine H_2 receptors.

4. Select a drug that increases gastric motility.

5. Which drugs might cause drug interactions by liver enzyme inhibition?

6. Which drug or drugs might be used to treat or prevent NSAID-induced ulceration?

Theme: Lower gastrointestinal disorders

Options

A. Diphenoxylate

B. Lactulose

C. 5-ASA

D. Infliximab

E. Mebeverine

F. Bisacodyl

G. Metoclopramide

For each of the questions below, choose the most appropriate options from the list above. Each option may be used once, more than once, or not at all.

1. Which drug or drugs would be best to treat opiate-induced constipation?

2. Which drug or drugs might cause diarrhoea?

3. Which drug or drugs might be used to treat Crohn's disease?

4. Which drug is most likely to be fatal in overdose (e.g. in children)?

5. Which drug or drugs can be used in irritable bowel syndrome?

Self-assessment on Chapter 11: answers

Multiple choice answers

1. a. **True.** Its association with gastric ulcers is less certain.
   b. **False.** Relapse is frequent since the cause of the peptic ulcer, the *H. pylori* infection, persists.
   c. **True.** This is how it protects itself from stomach acid.
   d. **True.** As a result of blockage of negative feedback on gastrin.
   e. **False.** Triple therapy with proton pump inhibitors, bismuth and antibiotics is successful in about 90% of cases, if the patent is compliant with therapy.

2. a. **True.** Very high but unpalatable doses can be used to heal ulcers also.
   b. **False.** Acid production is reduced by about 70–80%.
   c. **False.** Cimetidine, however, does, because of its effects on liver enzymes.
   d. **True.** Hence omeprazole is the most effective of all antisecretory drugs.
   e. **True.** Again, omeprazole is the most effective treatment.

3. a. **True.** By replacing the decreased mucosal prostaglandins.
   b. **False.** It is unnecessary in many patients, has adverse effects of its own and adds considerably to the costs.
   c. **True.** Less widely used today because it is less pleasant than alternatives and because we now know of the importance of treating *H. pylori*.
   d. **False.** There would be a serious risk of bismuth encephalopathy.
   e. **False.** Sucralfate tends to cause constipation.

4. a. **True.** For instance, used with paracetamol in patients with migraine.
   b. **True.** Especially in children or young women.
   c. **True.** Because dopamine inhibits prolactin release from the pituitary.

d. **False.** Domperidone may stimulate upper gastrointestinal motility, but not lower.
   e. **False.** Bisacodyl stimulates peristalsis and is used in the management of constipation.

5. a. **True.** A 5-HT$_3$ antagonist.
   b. **True.** Widely and perhaps excessively used.
   c. **False.** Bromocriptine is a dopamine agonist, and its adverse effects include nausea.
   d. **False.** Although the anticholinergic hyoscine is used.
   e. **True.** Especially after anticancer chemotherapy.

6. a. **True.** Anticholinergic, so may cause constipation.
   b. **True.** Diarrhoea.
   c. **True.** Diarrhoea (one of its most frequent effects), and so may many other antibiotics.
   d. **True.** Constipation.
   e. **True.** Constipation.

7. a. **True.** Often forgotten.
   b. **False.** Sulfasalazine is used to treat inflammatory bowel disease of the colon.
   c. **False.** A stimulant laxative is usually needed.
   d. **True.** Very important and often forgotten. High fibre diets and improving fluid intake can be very effective.
   e. **True.** Diphenoxylate is an opioid.

8. a. **True.** Either systemically or topically depending on the severity of the illness.
   b. **False.** Topical use will limit adverse effects and is desirable wherever possible but systemic steroids will need to be used in many cases.
   c. **False.** This is an adverse effect of sulfapyridine, part of sulfasalazine.
   d. **True.** For several reasons: firstly because the disease itself may cause bleeding or in the case of Crohn's nutritional problems, but also because many of the drugs used (e.g. 5-ASA or more powerful immunosuppressants) may affect the blood.

e. **False.** Infliximab is a monoclonal antibody, or protein; it will be digested if given orally. It is not absorbed across mucous membranes.

Case history answers

Case history 1

1. In general, current opinion is that he should not. The link between *H. pylori* and simple dyspepsia is not strong and anti-*H. pylori* treatment will benefit relatively few patients while causing adverse effects in some. There is an argument for endoscoping all patients with dyspepsia early to make a definitive diagnosis, especially in older patients (over 55) where the possibility of finding serious pathology is increased. However, in a young person like this, symptomatic treatment in the first instance is reasonable. However, once he is known to have a duodenal ulcer, more specific treatment is certainly warranted.

2. Triple therapy with omeprazole or other proton pump inhibitor, metronidazole, and amoxicillin or clarithromycin is the standard therapy at present: many other, perhaps more acceptable, regimens are also suitable.

3. The ulcer will heal if *H. pylori* is eradicated but more slowly. Giving a longer course of a proton pump inhibitor beyond the usual *H. pylori* course will speed healing up.

4. The recurrence rate at 1 year is 80–90%.

5. This is not usually necessary. Many would do a noninvasive hydrogen breath test to confirm eradication of the *H. pylori* and if not eradicated first time, treat again with an alternative regimen.

6. NSAIDs should be avoided wherever possible in patients with peptic ulcer disease, even if healed. Patients with osteoarthritis often need only analgesia and not an anti-inflammatory, so paracetamol used regularly might be sufficient. If the patient had a true inflammatory arthropathy, a Cox-2 selective NSAID or a standard NSAID might be necessary and prophylactic therapy with misoprostol or omeprazole should be considered.

Case history 2

1. Drug treatment would normally be an antacid with alginate, drugs to suppress acid secretion, or occasionally prokinetic agents – or combinations of these.

2. Metoclopramide increases the tone of the lower oesophageal sphincter and increases gastric emptying.

3. Drugs with an anticholinergic adverse effect decrease lower oesophageal tone, as do smooth muscle relaxants (e.g. calcium-channel blockers).

4. The drug of choice in severe cases is omeprazole, which is exceedingly effective and may be needed for long-term maintenance in some patients.

5. Omeprazole may cause headache, diarrhoea and drug interactions.

Case history 3

1. Drugs with anticholinergic adverse effects, such as tricyclic anticonvulsants or phenothiazines, also opiate analgesics.

2. Hypothyroidism and depression should be excluded. Other factors include poor diet (deficient in fibre), immobility and dehydration.

3. The first line of drug treatment is usually supplementation of fibre intake, either by diet or by use of a bulking agent, followed by an osmotic laxative and finally intermittent use of a stimulant laxative.

4. Atony of the bowel and laxative dependency.

5. Local treatment with suppositories (e.g. glycerin or bisacodyl) or by enema (e.g. phosphate enema) may be useful in acute severe cases: serious pathology, e.g. intestinal obstruction, should be excluded first.

Short note answers

1. This should mention regimens including 2 weeks with a proton pump inhibitor with two antibiotics. Reserve schemes should include mention of bismuth-based preparations in combination with antibiotics.

2. This should discuss histamine H_2-blockers, proton pump inhibitors and, for the very perceptive student, anticholinergics, although these are no longer used therapeutically.

3. This might describe antacids with alginates, histamine H_2-blockers and proton pump inhibitors (PPIs). Description of the drugs alone would not suffice here; a student would

also be expected to show an awareness of how the drugs are used, and which are the most effective approaches, etc. An alternative would be a step-up approach – using antacids, H_2-blockers if not resolved, and then PPIs if still not resolved – or a step-down approach – using high-dose PPIs to heal inflammation and then settling down to a maintenance dose, possibly given intermittently in mild cases. Both regimens have their advocates. In severely affected patients, PPIs are by far the most effective.

Extended matching items answers

Theme: Upper gastrointestinal disorders

1. A, C, E or F, C, and E. These are standard regimens, a proton pump inhibitor with two antibiotics, for 2 weeks.

2. G. Metoclopramide is a standard antiemetic.

3. B or D. (Loratadine binds to histamine H_1 receptors; see Ch. 10 on hypersensitivity.)

4. G or H (surprisingly). Metoclopramide increases gastric motility. So too does erythromycin, which seems to act at specific receptors. This is partly the basis of its common adverse effects. It is used as a gastric stimulant occasionally, for instance in patients with severe gastric stasis secondary to diabetic autonomic neuropathy.

5. A and B (and H). Omeprazole and cimetidine inhibit the metabolism of drugs such as warfarin and phenytoin, among others.

6. A or F would be best. B and D could be used but are less effective.

Theme: Lower gastrointestinal disorders

1. F. A stimulant laxative would be most useful.

2. B or F. This may seem incredibly obvious but is often overlooked.

3. C or D. C is used to treat mild Crohn's of the colon, just as it is in ulcerative colitis. D is used in refractory disease, especially where there are fistulas that fail to heal.

4. A. It is an opiate. A propriety preparation containing diphenoxylate and atropine is available over the counter and might be misused to treat diarrhoea in children – this is a problem for two reasons: first the proper treatment for diarrhoea in children is usually rehydration; second, the combination can be very dangerous in overdose in children.

5. A, B, E, D. The choice depends on what symptoms are the most prominent in individual patients: pain, diarrhoea or constipation.

Drugs for endocrine and metabolic disorders

Chapter 12

12.1 Diabetes mellitus	**165**
12.2 Thyroid disease	**169**
12.3 Corticosteroids	**171**
12.4 The reproductive steroids	**174**
12.5 Other pituitary hormones	**179**
12.6 Calcium metabolism and osteoporosis	**179**
Self-assessment on Chapter 12: questions	181
Self-assessment on Chapter 12: answers	186

Overview

The management of endocrine disorders can be complex because hormones can have widespread and diverse effects. Drugs can be used to replace deficiencies, to treat overactivity or to modulate secondary effects.

Diabetes mellitus is the most common endocrine disorder. Its complications are severe and can be reduced by good management. Patients with type 1 diabetes require insulin; patients with type 2 diabetes can be treated with oral antihyperglycaemic drugs and also sometimes with insulin. Both groups are prone to complications that can be reduced by good diabetic control.

The thyroid gland can be either over- or underactive. Treatment of overactivity depends largely on drugs, including radioiodine. Underactivity of the thyroid is generally easy to treat with thyroid replacement therapy.

Corticosteroids are widely used both as replacement therapy and as potent anti-inflammatory or immuno-suppressant drugs. The major drugs and their uses are described. Their adverse effects are common and serious.

Sex hormone steroids are used for contraception and for hormone replacement therapy after the menopause, both to relieve symptoms and to prevent osteoporosis. Other drugs can also be used to prevent and treat osteoporosis, such as vitamin D, calcium salts and bisphosphonates.

Lastly there are drugs to replace or modulate the range of peptide hormones from the pituitary gland.

12.1 Diabetes mellitus

Learning objectives

At the end of this section you should:
- be able to distinguish between the types of diabetes mellitus
- know the complications of diabetes mellitus
- understand the major elements of non-pharmacological treatment of diabetes mellitus
- be able to describe the drug regimens for type 1 and type 2 diabetes mellitus
- be able to describe the major drug classes used and give examples.

Diabetes mellitus (DM) is common, affecting about 1% of the population. In DM, the body becomes unable to regulate blood glucose, leading to hyperglycaemia, and the characteristic symptoms of polyuria, polydipsia and weight loss may occur. DM is really two distinct disorders. DM of either type is associated with serious long-term complications, including neuropathy (damage to nerves), retinopathy (damage to the retina), nephropathy (DM is the commonest cause of chronic renal failure) and arterial disease (DM is a major risk factor for ischaemic heart disease). The treatment of DM aims to control the blood glucose, relieve symptoms, and reduce the severity and frequency of the complications. Good control reduces the risk of complications in both types of DM.

Type 2 diabetes mellitus

Type 2 diabetes (T2DM), formerly classified as non-insulin-dependent diabetes mellitus (NIDDM):

- is more common (about 80% of all cases)
- usually occurs in middle-aged or elderly patients, although more cases are being

diagnosed in children and young adults, typically in the setting of obesity
- often has a family history
- is resistant at the cellular level to the effects of insulin.

A feature of the insulin resistance is the presence of high circulating concentrations of insulin. T2DM is associated with obesity and hypertension. The pathophysiology is that of a relative insulin deficiency with the pancreas secreting more insulin in an attempt to 'overcome' the insulin resistance of the tissues to achieve the same effect. Eventually the pancreas will fail to meet these demands.

Clinical sketch

A 66-year-old woman has a family history of T2DM. She complains of mild polyuria and thirst. She is obese and has recurrent low-grade fungal infections in the groin and under her breasts.

Comment: the incidence of T2DM is increasing with an ageing population and with increasing obesity. Family history is common. The onset is often slow and insidious and in many cases goes undiagnosed. These patients are more susceptible to infections.

The same patient is diagnosed as T2DM and a weight-reducing diet is advised. She is also prescribed metformin. This controls her condition for a period but gradually the blood sugar control deteriorates over the next 3–4 years.

Comment: T2DM is a progressive disease and even patients achieving good early control may go out of control later and the disease will progress. This does not necessarily imply that the patient is failing to comply with diet or therapy.

Management

Treatment of T2DM involves:

- patient education
- careful attention to diet (a diet which is low in fat and low in sugar)
- weight loss if there is obesity
- in some patients, the use of oral antihyperglycaemic drugs (OAHDs)
  — *metformin*
  — *sulphonylureas*
  — *glitazones/thiazolidinediones*
  — combinations of drugs commonly required
- insulin if oral medication is unsuccessful; however, these patients are not considered 'insulin dependent' in that if they discontinue their insulin, they are generally not at risk of ketosis
- careful treatment of other cardiovascular risk

factors: hypertension and dyslipidaemia particularly
- T2DM is a progressive disease: blood glucose control tends to deteriorate over time and requires an escalation in therapy.

Type 1 diabetes mellitus

Clinical sketch

A 20-year-old man presents with severe vomiting and a short history of weight loss, polyuria and severe thirst. On examination he is dehydrated and is considered to be hyperventilating.

Comment: type 1 diabetes mellitus tends to have a much more dramatic onset with the patient rapidly becoming dehydrated and acidotic. This is a medical emergency and requires urgent treatment.

Type 1 diabetes (T1DM), formerly known as insulin-dependent diabetes mellitus (IDDM) tends to occur in younger patients. It:

- is caused by the autoimmune destruction of the beta cells in the islets of the pancreas, which produce insulin
- involves an absolute insulin deficiency, which prevents most cells from taking up glucose and forces them to metabolise lipids
- leads to ketosis and acidosis
- requires insulin therapy in addition to diet control
- without insulin, will result in the patient rapidly falling ill and possibly dying
- necessitates careful patient education
- requires careful treatment of complications/cardiovascular risk factors (as in T2DM).

Insulin

Insulin is a peptide hormone normally produced by the islet cells of the pancreas. It has a range of actions which depend on the type of cell (Fig. 44). It:

- allows the active uptake of glucose and its utilisation in muscle and fat cells
- stimulates synthesis of glycogen in the liver
- inhibits formation of glucose (gluconeogenesis) in the liver
- inhibits breakdown of lipids
- stimulates protein synthesis
- stimulates some cell ion transport mechanisms (e.g. Na^+/K^+-ATPase).

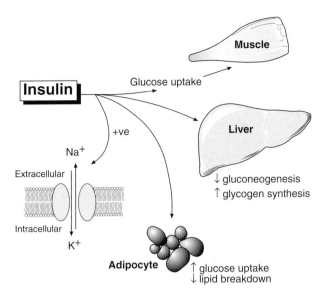

Fig. 44 Action of insulin.

Drugs used in the treatment of diabetes mellitus

Insulin

As insulin is a protein that would be broken down in the gut, insulin must be administered parenterally, usually by s.c. injection. It is metabolised by the liver and the kidney and has a half-life of 9–10 minutes. To extend its period of action, slow release preparations have been developed.

Formulations of insulin

Insulin preparations were originally derived from pigs (porcine insulin) or from cattle (beef insulin) and, as a result, antibodies sometimes developed. This was avoided by the development of highly purified porcine insulin. Now, however, most patients receive human insulin, produced either by biosynthesis (using genetic engineering to express the gene for human insulin in bacteria) or by chemical modification of the amino acid sequence of porcine insulin.

Human insulin is theoretically less immunogenic than porcine insulin but has no real advantage over the highly purified porcine insulins.

Insulins may be classified according to their duration of action as short, intermediate or long acting. Mixtures of these insulins are also available.

Short-acting preparations (e.g. soluble insulin) have a peak effect at about 1–2 hours when given s.c. and a duration of action of about 4–8 hours. They may also be given i.v.

Intermediate acting preparations (e.g. amorphous insulin zinc suspension) have insulin complexed with a zinc salt so that particles form. Insulin is then slowly released from these particles. The peak effect is at about 3–6 hours and the duration of action is about 12–24 hours.

Long-acting preparations (e.g. crystalline insulin zinc suspension) have the insulin–zinc complex formed as crystals, which break down more slowly still. The peak action is at 5–12 hours and the duration of effect is 16–30 hours.

New very short- and very long-acting insulin analogues are becoming available. The former are used to avoid postprandial surge in blood sugar. The latter provide a more reliable and consistent 24 hour control of blood glucose than achieved with the existing long-acting formulations. *Insulin lispro* and *insulin aspart* are short-acting analogues; *insulin glargine* is a long-acting preparation.

Insulin regimens

The dose and choice of preparations must be determined for each patient individually. Patients may use a short-acting and an intermediate- or long-acting preparation twice a day (before breakfast and the evening meal). Another popular regimen is a long-acting insulin once a day, supplemented around meal times with injections of soluble insulin, three times per day. Many patients will monitor their blood glucose at home and make minor adjustments in dose accordingly. Patients need to be educated about how to do this.

Clinical sketch

A 27-year-old man has been an insulin-dependent diabetic for the past 10 years. His control has never been particularly good. He is arrested by the police in the city centre one night, apparently confused and aggressive.

Comment: hypoglycaemia is the most common adverse effect of insulin. The patient may be confused and aggressive or become rapidly unconscious. Failure to treat adequately can result in permanent brain damage or death. Knowledge of the previous history of diabetes mellitus in this patient gives the game away, but in any confused or unconscious patient, blood sugar should be checked as soon as possible.

Adverse effects

Hypoglycaemia is the most common and serious adverse effect; it is the result of an imbalance between glucose intake (e.g. missing a meal), glucose utilisation (e.g. an unusual level of exercise) and insulin dose. The result is sympathetic activation (palpitations, anxiety and sweating) and neuroglycopaenia (visual disturbance, drowsiness or aggression, coma). Treatment is by administration of carbohydrate orally to a conscious patient, or i.v. glucose or i.m. *glucagon* (a peptide hormone and physiological antagonist of insulin). Patients and their families should be trained to spot the warning signs and how to treat hypoglycaemia, including possibly administration of glucagon if the patient loses consciousness.

Lipodystrophy is the atrophy or hypertrophy of fat at the site of injection. This is less common with the newer insulin preparations, but may result in variable insulin absorption from the injection site and hence unpredictable effects on blood sugar.

Acute diabetic ketoacidosis may occur in newly diagnosed T1DM or may arise in T1DM if the insulin dose is inadequate for needs, e.g. during infection or other physiological stress. The patient will become seriously dehydrated, hyperglycaemic and acidotic. This is a serious condition and its treatment is described in Box 6.

Oral antihyperglycaemic drugs

Biguanides

The biguanides are orally active agents that do not require functioning beta cells. They act by increasing peripheral utilisation of glucose and decreasing absorption of glucose from the gastrointestinal tract and gluconeogenesis. On their own, although they are antihyperglycaemic, they do not cause hypoglycaemia and are excreted unchanged by the kidney. *Metformin* is the only drug of this class in use.

Adverse effects

- gastrointestinal upsets are common; nausea, vomiting and anorexia. These can be reduced by reducing the dose or using a modified-release preparation
- vitamin B_{12} deficiency
- lactic acidosis is rare but can occur if metformin is used in patients with coexisting liver or renal disease or congestive cardiac failure. It is fatal in approximately half of all cases.

Sulphonylureas

The sulphonylureas stimulate release of endogenous insulin from the pancreas and so are only effective if the beta cells are functional. They may also have an extrapancreatic effect in decreasing breakdown of insulin and increasing the density of insulin receptors on the cell, improving insulin sensitivity.

Several sulphonylureas are available. The choice of drug is determined by the patient's age, the pres-

ence of other medical problems (such as renal dysfunction) and the intended duration of action. *Chlorpropamide* and *glibenclamide* are associated with a greater risk of hypoglycaemia because of their long duration of action. *Gliclazide* and *glimepiride* are commonly used agents.

Repaglinide and *nateglinide* are not chemically sulphonylureas but act in a similar way to stimulate insulin release. Their action is very rapid but short-lived. They are used to minimise the postprandial surge in blood glucose and are taken three times a day with main meals.

Adverse effects

- hypoglycaemia
- gastrointestinal upsets
- hypersensitivity: rashes, etc.
- weight gain: stimulation of appetite can be a problem in obese patients.

Drug interactions. Sulphonylureas are heavily protein bound and their actions may be increased by other drugs (e.g. sulphonamides) that compete for the binding sites.

Glitazones

The glitazones (or more correctly, the thiazolidinediones) are a relatively new class of oral antihyperglycaemic drug. They act by increasing cell sensitivity to insulin. They are used in combination with either a sulphonylurea or metformin when either of these alone is insufficient to control blood glucose. The long-term effects of these drugs are not yet known. Examples of glitazones are pioglitazone and rosiglitazone.

Box 6 Treatment of acute diabetic ketoacidosis

It is important to carefully monitor the clinical state and serum biochemistry and to consider why the ketoacidosis might have occurred (e.g. infection, myocardial infarction, etc.). Treatment involves:

- rehydration: the fluid deficit may be as much as 5–12 litres
- insulin given as a slow i.v. infusion
- it is not usually necessary to treat the acidosis separately
- monitor serum K^+ level: may be high initially but supplementation needed as rehydration proceeds: insulin pushes potassium into cells so the serum K^+ level will soon drop
- treat any underlying cause
- beware of aspiration from gastric stasis.

Adverse effects

- hepatitis (a previous drug, troglitazone, was withdrawn from the market because of serious liver toxicity)
- weight gain
- fluid retention and heart failure.

12.2 Thyroid disease

Hyperthyroidism

Excessive activity of the thyroid gland most often results from an autoimmune condition, *Graves' disease*, in which autoantibodies stimulate the thyroid cells. Graves' disease tends to undergo spontaneous remission in time, and treatment does not cure the condition but rather suppresses the hyperthyroidism until a remission occurs. Some patients will experience only one episode: about half will experience repeated episodes and may need a more definitive procedure such as radioactive iodine or surgery (see Fig. 45).

Hyperthyroidism can also result (in older patients) from autonomous overactivity of a single toxic adenoma, or from a toxic multinodular goitre. In these cases, remission is less likely and long-term therapy or definitive procedure will probably be needed.

High circulating concentrations of thyroxine:

- suppress the release of thyroid-stimulating hormone (TSH) from the pituitary
- increase metabolism: causing weight loss, anxiety, tremor, palpitations and diarrhoea.

In the elderly, these symptoms may be less clear and hyperthyroidism more difficult to diagnose.

Clinical sketch

A 58-year-old woman presents with weight loss, tremor and palpitations. She is diagnosed as being hyperthyroid based on raised plasma thyroxine concentrations and low thyroid-stimulating hormone (TSH). She is treated initially with carbimazole for 6 months. This initially achieves control, but when the drug is withdrawn she relapses.

Comment: Graves' disease is an autoimmune cause of hyperthyroidism. Long courses of carbimazole (12–18 months) are often adequate to treat this. However, in an older patient, the more likely cause is a toxic nodule and although carbimazole will control the thyroid while it is taken, remission of the underlying disease is unlikely. This patient is likely to need radioiodine, surgery or long-term carbimazole.

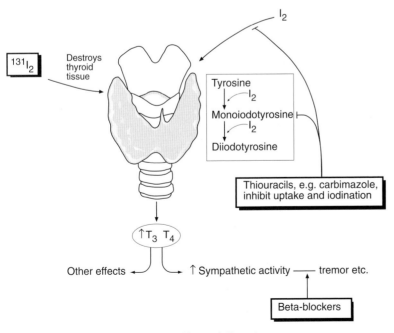

Fig. 45 Hyperthyroidism. T_4, thyroxine; T_3, triiodothyronine.

Thyroid crisis

Thyroid crisis is severe sudden hyperthyroidism perhaps precipitated by physiological stress, surgery, etc. It comprises fever, tachycardia, dehydration and encephalopathy. Treatment is outlined in Box 7.

Box 7 Treatment of thyroid crisis

Clinical features:
- fever
- tachycardia
- dehydration
- encephalopathy.

Treatment:
- i.v. fluids
- beta-blockers
- iodine solution
- corticosteroids
- carbimazole or propylthiouracil

Drugs used to treat hyperthyroidism

Thiouracils

The thiouracils inhibit the formation of thyroxine by inhibiting the uptake of iodine by the thyroid, the iodination of tyrosine and the coupling of iodinated tyrosine to form thyroxine (Fig. 45).

Carbimazole may have additional properties, influencing the immunological disorder in Graves' disease and increasing the likelihood of remission. Carbimazole is metabolised to methimazole (which is used widely to treat hyperthyroidism in the USA and Europe). If it is given to pregnant women, carbimazole can cross the placenta and may result in fetal hyperthyroidism or goitre.

Carbimazole is given in high doses initially until the patient becomes euthyroid (usually 4–8 weeks) then gradually reduced over 12 months, while monitoring symptoms and thyroid function tests. Repeated courses or continuous therapy will be necessary in some patients.

Some endocrinologists combine thyroxine with carbimazole once the patient is euthyroid (blocking-replacement regimen), which may achieve better results than with carbimazole alone.

Adverse effects

- *neutropenia*: carbimazole may cause neutropenia which, if treatment is not stopped, may develop into full agranulocytosis. This may arise suddenly, and patients must be carefully warned to report any evidence of infection, such as a sore throat, immediately. A full blood count should then be checked straightaway and if there is any evidence of neutropenia, the carbimazole should be withdrawn
- allergy with rash and fever can occur
- hepatitis and arthralgia may rarely occur.

Propylthiouracil is similar to carbimazole but is less likely to cause agranulocytosis.

Nonspecific beta-blockers

Nonspecific beta-blockers, such as *propranolol* (Ch. 3) are usually given (if there are no contraindications) to improve many of the sympathetically mediated symptoms at the start of treatment before the thiouracils have reached their full effect. This is symptomatic treatment only and does not have any disease-modifying activity.

Potassium iodide or iodine solution

Paradoxically, iodide/iodine causes an immediate reduction in the plasma thyroid hormone concentrations, as well as inhibiting thyroxine formation. The vascularity of the gland is also decreased. The effect is transient, lasting only 3–4 weeks, but is valuable in managing patients awaiting thyroid surgery or in thyroid crisis (see Box 7).

Radioactive iodine

Isotopic ^{131}I is well absorbed and concentrated in the thyroid where it causes permanent damage to the hormone-producing tissue. A single oral dose is usually effective. Standard antithyroid therapy is used before and after ^{131}I administration since ^{131}I takes 4–6 weeks to work. Radioactive iodine is used in patients who have failed to respond to medical therapy or who have relapsed, or increasingly as first line therapy for hyperthyroidism, especially in the elderly.

There is a very high incidence of hypothyroidism subsequently, but treating hypothyroidism is easier than treating hyperthyroidism. There is no evidence of any risk of later malignancy or of genetic damage.

Hypothyroidism

Hypothyroidism may result from autoimmune thyroiditis (Hashimoto's), thyroidectomy, radioiodine treatment or, in some parts of the world, from iodine deficiency. Rarely, it may be part of hypopituitarism.

The patient is most often elderly and female and may have:

- tiredness and lethargy
- coarsening of the skin and hair
- bradycardia
- constipation
- menorrhagia
- slowly relaxing tendon reflexes.

The concentration of free thyroxine in the blood is reduced, while that of thyroid-stimulating hormone from the pituitary is usually greatly increased.

Drugs used to treat hypothyroidism

Treatment is by levothyroxine, given orally. The dose is adjusted according to patient symptoms and in response to the concentration of thyroid-stimulating hormone, which should be maintained within the low normal range.

Adverse effects

The adverse effects are those of overdose, mimicking hyperthyroidism.

In patients with ischaemic heart disease, levothyroxine should be started in a low dose and should be increased very slowly; otherwise, an attack of angina or a myocardial infarction may be precipitated.

12.3 Corticosteroids

Learning objectives

At the end of this section you should be able to:
- describe the indications for glucocorticoid and mineralocorticoid drugs and know their adverse effects
- name examples of the major glucocorticoids and mineralocorticoids used.

Corticosteroids are hormones produced in the cortex of the adrenal gland: they may be broadly defined as *glucocorticoids* (major effect on inflammation and glucose metabolism) or *mineralocorticoids* (major effect on Na^+/K^+).

Glucocorticoids. The natural glucocorticoid is hydrocortisone (cortisol), produced under the control of the hypothalamus, which secretes corticotrophin-releasing factor to stimulate the pituitary to secrete *adrenocorticotrophic hormone* (ACTH). This is termed the hypothalamic–pituitary–adrenal (HPA) axis (Fig. 46).

Mineralocorticoids. Although hydrocortisone has some mineralocorticoid effects, the major natural mineralocorticoid is *aldosterone*, produced in response

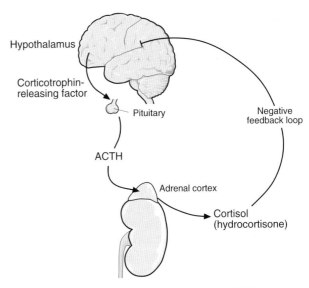

Fig. 46 The hypothalamic–pituitary–adrenal axis. ACTH, adrenocorticotrophic hormone.

to the renin–angiotensin–aldosterone (RAA) axis (see Ch. 3).

These hormones or synthetic derivatives can be given as drugs. These are powerful drugs with serious adverse effects and should be reserved for conditions where replacement is necessary, where other drugs have failed or where the illness is so severe that the benefits of treatment outweigh the risks. Corticosteroid drugs often show a mixture of both glucocorticoid and mineralocorticoid activity.

Glucocorticoids

Glucocorticoids bind to receptors in the cytoplasm. The complex is transported into the cell nucleus, where it binds to steroid-responsive elements on DNA to encourage new protein synthesis. The protein produced may have several effects; the best described is *lipocortin*, which in turn inhibits phospholipase A_2 and hence the release of *arachidonic acid*. This decreases activity in the cyclo-oxygenase and lipo-oxygenase pathways of production of inflammatory mediators. Corticosteroids do not appear to act for 12–18 hours after they are started and their action lasts for 24–48 hours after they are stopped.

Roles of glucocorticoids

Glucocorticoids are released in times of physiological stress. If absent, the patient may experience an Addisonian crisis, with hypotension, shock and death, when faced with physiological stress such as infection, etc.

Glucocorticoids are important in carbohydrate and protein metabolism; they promote gluconeogenesis, the formation of glycogen in the liver. Peripheral utilisation of glucose is decreased and the blood glucose may increase. Protein catabolism is increased, breaking down muscle and the matrix of bone.

Therapeutic uses

- Replacement therapy. In patients with adrenocortical insufficiency either caused by disease of the adrenal gland (autoimmune, Addison's disease), destruction or removal of the gland or pituitary failure. The doses of steroids used tend to be very low, as mimicking physiology as much as possible.
- Anti-inflammatory effect. Glucocorticoids may be used (systemically or topically) to reduce inflammation in many conditions (e.g. asthma, inflammatory bowel disease, eczema and other skin conditions, glomerulonephritis, treatment of hypersensitivity, arteritis). They are usually started at high doses and then reduced to the lowest level at which disease activity is suppressed, or withdrawn altogether if possible. Wherever possible, topical treatment is preferable to systemic so that adverse effects are minimised.
- Chemotherapy. Glucocorticoids are also used as part of chemotherapy for acute leukaemias and Hodgkin's lymphoma (see Ch. 15).

Clinical sketch

A 26-year-old woman presents with acute ulcerative colitis with rectal bleeding and extensive mucus production and diarrhoea.

Comment: immediate treatment of such a patient includes supportive therapy (i.v. fluids, transfusion, etc. as required) and immunosuppression with corticosteroids. These will be administered systemically initially, but as the patient improves there may be a change to topical application in the form of enemas. Topical application limits (but does not prevent) systematic exposure and reduces the risk of systemic side-effects.

Glucocorticoid drugs

Glucocorticoids are well absorbed after oral administration and broken down by liver metabolism. Because of the time to achieve any clinical effect, the use of i.v. rather than oral glucocorticoids is often unnecessary.

Hydrocortisone is used orally in low doses (approximately 20 mg/day) for replacement therapy in adrenal insufficiency. It is used in high doses (400–1200 mg/day) parenterally to treat severe acute allergy or asthma or in inflammatory bowel disease. It is used topically as enemas in inflammatory bowel disease and as creams in skin conditions such as eczema.

Prednisolone is about five times more potent than hydrocortisone as a glucocorticoid but has less mineralocorticoid action. It is used orally for acute asthma, hypersensitivity or other serious systemic inflammatory conditions (40–60 mg/day initially, reducing to 5–10 mg/day for maintenance).

Methylprednisolone is a derivative of prednisolone that can also be given parenterally and is used especially in treating transplant rejection.

Dexamethasone is about 20 times more potent than hydrocortisone but with little mineralocorticoid effect. It is given orally or parenterally for its anti-inflammatory effects, particularly in the treatment of cerebral oedema.

Beclometasone and *budesonide* are very potent glucocorticoids used topically by inhalation to treat asthma (Ch. 10). Many other potent fluorinated glucocorticoids are used in skin conditions.

Tetracosactide, a synthetic analogue of ACTH, was used by injection in the hope that the adrenals would not be suppressed. In practice, this advantage was slight and the clinical response to tetracosactide was so variable that it has been largely abandoned. It is used in tests of pituitary–adrenal function.

Mineralocorticoids

Mineralocorticoids affect Na^+ balance and cause Na^+ and water retention and increase Na^+ reuptake in the distal tubule in exchange for K^+.

Aldosterone is not used therapeutically. An analogue, *fludrocortisone*, is used in replacement therapy for patients with adrenal insufficiency. It has effectively no glucocorticoid activity.

Adverse effects of corticosteroids

The adverse effects of corticosteroids (Fig. 47) are serious and common in clinical use. The frequency of adverse effects is related to the dosage, duration of use and relative glucocorticoid/mineralocorticoid effects, e.g. hydrocortisone will have few adverse effects when used in low doses for replacement

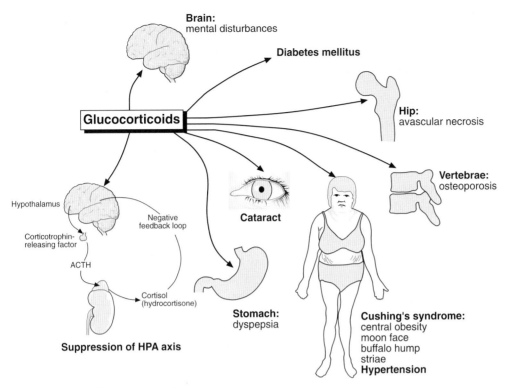

Fig. 47 Adverse effects of glucocorticoids.

therapy but will have both glucocorticoid and mineralocorticoid adverse effects when used in high doses. Dexamethasone, however, will have mostly glucocorticoid adverse effects. Topical therapy should be used wherever possible to minimise systemic adverse effects.

Clinical sketch

A 66-year-old man has chronic obstructive pulmonary disease. He has been treated with a range of medication including oral corticosteroids for many years. He presents with sudden onset of severe back pain. On examination, he is centrally obese with high blood pressure and bruising of the skin.

Comment: this patient demonstrates many of the adverse effects of long-term corticosteroids. The immediate diagnosis is probably a crush vertebra owing to osteoporosis caused by the corticosteroids. The other manifestations are the hypertension, the truncal obesity and easy bruising. The risks and benefits of long-term corticosteroid therapy need to be weighed carefully. Any patient on long-term steroid therapy should have their bone mineral density monitored and if appropriate should receive bisphosphonate therapy.

Glucocorticoid adverse effects

- impaired glucose tolerance or sometimes diabetes mellitus
- osteoporosis, especially of the vertebrae and in the elderly
- Cushing's syndrome, with characteristic appearance of moon face, buffalo hump, striae, as well as muscle wasting and thinning of the skin and poor healing
- immune suppression: there may be reduced resistance to infections such as tuberculosis
- growth suppression in children: the original disease state may be more relevant in causing growth suppression than the glucocorticoid
- mental disturbances: euphoria, agitation or depression
- cataracts
- striae and thinning of the skin: this may be a particular problem with topical use of potent glucocorticoids
- dyspepsia: common; peptic ulceration may occur but whether this is caused by glucocorticoids is not certain
- avascular necrosis of the hip
- adrenal suppression: administering glucocorticoids suppresses the HPA axis; if used

in high doses for prolonged periods, the adrenal glands may atrophy. This is also possible but less likely after topical use. To avoid this, it is important to use low doses for as short a time as possible.

Withdrawal of treatment after long-term gluco-corticoid use. This must be gradual (perhaps over several months) to allow the HPA to recover. Otherwise the patient may experience an Addisonian crisis. Similarly, in patients who have received glucocorticoids for prolonged periods, adrenal insufficiency may occur during physiological stress, e.g. during surgery or after an accident. If such a reaction is suspected, an increased dose of hydrocortisone should be administered. All patients prescribed glucocorticoids should be warned of these dangers and should be issued with a 'steroid card', giving details of dosage and possible complications.

Mineralocorticoid adverse effects

- sodium and water retention, leading to hypertension.
- hypokalaemia.

12.4 The reproductive steroids

> **Learning objectives**
>
> At the end of this section you should be able to describe:
> - the use of combined and progestogen-only contraceptives
> - the adverse effects and contraindications of each type of drug used, and give examples
> - the problems that may occur as a result of the menopause
> - the use of hormone replacement therapy and the drugs used (including the selective oestrogen receptor modulators)

The steroid hormones of the reproductive system are of three broad types:

- oestrogens, produced by the ovary and also in adipose tissue
- progesterone, also produced by the ovary
- testosterone, produced by the testis.

Contraception and steroid hormones

The most common therapeutic use of the sex hormones is in oral contraceptives. These are of two types (Fig. 48):

- oestrogen–progestogen combinations (the combined pill)
- progestogen-only pill (mini-pill).

Oestrogen–progestogen combinations

These act by inhibiting ovulation. Oestrogen inhibits release of follicle-stimulating hormone (FSH) from the pituitary; progestogen blocks luteinising hormone (LH) release. Both are taken for 21 days and then stopped for 7 days before resuming the cycle. During the withdrawal period, there is uterine bleeding similar to menstruation. The tablet should be taken at the same time every day; if missed for more than 12 hours, the contraceptive effect may be lost. Therapy should be started on the first day of a cycle so as to provide contraceptive cover for that cycle; if started later, barrier contraceptives should also be used for that cycle. The failure rate is about 1 per 100 woman years or less.

Examples

There is a wide variety of preparations available.

The oestrogen most commonly used is the synthetic *ethinylestradiol* in doses between 50 and 20 μg (the natural oestrogens undergo extensive first pass metabolism and are unsuitable). Lower dose pills are now recognised as being as effective and have fewer adverse effects.

The progestogen is usually *norethisterone* or *levonorgestrel*. These are derivatives of nortestosterone and may also have androgenic effects. Other progestogens without androgenic effects are also used including gestodene and desogestrel.

These synthetic steroids are all:

- absorbed well
- eliminated by conjugation with glucuronide
- excreted in bile.

There is enterohepatic circulation, i.e. the conjugated oestrogen is broken down in the gut by bacteria and the free oestrogen is reabsorbed. This means that if broad spectrum antibiotics are co-administered, gut bacteria may be reduced with a reduced amount of oestrogen being reabsorbed. A diminished contraceptive effect may result, thus requiring additional contraceptive methods during this time. Similarly, the simultaneous use of enzyme-inducing drugs such as carbamazepine or rifampicin accelerates the metabolism of oestrogen, potentially leading to follicle development and ovulation.

Action

Other effects

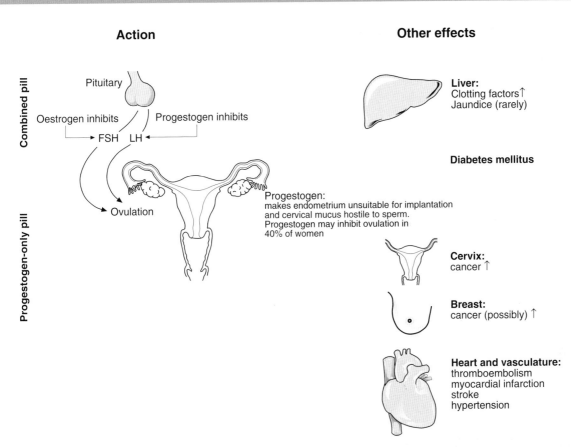

Combined pill

Pituitary

Oestrogen inhibits   Progestogen inhibits

FSH   LH

Ovulation

Progestogen-only pill

Progestogen:
makes endometrium unsuitable for implantation
and cervical mucus hostile to sperm.
Progestogen may inhibit ovulation in
40% of women

Liver:
Clotting factors↑
Jaundice (rarely)

Diabetes mellitus

Cervix:
cancer ↑

Breast:
cancer (possibly) ↑

Heart and vasculature:
thromboembolism
myocardial infarction
stroke
hypertension

Fig. 48 Action of the combined and progestogen-only oral contraceptives.

Other uses

The combined pill is sometimes used for cycle regulation in women with dysmenorrhoea or dysfunctional uterine bleeding (see below).

Clinical sketch

A 22-year-old woman wishes to go on the combined oral contraceptive. There is a family history of thromboembolic disorders in that her mother died from a pulmonary embolus postoperatively.

Comment: the risk of thromboembolic disorders is increased in women taking combined oral contraceptives by a factor of 3 or more. This is even higher in women who have a familial predisposition to thromboembolic disorders, possibly as a result of mutations in factor V or antithrombin III. It might be wise to screen this patient for such predispositions before initiating a combined oral contraceptive. There are alternatives available such as progestogen-based pills, implants or IUDs (intrauterine devices) which do not carry an increased risk of thromboembolic disorders.

Adverse effects

The most serious adverse effects involve the cardiovascular system:

- venous thromboembolic disease, i.e. deep venous thrombosis or pulmonary embolism: the risk is approximately trebled by the combined pill to approximately 15/100 000 woman years
  — more common with the higher oestrogen dose pills initially used and caused by a decrease in antithrombin III production and increase in fibrinogen production by the liver; this may be a particular risk around the time of surgery, and women having elective operations should discontinue the combined pill for 4 weeks before the operation and for 2 weeks after
  — also more common with use of the newer progestogens, e.g. *gestodene* and *desogestrel*: about 25/100 000 woman years.

Twelve

- myocardial infarction and stroke: these are more common with higher oestrogen dose pills, in older women (>35 years), and smokers, probably because of the alteration of clotting factors and increased platelet aggregation.
- hypertension: many women will experience a slight rise in blood pressure of little significance. In about 5–10%, the rise is greater and withdrawal of the combined pill may be necessary.

Other adverse effects are:

- malignant disease: the combined pill protects against endometrial and ovarian malignancy but is associated with an increased risk of cervical carcinoma and possibly breast carcinoma
- glucose intolerance and diabetes
- headache
- menstrual irregularity in the first months of treatment
- cholestatic jaundice, hepatic tumours: rarely.

Contraindications to the combined pill

- history of thromboembolic disease
- liver disease
- undiagnosed vaginal bleeding
- hyperlipidaemia
- breast, endometrial or hepatic carcinoma.

Use with caution

- diabetes mellitus
- smokers
- older patients (aged over 35 years)
- hypertensives
- migraine sufferers.

The progestogen-only pill

The progestogen-only pill works by altering the cervical mucus and the endometrium so that fertilisation or subsequent implantation is unlikely. Ovulation is also inhibited in about 40% of women. The failure rate is higher than with the combined pill (about 2/100 woman years) but it may be more suitable for patients with contraindications to oestrogens.

The tablets are taken constantly with no breaks. They should be taken at exactly the same time every day: if there is delay for more than 3 hours, the contraceptive effect may be lost.

Examples

The progestogens used are the same as in the combined pill, but in a lower dose, e.g. in the combined pill, *norethisterone* may be given in doses of 500–1000 µg/day while in progestogen-only pills, the dose is 350 µg/day.

Medroxyprogesterone is a depot progestogen given by injection: a single dose may provide contraception for 3 months. Levonorgestrel-releasing silastic rods are available, providing protection for up to 3 years. Levonorgestrel-releasing intrauterine devices provide very effective contraception for up to 5 years, reduce uterine bleeding and avoid systemic adverse effects.

Adverse effects of progestogens

- menstrual irregularities
- nausea and vomiting
- breast discomfort.

Emergency contraception

Levonorgestrel in high dose is used as emergency hormonal contraception, taking the drug within 72 hours of unprotected intercourse; efficacy decreases with time. The insertion of intrauterine devices (IUDs) is also used in the event that postcoital contraception is required.

Dysfunctional uterine bleeding

The combined pill is sometimes used for cycle regulation in women with dysmenorrhoea or dysfunctional uterine bleeding.

Tranexamic acid reduces blood loss (see Ch. 5).

Danazol inhibits the release of pituitary gonadotrophins and is anti-oestrogen, anti-androgen and anti-progestogen. It is used to treat endometriosis and menorrhagia.

Adverse effects include gastrointestinal upsets and virilisation.

In severe cases of endometriosis, gonadotrophin releasing hormone (gonadorelin, GnRH) analogues may be used (see below).

Hormone replacement therapy

The menopause occurs at widely varying ages with a mean of 53 years. It is primary ovarian failure resulting in a fall in serum oestrogen levels and increased release of FSH/LH, the attempt by the pituitary to overcome increasing ovarian failure – an example of negative feedback.

Clinical sketch

A 56-year-old woman presents to her GP complaining of hot flushes and vaginal dryness. It is 18 months since her last period. She is concerned about osteoporosis since she thinks she is menopausal.

Comment: the patient is probably menopausal, based on the symptoms and her age. It would be reasonable to prescribe hormone replacement therapy (HRT) for a period of 12–18 months to relieve her menopausal symptoms. However, if she is to be protected from osteoporosis she will need much longer therapy than this, at least 5 years. To achieve significant protection against hip fracture at its most common age in the early 80s, much longer than that is required. The patient should be given general lifestyle advice about what she can do to reduce her risk of osteoporosis, e.g. reducing smoking, increasing vitamin D and calcium intake and exercise in addition to considering long-term HRT. The benefits of long-term HRT need to be weighed against its possible risk. All types of HRT increase the risk of breast cancer within 1–2 years of initiating treatment. There is also an increased risk of venous thromboembolism and stroke.

The loss of sex hormone-dependent bone production hastens osteoporosis and there is also an increased risk of cardiovascular disease.

The main symptoms are vasomotor: hot flushes, vaginal dryness. The use of hormone replacement therapy (HRT):

- treats symptoms (treatment needed for 6–12 months)
- avoids osteoporosis (treatment needed for 5–10 years or longer). However, other drugs are preferred for this (see below).

Treatment

HRT is given as once daily oral doses, e.g. *conjugated equine oestrogens* or *estradiol*.

Progestogens are unnecessary in women who have had a hysterectomy. However, a progestogen must be given to all women with an intact uterus. HRT does not provide contraception. Ovulation may still occur.

In women whose major problem is vaginal dryness, an oestrogen cream applied to the affected area intermittently may be more appropriate than systemic therapy.

Adverse effects

- increase in the risk of endometrial carcinoma: this can be avoided by giving progestogens in addition to the oestrogen for 10–12 days in every 28. This will cause a withdrawal bleed. Alternatively, continuous progestogen can be given – this usually results in amenorrhoea
- a probable increase in the risk of breast cancer in women who use long-term HRT (by 10–30%)
- increased risk of thromboembolic disorders (despite the low dose of oestrogen used)
- other oestrogen-related effects as described above.

Contraindications

Contraindications to HRT are fewer than to the use of higher-dose oestrogens as contraceptives:

- thromboembolic disorders
- liver disease
- oestrogen-sensitive malignancy.

Hormone modulating therapy

Drugs that reduce the effects of oestrogens or progestogens in certain tissues are used in a number of indications: cancer, infertility, termination of pregnancy.

Selective oestrogen receptor modulators

The selective oe/estrogen receptor modulators (SERMs) have some oestrogen-like effects and some anti-oestrogen effects in different tissues. Examples are *tamoxifen, raloxifene*.

Tamoxifen

Breast cancer cells may have oestrogen receptors. Reducing oestrogen levels (by oophorectomy) is beneficial in about 60% of such cases, as well as in about 10% where oestrogen receptors are not identified.

Tamoxifen is an oestrogen receptor antagonist in breast tissue and is used to treat breast cancer. It may cause a response in about 30–40% of women. In other tissues, it has oestrogen-like activity: it can reduce osteoporosis, and stimulates the endometrium but is not used for these indications.

Adverse effects include hot flushes and gastrointestinal upsets. It may prevent development of breast cancer in high-risk patients.

Anastrozole

Anastrozole prevents the formation of oestrogens from androgens in peripheral tissue by inhibiting aromatase enzymes. Anastrozole is licensed for the adjuvant treatment of oestrogen-receptor positive early breast cancer in post-menopausal women unable to take tamoxifen, either because they have a high risk of thromboembolism or because of endometrial abnormalities contraindicating its use.

Raloxifene

Raloxifene has oestrogen-like activity in bones and is used to prevent osteoporosis but does not stimulate the endometrium. It may reduce the risk of breast cancer and possibly heart disease, though this is not yet proven. It does not treat menopausal symptoms. It may cause thromboembolic disease.

Gonadotrophin-releasing hormone (gonadorelin) and its analogues

Gonadorelin (GnRH) is a peptide released in a pulsatile fashion by the hypothalamus. Initially it stimulates the release of both FSH and LH (and hence oestrogen production in females or testosterone in males). Continued administration of GnRH analogues downregulate the GnRH receptors so that, after the initial surge of gonadotrophins, FSH and LH release falls off and oestrogen or testosterone fall to very low levels.

Long-acting analogues of GnRH (e.g. *goserelin*) can be given in slow-release depot injections to provide constant stimulation. *Buserelin* can also be administered intranasally.

GnRH analogues are used in a variety of different clinical scenarios: from the treatment of prostatic and breast cancer to the management of infertility and endometriosis.

Adverse effects include promotion of artificial menopause in male and female with secondary effects on bone, etc. and tumour 'flush' on first administration in metastatic prostatic cancer.

Hormone modulation in infertility

Clomifene

Clomifene is an oestrogen antagonist at central receptors in the hypothalamus. By blocking these receptors, the normal negative feedback control on FSH and LH release is prevented. FSH/LH levels rise, stimulating ovulation and increasing the potential for fertilisation. The main adverse effect is the risk of overstimulation, with multiple follicles being developed and ovulated, and potentially therefore multiple pregnancy.

Gonadorelin

Gonadorelin given by intermittent injection simulates the physiological pulsatile secretion to cause FSH and LH release in the treatment of infertility.

Hormone modulation in pregnancy or its termination

Oxytocin

Oxytocin is a peptide hormone from the posterior pituitary (neurohypophysis). It stimulates the uterus during labour. It is given i.v. to stimulate contractions during the active management of labour. It is given in combination with ergometrine i.m. during the third stage of labour to reduce the risk of postpartum haemorrhage.

Mifepristone

Mifepristone is a semisynthetic steroid used with prostaglandins to cause termination of pregnancy at up to 9 weeks. It acts as a progestogen antagonist, preventing endometrial maturation and increasing activity of the myometrium. The combination is effective in 95% of patients but may cause severe uterine pain and hypotension.

Prostaglandins

Prostaglandins have significant effects on the uterus, causing vasoconstriction and muscle contraction. *Dinoprostone* and *gemeprost* are used to cause abortion. *Carboprost* can be used to treat postpartum haemorrhage.

Androgens and antiandrogens

Testosterone is normally produced by the testis. Synthetic testosterone can be given in cases of deficiency: after orchidectomy or in primary deficiency states. In these patients, it will prevent osteoporosis and increase the libido. It is available in a number of different preparations, including as depot injections, gels or patches applied to skin.

Hormonal treatment of prostatic cancer

Prostatic cancer is treated using drugs or surgery to reduce the action of androgens:

- androgen production suppression
  - castration
  - long-acting GnRH analogue (risk of tumour 'flare' when first used). Tumour flare is caused when an initial surge in testosterone production may be associated with progression of the prostate cancer, leading to problems such as spinal cord compression or increased bone pain
  - *flutamide*: blocks androgen formation probably by inhibiting androgen uptake or androgen binding to cytoplasmic/nuclear

receptors; consequently it is a 'pure' antiandrogen with virtually no other hormonal effects

- testosterone receptor blocker: *cyproterone acetate*
- combinations sometimes used
  — to prevent tumour flare
  — for long-term treatment in selected patients.

12.5 Other pituitary hormones

Learning objectives

At the end of this section you should be able to:
- list the major hormones produced by the pituitary gland (adeno- and neurohyophysis)
- describe drugs used to replace or oppose them.

Antidiuretic hormone

Cranial diabetes insipidus (DI) is caused by a deficiency of antidiuretic hormone (ADH, also known as vasopressin). This is a peptide that is secreted from the posterior pituitary (cranial DI). It reduces the resabsorption of water in the renal collecting tubules and its absence leads to polyuria, polydipsia and dehydration with hypernatraemia.

Analogues of antidiuretic hormone

Treatment of deficiency of antidiuretic hormone is by synthetic analogues. *Desmopressin* is given as a nasal spray. The dose is adjusted according to effect. The major adverse effect is water intoxication if too much is used. *Arginine vasopressin* may be used parenterally. It may cause severe vasoconstriction and is used for this purpose in the treatment of bleeding from oesophageal varices.

Growth hormone disorders

Somatropin is a peptide analogue of human growth hormone. It is used parenterally in the treatment of short stature in growth hormone-deficient children and in certain growth hormone-deficient adults (e.g. following pituitary surgery).

Octreotide is a peptide analogue of somatostatin, a naturally occurring growth hormone antagonist. It is used to treat growth hormone excess in acromegaly and in gastrointestinal disease (Ch. 11).

Bromocriptine (dopamine agonist; see Ch. 6) can also be used to reduce secretion of growth hormone (and to reduce prolactin secretion in prolactinomas). *Cabergoline* has actions similar to bromocriptine.

12.6 Calcium metabolism and osteoporosis

Learning objectives

At the end of this section you should be able to describe:
- the role of vitamin D in the metabolism of calcium in the body
- the drugs used in the management of calcium and related bone disorders
- the management of osteoporosis.

Vitamin D_2 (*ergocalciferol, calciferol*) is a fat-soluble vitamin that is formed in the skin on exposure to UV light. It may also be derived from the diet (dairy products). It is activated first in the liver and then in the kidney to 1,25-dihydroxycholecalciferol. It acts to:

- increase the serum Ca^{2+} by enhancing the absorption of Ca^{2+} from the gastrointestinal tract and the reabsorption of Ca^{2+} and phosphate from the renal tubule
- stimulate osteoclasts to increase bone turnover and release Ca^{2+}.

Deficiencies of vitamin D may be dietary (especially in vegetarians and the elderly) or be the result of malabsorption, liver disease or renal disease. The clinical result is *osteomalacia* (known in children as rickets).

Ergocalciferol

Ergocalciferol is used orally in vitamin D-deficiency states, malabsorption, liver and renal disease (in which very high doses may be required) and hypoparathyroidism. Its use in osteoporosis is controversial. *1α-hydroxycholecalciferol* is a more potent analogue.

Adverse effects

Hypercalcaemia may occur; careful monitoring of serum Ca^{2+} is necessary.

Osteoporosis

Osteoporosis is the loss of trabecular bone, leading to weakening of bone and possible fractures. It can occur as an adverse effect of some drugs (e.g. corticosteroids, heparin) but more commonly is a result of age. Peak bone density occurs in the mid to late 20s; thereafter bone density declines. In women, sex

Twelve

hormone-dependent bone (approximately 15% of bone in vertebrae, hip, wrist) declines rapidly at the menopause. Women are, therefore, more vulnerable to osteoporosis than men. This may be avoided by oestrogen replacement. Other factors predisposing to osteoporosis are cigarette smoking, alcohol abuse and liver or renal disease. Weight-bearing exercise is protective.

Patients at high risk

- elderly
- women, especially if in early menopause
- smokers
- alcohol abusers
- long-term steroid users (more than 7.5 mg prednisolone/day for 6 months).

Prevention

- exercise, prevent any preventable risk factors
- calcium intake and vitamin D: dietary intake often inadequate in the elderly; supplementation trials (approximately 1200 mg calcium in the form of calcium carbonate and 800 units ergocalciferol) show reduced risk of fracture
- HRT or raloxifene therapy in women
- bisphosphonates may be used.

Treatment of established osteoporosis

- calcium/vitamin D
- HRT
- bisphosphonates.

Bisphosphonates

The bisphosphonates bind to hydroxyapatite crystals in bone and reduce the breakdown of bone. Some inhibit osteoclasts (break down bone) and osteoblasts (build up bone) (e.g. *etidronate*); others are just selective for osteoblasts (e.g. *alendronate*).

Bisphosphonates are used to treat:

- Paget's disease of the bones
- hypercalcaemia of malignancy
- severe osteoporosis complicated by vertebral fractures
- corticosteroid-induced osteoporosis (in combination with calcium salts).

Examples: *etidronate* (oral or i.v.), *pamidronate* (i.v. only), *clodronate* and *alendronate* (oral only).

Adverse effects

- gastrointestinal upsets
- oesphageal ulceration (alendronate only)
- hypocalcaemia.

Some drugs also inhibit osteoblasts and fractures may occur. Etidronate is used intermittently in osteoporosis to avoid this.

Calcitonin

Calcitonin is a peptide secreted by the C cells of the thyroid that lowers serum Ca^{2+} by decreasing bone turnover and increasing excretion of Ca^{2+} through the kidneys. It is used to treat Paget's disease. Its adverse effects include flushing of the face and nausea.

Self-assessment on Chapter 12: questions

Multiple choice questions

1. Drugs that may impair glucose tolerance include:
   a. Bendroflumethiazide
   b. Prednisolone
   c. Oral contraceptives
   d. Enalapril
   e. Benzylpenicillin

2. Carbimazole:
   a. Is a prodrug
   b. May cause hypothyroidism
   c. May cause thrombocytopenia
   d. Blocks iodine uptake in the gastrointestinal tract
   e. Treatment is rarely followed by relapse

3. In treating hyperthyroidism:
   a. High-dose potassium iodide is useful in the long-term treatment of hyperthyroidism
   b. Patients may be treated with ^{131}I while still taking carbimazole
   c. There is a high risk of hypothyroidism in patients treated with ^{131}I
   d. Hypothyroidism may be treated with dietary iodine supplements
   e. Treatment of hypothyroidism is best monitored by measuring serum thyroxine

4. Insulin:
   a. Is formed in the liver
   b. Tends to increase body weight
   c. In patients treated with insulin, diet is unimportant
   d. Human insulin is more likely to cause hypoglycaemia than porcine insulin
   e. Good control of type 1 diabetes mellitus (T1DM) results in a decreased risk of serious complications

5. The following statements are correct:
   a. T1DM is more common than type 2 diabetes (T2DM)
   b. Patients with T1DM should change their treatment only on the advice of their doctor
   c. Hypoglycaemia is the most common adverse effect of insulin
   d. Soluble insulin may be given i.v.
   e. In hypoglycaemia, high-dose, i.m. glucose should be given

6. The following statements are correct:
   a. In diabetic ketoacidosis, dehydration may be life-threatening
   b. Acidosis always requires urgent treatment with i.v. sodium bicarbonate
   c. Crystalline insulin is used for its long duration of action
   d. Patients treated with insulin can monitor their own blood glucose
   e. Antibodies to insulin are more common with porcine than with human insulin

7. Concerning oral antihyperglycaemic therapy in T2DM:
   a. Sulphonylureas can be used to treat a patient who has developed diabetes mellitus because of pancreatitis
   b. Chlorpropamide is appropriate for elderly patients
   c. Sulphonylureas are not the drug of choice in obese patients with T2DM
   d. Metformin may cause lactic acidosis in some patients
   e. Hypoglycaemia is a common adverse effect of oral antihyperglycaemic drugs

8. Concerning calcium metabolism:
   a. Vitamin D causes calcium reabsorption from the kidney
   b. Vitamin D can be manufactured in the body
   c. Vitamin D is found in fresh fruit and vegetables
   d. Vitamin D and Ca^{2+} are used to treat hypoparathyroidism
   e. Etidronate stabilises bone and reduces hypocalcaemia in malignant disease

9. Systemic glucocorticoids may cause:
   a. Psychosis
   b. Opportunistic infections

c. Osteomalacia

d. Suppression of the renin–angiotensin–aldosterone axis

e. Skin changes

10. Corticosteroids:

a. Hydrocortisone has no mineralocorticoid effects

b. Glucocorticoids are potent anti-inflammatory drugs

c. Hydrocortisone is a naturally occurring hormone

d. Adrenocorticotrophic hormone (ACTH) is often used to treat inflammatory disease

e. Aldosterone can be given to treat adrenal insufficiency

11. Diseases in which corticosteroids are used include:

a. Addison's disease

b. Conn's syndrome

c. Asthma

d. Cellulitis

e. Lymphoma

12. In contraception:

a. The combined oral contraceptive pill (COCP) may cause ischaemic heart disease

b. The failure rate for the progestogen-only pill is lower than for the COCP

c. The progestogens used in the COCP may have androgenic effects

d. Enterohepatic circulation of oestrogen occurs

e. COCP may be involved in a variety of drug interactions

13. In contraception:

a. Low-dose oestrogen COCPs are less likely to cause thromboembolic disease than older high-dose preparations

b. COCP should never be used in women over the age of 35

c. COCP decreases the risk of uterine carcinoma

d. COCP should not be used in women who smoke

e. The progestogen-only pill is safe in women with a history of thromboembolic disease

14. Postmenopausal hormone replacement therapy:

a. Is contraindicated in women with ischaemic heart disease

b. If given to patients with a uterus, should include a progestogen as well as an oestrogen

c. If given long term, may decrease the risks of osteoporosis

d. Decreases the risks of breast cancer

e. Should not be started for at least a year after the last period

Case history questions

Case history 1

A 28-year-old woman presents with hyperthyroidism caused by Graves' disease.

1. What treatment or treatments would be appropriate as first line?

2. What possible adverse effects of treatment must she be warned about?

While being treated for hyperthyroidism, she becomes pregnant.

3. What are the risks to the fetus?

She is treated for 12 months, but on stopping therapy, she quickly relapses.

4. What treatment options should be considered now?

5. What drugs may interfere with the interpretation of thyroid function tests?

Case history 2

An obese 68-year-old woman with hypertension complains of thirst and polyuria and is noted to have glycosuria. Blood sugar analysis confirms that she is diabetic.

1. What are the main lines of treatment to recommend to this woman?

2. What maintenance drug treatment should be considered first line?

3. If this fails, what should be second line?
4. What drugs may have precipitated her diabetes?
5. When might insulin therapy be considered in such a patient?

Case history 3

A 25-year-old man presents with a 3-day history of vomiting, polyuria and thirst. There is no previous history. Urinalysis shows glycosuria and ketonuria, and blood glucose is high.

1. What is the diagnosis?
2. What treatment should he be given?
3. How are insulins administered?

He is treated for diabetes mellitus over the next 3 years. However, one day he is found unconscious.

4. What diagnosis should be considered first?
5. How should he now be treated?

Case history 4

A 58-year-old woman is given high-dose prednisolone for several months because of giant cell arteritis, an inflammatory disease. Her condition responds well to this.

1. What problems may arise if her prednisolone is suddenly stopped?
2. She complains of swollen ankles: why might this be?
3. What musculoskeletal changes might she experience?
4. What other adverse effects might she experience?

She fractures her hip in a fall and requires surgery.

5. What complications might she suffer because of her therapy around the time of operation?

Case history 5

A 19-year-old woman wishes to go on an oral contraceptive.

1. She is worried because she has heard that the combined oral contraceptive pill (COCP) can cause cancer: what can you tell her?
2. She smokes: is this a particular problem?

She is started on a combined oestrogen–progestogen pill: she telephones you 6 months later to say that she forgot to take her pill yesterday and to ask what she should do.

3. What is your advice?

She complains of pleuritic chest pain 6 months later again.

4. What drug-related diagnosis should be considered?

She later develops epilepsy and is treated with carbamazepine; she wishes to continue using an oral contraceptive.

5. Are there any problems with this?

Case history 6

A 50-year-old woman develops irregular periods. She complains of hot flushes, about 3 months after her last period, as well as feeling tired and irritable. She asks whether she should have hormone replacement therapy (HRT).

1. What are the likely benefits to this patient of short-term (6 months) treatment with HRT?
2. She asks about osteoporosis, since there is a family history of fractured hips; what should you tell her about this and HRT?
3. There is also a strong family history of ischaemic heart disease. Would you expect HRT to increase or decrease the risks of this?
4. Are doses of oestrogen in HRT higher than in combined oral contraceptives?
5. She is concerned particularly about vaginal dryness. Will HRT help this?

Short note questions

Write short notes on:

1. The adverse effects of corticosteroids
2. The management of hyperthyroidism

3. Insulin regimens in the treatment of T1DM

4. The treatment of established osteoporosis

Extended matching items questions

Theme: Drug selection in endocrinology

Options

A. Ethinylestradiol

B. Gestodene

C. Flutamide

D. Levonorgestrel

E. Hydrocortisone

F. Aldosterone

G. Testosterone

H. Tamoxifen

I. Estradiol

J. Clomifene

K. Goserelin

L. Finasteride

For each of the requirements below, choose the most appropriate option from the list above. Each option may be used once, more than once, or not at all.

1. An oestrogen used in postmenopausal hormone replacement therapy.

2. A drug to decrease oestrogen production.

3. A drug with mineralocorticoid effect.

4. A drug used in contraceptive implants and intrauterine devices.

5. A drug used as an oestrogen antagonist in the treatment of breast cancer.

6. A drug used as an oestrogen in combined oral contraceptives.

7. A drug used as a progestogen in combined oral contraceptives.

8. A drug used to treat benign prostatic hypertrophy.

Theme: Making a diagnosis in endocrine disorders

Options

A. Addison's disease

B. Conn's syndrome

C. Cushing's syndrome

D. Diabetes insipidus

E. Hyperlipidaemia

F. Hyperthyroidism

G. Hypoglycaemia

H. Hypothyroidism

I. Osteoporosis

J. Type 1 diabetes mellitus

K. Type 2 diabetes mellitus

From the list of options above select the most likely diagnosis for each of the patients described below.

1. A 36-year-old woman complains of weight loss with palpitations and diarrhoea. Her previous doctor felt she was very anxious. She has a fine tremor on examination and is tachycardic.

2. An 82-year-old woman is brought into hospital hypothermic and bradycardic. Over the preceding few months she has been complaining of cold intolerance.

3. A 25-year-old man presenting to his GP with a 6-month history of polydipsia and polyuria and weight loss of 6 kg. Urinalysis reveals 3$^+$ glucose and his random blood sugar is 19 mmol/L.

4. A 75-year-old woman living on her own is found confused, sweaty and tachycardic by her carers. Her list of medication prescribed by her GP includes tolbutamide.

5. A 46-year-old man has hypertension that is very difficult to control with four different drugs. His blood results persistently show hypokalaemia.

Theme: Management of diabetes mellitus

Options

A. Acarbose

B. Dietary modification

C. Glimepiride

D. Intravenous insulin

E. Intravenous insulin, and intravenous 0.9% saline

F. Metformin

G. Pioglitazone

H. Subcutaneous insulin (any regimen)

From the list of options above select the optimal management for each of the patients described below.

1. A 60-year-old obese woman with a BMI of 34 is diagnosed by her GP as having type 2 diabetes mellitus. Dietary modification over a period of 6 months has failed to control her symptoms or hyperglycaemia.

2. A 25-year-old man presenting to the A&E department with a 4-month history of polydipsia and polyuria and weight loss of 5 kg. Urinalysis reveals 3[+] glucose and 3[+] ketones. His random blood sugar is 25 mmol/L. He is very dehydrated clinically and biochemically (with a urea of 14 mmol/L) and his serum potassium is 5.8 mmol/L (normal range 3.5–5.0 mmol/L). Arterial pH is 7.1.

3. A 25-year-old man presenting to his GP with a 4-month history of polydipsia and polyuria and weight loss of 5 kg. Urinalysis reveals 3[+] glucose and 3[+] ketones. His random blood sugar is 17.9 mmol/L. There is no ketoacidosis.

4. A 60-year-old obese man with type 2 diabetes mellitus and a combination of renal failure and congestive cardiac failure (following a previous myocardial infarction). Treatment with a sulphonylurea has not been successful.

5. A 50-year-old woman has attended her GP following a recent oral glucose tolerance test that has confirmed the suspected diagnosis of T2DM. She is asymptomatic.

Theme: Mechanism of action of endocrine drugs

Options

A. Acarbose
B. Alendronate
C. Carbimazole
D. Gliclazide
E. Insulin glargine
F. Metformin
G. Rosiglitazone
H. Porcine insulin
I. Propylthiouracil
J. Thyroxine

From the list of options above select the drug that best fits the description of its mechanism(s) of action.

1. Increased peripheral utilisation of glucose, reduced gluconeogenesis without weight gain.

2. Inhibition of iodination of tyrosine and immunological modification.

3. Stimulation of pancreatic β cells.

Self-assessment on Chapter 12: answers

Multiple choice answers

1. a. **True.** This is a thiazide diuretic.
   b. **True.** Glucocorticoids cause a rise in blood glucose by several mechanisms.
   c. **True.** But this is not usually clinically significant.
   d. **False.** ACE inhibitors may even increase insulin sensitivity.
   e. **False.** No effect on the pancreas or peripheral cells.

2. a. **True.** Converted to thiamazole.
   b. **True.** If used in high doses for prolonged periods.
   c. **False.** May cause agranulocytosis.
   d. **False.** Blocks iodine uptake by the thyroid gland.
   e. **False.** Carbimazole does not reverse the underlying cause and relapse is common.

3. a. **False.** Short-term use only.
   b. **False.** Carbimazole would impede uptake of ^{131}I into the thyroid. The patient should be off carbimazole for several days beforehand.
   c. **True.** Whether caused by the ^{131}I or the natural history of the condition.
   d. **False.** Thyroxine is needed.
   e. **False.** Thyroid-stimulating hormone is the best measure.

4. a. **False.** Insulin is formed in the pancreas.
   b. **True.** Insulin tends to stimulate appetite.
   c. **False.** Diet is exceedingly important in all patients with diabetes.
   d. **False.** There is no evidence of this.
   e. **True.** Although many patients, even those with poor control, do not develop complications: there is still much to be understood about the cause of diabetic complications.

5. a. **False.** T2DM is far more common.
   b. **False.** Patients should be sufficiently knowledgeable about their condition to adjust their dose of insulin by themselves.

   c. **True.** This may be life threatening.
   d. **True.** This is the only insulin that may be given in any way other than subcutaneously.
   e. **False.** High concentrations of glucose are very hyperosmolar and severe tissue necrosis would be likely. Glucose should be given either orally or, if the patient is unconscious, i.v.

6. a. **True.** The extent of the dehydration is commonly underestimated.
   b. **False.** Acidosis usually corrects itself when dehydration and hyperglycaemia are treated. Sodium bicarbonate should only be given in extreme circumstances only and by doctors who are expert in giving this, as it can make the intracellular acidosis worse.
   c. **True.** Often in combination with a short-acting insulin.
   d. **True.** And may adjust their dose of insulin accordingly.
   e. **True.** But with purified porcine insulins, this is of little clinical importance.

7. a. **False.** Because sulphonylureas depend mainly for their action on stimulating release of endogenous insulin.
   b. **False.** Its half-life is so long that it may accumulate and cause dangerous hypoglycaemia in the elderly.
   c. **True.** Because by stimulating insulin release they may increase the appetite. Metformin is the drug of choice.
   d. **True.** In patients with liver or renal disease.
   e. **True.** For the sulphonylureas.

8. a. **True.** One of its major actions.
   b. **True.** In the skin, vitamin D can be formed from cholesterol by the action of UV light.
   c. **False.** Milk and other dairy products are the best sources.
   d. **True.** Since the effect of hypoparathyroidism is hypocalcaemia.
   e. **True.** Its major use.

9. a. **True.** Usually depression, occasionally mania.

b. **True.** Because of immune suppression.

c. **False.** Osteoporosis, not osteomalacia.

d. **False.** This axis is not dependent on corticotrophin-releasing factor or adrenocorticotrophic hormone.

e. **True.** Striae and easy bruising.

10. a. **False.** Fluid retention is a common adverse effect of hydrocortisone.

b. **True.** Their major use.

c. **True.** Usually known as cortisol, for some reason.

d. **False.** In the past, yes, but rarely used today.

e. **False.** If mineralocorticoid replacement is needed, fludrocortisone is used.

11. a. **True.** This is adrenocortical insufficiency.

b. **False.** This is primary hyperaldosteronism caused by tumour-secreting aldosterone.

c. **True.** Usually by inhalation.

d. **False.** Might even exacerbate this by causing immune suppression.

e. **True.** For Hodgkin's and some other types.

12. a. **True.** But less likely with low-dose oestrogen types used today.

b. **False.** About 2/100 as opposed to 1/100 for the COCP.

c. **True.** Some are testosterone derivatives, such as norethisterone or levonorgestrel. This is less likely for desogestrel or gestodene.

d. **True.** Important for its action.

e. **True.** With enzyme inducers and broad spectrum antibiotics for instance.

13. a. **True.** Hence their widespread use today, while the high-dose pills are reserved for special circumstances.

b. **False.** However, the risks are undoubtedly increased, and other risk factors should be considered before using them in older women.

c. **True.** But may increase the risk of cervical and possibly breast cancer.

d. **False.** Although again the risk is increased and women should be warned against smoking, particularly in combination with other risk factors.

e. **True.** Although this is still mentioned as a contraindication in the data sheets of most of these drugs.

14. a. **False.** Probably even decreases risk of progression of ischaemic heart disease.

b. **True.** Otherwise there is a risk of endometrial carcinoma.

c. **True.** But therapy for 5–10 years is needed.

d. **False.** The evidence is that HRT increase the risks of breast cancer.

e. **False.** Vasomotor symptoms may start even before the last period and may be treated.

Case history answers

Case history 1

1. Carbimazole (perhaps with thyroxine added at a later stage when euthyroid again) and a nonspecific beta-blocker (if not contraindicated).

2. The risks of agranulocytosis on carbimazole: she must be warned to return immediately if she develops any signs of infection, such as a sore throat, so that her white cell count can be checked.

3. The antibodies that cause hyperthyroidism in Graves' disease can cross the placenta and cause neonatal hyperthyroidism: carbimazole may cause goitre in a fetus and this may lead to complications in the delivery.

4. The options are long-term carbimazole, surgery or radioiodine (even in someone so young, this is a safe treatment).

5. Oral contraceptives increase production of thyroid-binding globulin, giving rise to increased serum total thyroxine concentrations (but not free thyroxine or thyroid-stimulating hormone, which remain normal). Some heavily protein-bound drugs (such as phenytoin) can cause displacement of thyroxine from protein-binding sites and lower total (but not free) thyroxine.

Case history 2

1. Weight loss, diet and perhaps oral antihyperglycaemics. She should be educated about lifestyle, smoking, etc.

2. Metformin is most appropriate drug as first line in a patient with T2DM, particularly in an obese patient.

3. Sulphonylureas might be considered second line, in addition to metformin. They should probably not be used alone, if avoidable, in an

obese patient since they tend to stimulate the appetite.

4. Since she is hypertensive, thiazide diuretics might have been a precipitant; many other drugs, e.g. corticosteroids, are also possible. However, hypertension and diabetes are associated even in the absence of drug therapy.

5. Insulin should be considered if oral drugs fail to control her blood sugar, or during periods of intercurrent illness (e.g. infections, etc.) or surgery, when her diabetes is likely to go out of control.

Case history 3

1. Diabetic ketoacidosis.

2. Intravenous fluids to rehydrate, i.v. insulin to lower the blood sugar and K^+ supplements as appropriate, depending on the serum K^+. The precipitating cause should be identified and treated where possible.

3. Soluble insulin may be given i.v., i.m. or s.c.; all others are given s.c. only. In the future, insulin by inhaler may be available.

4. Hypoglycaemia.

5. He should be treated without delay, even if the diagnosis cannot be immediately confirmed: i.v. glucose can be given by trained staff, but in the absence of these, i.m. glucagon can be given by someone with very little training.

Case history 4

1. She might experience an Addisonian crisis with hypotension, collapse and death, since her hypothalamic–pituitary–adrenal axis is almost certainly suppressed and will need some time to recover. She might also experience a flare up of disease activity.

2. Prednisolone has some mineralocorticoid effects and will cause Na^+ and fluid retention.

3. She is at risk of osteoporosis and muscle wasting.

4. Impaired glucose tolerance, Cushingoid appearance, immune suppression are the most common.

5. Risk of an Addisonian crisis unless given additional parenteral steroids before operation; poor healing of wounds, which may delay recovery afterwards.

Case history 5

1. The COCP protects against endometrial and ovarian carcinoma but is associated with an increased incidence of cervical carcinoma. This may be caused by lifestyle rather than a direct drug effect. There may also be an increase in the incidence of breast carcinoma, although this is controversial.

2. She is at higher risk of myocardial infarction or cerebrovascular accident while taking a COCP and smoking: she should be advised to stop smoking. However, in a young woman this would not be a contraindication to the COCP.

3. If she is less than 12 hours late, she should take the pill as soon as possible and the next pill at the usual time. If more than 12 hours late, the pill may be ineffective: she should continue taking the pill as usual, but use additional barrier contraceptive methods for the next 7 days. If there were less than seven tablets left in the pack, she should begin the next pack without the usual 7-day break.

4. Pulmonary embolism.

5. Carbamazepine may induce liver enzymes and reduce the efficacy of the COCP. She may need a high-oestrogen dose pill.

Case history 6

1. Improvement in vasomotor and other symptoms of the menopause: no prophylactic effects can be anticipated in such short-term therapy.

2. Osteoporosis is common in women as there is increased bone loss after the menopause. HRT given for periods of 5–10 years reduces this but there are concerns that there may be an increased bone loss when HRT is stopped.

3. HRT probably decreases the risks of ischaemic heart disease.

4. The doses of oestrogen used in HRT are lower than in COCP and, therefore, fewer adverse effects are to be expected.

5. Systemic HRT will improve vaginal dryness, but if this is the predominant symptom, the patient may prefer to use just a local vaginal oestrogen ointment.

Short note answers

1. This should include hypertension, impaired glucose tolerance and possibly diabetes mellitus. Also cover skin changes, truncal obesity, immunosuppression, mental disturbances, cataract and suppression of the hypothalamic–pituitary–adrenal axis as well as the potential problems that may arise if the steroid is withdrawn suddenly.

2. This should include drugs such as carbimazole and propylthiouracil, including their possible adverse effects, and also discuss the role of surgery and radioiodine in long-term treatment of resistant disease.

3. This should consider the use of a long-acting insulin once or twice a day with short-acting insulin two or more times a day, in particular to cover mealtimes (expand on this a little bit).

4. This should include consideration of:
   a. vitamin D and calcium
   b. bisphosphonates if the patient is high risk and has demonstrated this, for instance by having an osteoporotic-related fracture
   c. hormone replacement therapy in women or use of selective oestrogen receptor modulator. Calcium and vitamin D can be considered for all patients, bisphosphonates for the high-risk patients and HRT or SERM for female patients who have other indications for these therapies as well.

Extended matching items answers

Theme: Drug selection in endocrinology

1. I. Oestradiol, a naturally occurring oestrogen, is the most commonly used. Synthetic oestrogens such as ethinylestradiol are avoided as it is thought that they might cause excessive stimulation of breast tissue.

2. K. Goserelin is a long-acting LHRH analogue which decreases oestrogen (and testosterone) production by causing down-regulation and loss of sensitivity of LHRH receptors.

3. E. Hydrocortisone (aldosterone is a hormone and not a drug).

4. D. Levonorgestrel.

5. H. Tamoxifen is an oestrogen antagonist in breast tissue but an oestrogen agonist in some other areas such as bone and endometrium.

6. A. Ethinylestradiol, a synthetic oestrogen.

7. B or D. Levonorgestrel or gestodene are both used. Gestodene-containing pills are associated with an increased risk of thromboembolic disorders compared with pills containing the older progestogens such as levonorgestrel.

8. L. Finasteride inhibits formation of the active dihydrotestosterone and has anti-androgenic effects in the prostate (and some other tissues such as the scalp). Some other drugs named here (goserelin, flutamide) have anti-androgenic effects and are used in prostatic cancer but not in benign prostatic hypertrophy.

Theme: Making a diagnosis in endocrine disorders

1. F. The patient demonstrates many of the classical clinical features of hyperthyroidism, often mistaken for anxiety in its early stages and ignored by patients and doctors alike.

2. H. This is hypothyroidism at its most extreme. It is rare to see such presentations but you should be aware of classical presentations of common disorders.

3. J. This is type 1 diabetes. He demonstrates the osmotic symptoms with weight loss. He should be tested for ketosis, and if positive significant ketoacidosis should be excluded.

4. G. This is a medical emergency.

5. B. Patients with severe hypertension refractory to treatment should be investigated for secondary causes. The presence of hypertension and hypokalaemia should alert you to the possibility of Conn's syndrome.

Theme: Management of diabetes mellitus

1. F. In the absence of any contraindications such as renal failure, metformin should be used as first line therapy in the management of T2DM following a trial period of dietary modification.

2. E. This is diabetic ketoacidosis. This is a medical emergency. He should be given an

intravenous insulin infusion and aggressive fluid resuscitation. He is very dehydrated.

3. H. This is a new diagnosis of presumed T1DM (if the patient is not obese). He will need to be started on insulin therapy, but this can be a subcutaneous regimen if he is not acutely unwell.

4. H. There are contraindications to many further oral agents: renal failure (metformin) and cardiac failure (pioglitazone). Insulin therapy will need to be started without further delay.

5. B. It would be appropriate to have a trial period of dietary modification in the first instance. This patient needs referral to a dietician.

Theme: Mechanism of action of endocrine drugs

1. F. The exact mechanism of action is unknown. It is essentially insulin-sensitising.

2. I. Carbimazole and propylthiouracil have these properties.

3. D. Sulphonylureas thus require some β cell function being left in order to work.

Antibiotics (antimicrobials)

13.1	Action and use of antibiotics	191
13.2	Major antibiotics	194
13.3	Antibiotics for mycobacterial infections	200
	Self-assessment on Chapter 13: questions	202
	Self-assessment on Chapter 13: answers	206

Overview

Antibiotics are substances that kill or inhibit the growth of microorganisms. The first antibiotics were produced by and isolated from microorganisms but subsequently knowledge of these agents has been used to synthesise chemotherapeutic agents. Biochemical differences between the host and the pathogen have also been exploited to produce drugs with selective toxicity.

In this chapter the major antibiotics are described in terms of their mode of action, their therapeutic use and their adverse effects. The effect of microbial resistance to drugs is also covered. The antibiotic regimens used for tuberculosis and leprosy are also discussed.

13.1 Action and use of antibiotics

Learning objectives

At the end of this section you should:
- understand the broad principles governing use of antibiotics
- be able to describe the common mechanisms by which antimicrobials work
- know examples of an antibiotic working by each mechanism
- be able to outline mechanisms of microbial resistance to antibiotics and the implications of this for prescribing.

Antimicrobials are drugs used to treat infection. They may be:

- antibacterial (often called antibiotics, since many are derivatives of naturally produced chemicals)
- antiviral (Ch. 14)
- antifungal (Ch. 14)
- antiprotozoal (Ch. 14)
- anthelmintic (Ch. 14).

Antibiotics may either kill the microorganism (bactericidal) or may retard their growth (bacteriostatic) so that the body's own immune system can overcome the infection. In clinical use, this distinction is usually not important, but bacteriostatic drugs should not be used in immunosuppressed patients, nor in life-threatening diseases such as endocarditis or meningitis.

Clinical sketch

A man presents with weight loss and fever, present for about 3 weeks. Examination reveals no clear cause of this and initial investigations including a chest radiograph are normal. The full blood count shows a slightly raised white cell count at 13×10^9/litre (normal 4–11) and the erythrocyte sedimentation rate (ESR) is raised at 52 mm/h (normal is up to 12). It is not clear what is wrong but the doctor prescribes broad spectrum antibiotics.

Comment: This is bad practice. Patients such as this require investigation to identify the cause of the fever. The ESR and full blood count are nonspecific markers of inflammation, most often caused by infection but a range of other causes are possible, such as malignancy or autoimmune disease. The prescription of broad spectrum antibiotics will muddy the water and will delay diagnosis of the true cause. It might also lead to disastrous partial treatment of a condition such as infective endocarditis. A patient with a fever for this long requires thorough investigation and a definitive diagnosis.

A 30-year-old patient who previously had rheumatic fever presents with fever, clubbing and splinter haemorrhages. The patient has the murmur of aortic incompetence. Blood cultures grow *Streptococcus viridans*.

Comment: This patient has infective endocarditis and will require intensive antibiotic therapy, typically (given the organism) for a prolonged period, and may even need surgery. A typical regimen (depending on antibiotic sensitivities of the organism and local policies) would be benzylpenicillin i.v. for 2 weeks, followed by oral amoxicillin for a further 2 weeks or longer. For the first week, the patient might also be prescribed gentamicin, with monitoring of plasma concentrations. Infectious endocarditis is a serious illness, which will be fatal if not adequately treated.

Principles of prescribing antibiotics

Antibiotics are often abused, i.e. used excessively or inappropriately, for example to treat minor viral infections (especially in childhood). Broad principles for the use of antibiotics, therefore include:

1. Make a diagnosis of bacterial infection (fever alone does not always imply bacterial infection) and its site and consider the likely organisms, e.g. in lobar pneumonia, the likely organism is *Streptococcus pneumoniae*.
2. Wherever possible, and particularly in all serious infections, take appropriate specimens (blood, sputum, pus, urine, swabs) for culture and antibiotic sensitivity testing, and perhaps for microscopy and Gram staining. It is not always practical to do this.
3. Consider the need for antibiotic therapy at all, e.g. antibiotics are usually inappropriate in gastroenteritis or many skin infections.
4. If cultures have been taken, is there a need for urgent therapy before results are available? Empirical antibiotic therapy may be necessary in seriously ill patients but may prevent the confirmation of the diagnosis of infection later or the identification of the infecting organism. This may be particularly important when there is a subsequent failure to respond or only partial response to the chosen antibiotic.

5. Select the most appropriate drug, its dose and route of administration. Consider the following factors.
   a. The organism: what antibiotics is it sensitive to? This would ideally be based on microbiological sensitivity testing but may have to be a 'best guess' if the organism or its sensitivities are not known.
   b. The patient: age, allergy, renal or hepatic function, diminished resistance to infection (malnutrition, malignant disease, immunosuppression, including by drugs such as corticosteroids), pregnancy or genetic factors (may all influence choice of or response to antibiotics).
   c. The severity of the infection: this will influence the choice of drug and route of administration. Some antibiotics are not absorbed when given orally (e.g. aminoglycosides). In seriously ill patients, parenteral administration is more reliable.
   d. The site of infection: antibiotics often do not penetrate abscess cavities well, and abscesses in general require drainage in addition. Some antibiotics may not penetrate to the site of infection (e.g. aminoglycosides are inappropriate for meningitis).
   e. The presence of foreign bodies: such as a prosthetic heart valve or a piece of glass in a skin wound, again likely to diminish or prevent response to antibiotics.
6. Monitor success of therapy clinically, or microbiologically by repeated cultures as appropriate. Some antibiotics with serious concentration-related toxicity also require monitoring of plasma concentrations (e.g. gentamicin).
7. Combinations of antibiotics are occasionally used:
   a. where there is a mixed infection, e.g. in peritonitis
   b. where the two antibiotics can produce a greater effect than one alone (synergism), e.g. penicillin and gentamicin in treating infective endocarditis
   c. where the infecting organism is not known and broad spectrum cover is required urgently, e.g. septicaemia
   d. to prevent the development of resistance to one antibiotic, e.g. in tuberculosis.
8. Antibiotics may also be used occasionally for prophylaxis, i.e. to prevent the development of

infection rather than to treat established infection. Examples are in some abdominal or orthopaedic surgery, in dental procedures for patients at risk of infective endocarditis, or in the close contacts of patients who have meningococcal meningitis. The duration of prophylactic use is brief (usually 24 hours or less), and the choice of drug is based on previous experience of what organisms are likely to be responsible.

Reasons not to use antibiotics without consideration:

- risk of missing alternative diagnosis
- adverse reactions
- promotion of antibiotic resistance
- expense.

Sites of action

Antibiotics may act at different sites (Fig. 49):

- by inhibiting formation of the bacterial cell wall, e.g. penicillin and cephalosporins
- by inhibiting bacterial protein synthesis, e.g. tetracyclines, aminoglycosides, erythromycin, chloramphenicol
- by inhibiting nucleic acid synthesis, either at an early stage, e.g. sulphonamides, trimethoprim, or later, e.g. ciprofloxacin, rifampicin
- by altering the permeability of cytoplasmic membranes, e.g. amphotericin (an antifungal, see Ch. 14).

Protein synthesis inhibited e.g. aminoglycosides

Formation of cell wall impaired e.g. penicillin

Cell membrane permeability altered e.g. amphoteracin

Nucleic acid synthesis or DNA formation inhibited e.g. sulphonamides

Fig. 49 Modes of action of antibiotics.

Clinical sketch

A patient is found to have septicaemia with the methicillin resistant *Staphylococcus aureus (MRSA)*. The doctor seeks advice from the microbiologist as to the most appropriate treatment.

Comment: This organism is becoming increasingly common in hospitals. While it is often a harmless commensal, its spread between patients and staff in hospitals should be limited as much as possible by barrier nursing techniques and basic hygiene. Specific treatment is often not necessary unless it causes serious illness, as in this case. If the organism is resistant to flucloxacillin, treatment may involve the following antibiotics: vancomycin or teicoplanin, gentamicin, fusidic acid, rifampicin. These drugs may need to be used in combinations depending on the patient's response and the severity of illness. Organisms resistant to each and even all of these drugs are reported.

Antimicrobial resistance

The increased use of an antibiotic encourages the emergence of resistant strains of bacteria. There are geographic variations in antibiotic resistance depending on local prescribing trends. For safe empirical therapy, it is important to know the local patterns of resistance and help should be sought from a microbiologist. The reasons for resistance vary. Some antibiotics would never affect an organism because of its structure and their site of action. For example, Gram-negative bacilli are resistant to benzylpenicillin.

Mechanisms of resistance

Some bacteria acquire resistance. These traits may arise as new mutations or may be transferred from organism to organism by plasmids (DNA packages) either by conjugation or transduction, or by bacteriophage viruses.

Resistance can occur through a number of mechanisms:

- the production of an enzyme that breaks down the antibiotic, e.g. β-lactamase and many penicillins. Some penicillins are designed to be resistant to this, e.g. methicillin or flucloxacillin, but resistance may also occur by other routes
- the cell membrane becomes impermeable to a drug, e.g. tetracyclines
- structural or biochemical alteration within the organism makes it less susceptible, e.g. alteration

of ribosomal structure may lead to erythromycin resistance

- development of a pathway that bypasses the reaction inhibited by the antibiotic, e.g. a dihydrofolate reductase that is insensitive to trimethoprim inhibition.

13.2 Major antibiotics

Learning objectives

At the end of this section you should:
- be able to list the major classes of antibiotics, giving examples
- know their spectrum of activity
- know their adverse effects.

Clinical sketch

A 25-year-old woman presents with dysuria and frequency. Dip stick testing of the urine shows blood and leucocytes. A midstream urine (MSU) specimen is sent to the laboratory. The doctor starts empirical treatment immediately with trimethoprim, and tells the patent to drink plenty of fluids.

Comment: The clinical features here are consistent with a urinary tract infection. A purist argument might be to wait until the results of the MSU are sent back from laboratory but this will take 3–4 days typically. The organisms that cause urinary tract infection are well known (most often Escherichia coli*) and in simple presentation such as this, empirical treatment is reasonable. It is, however, wise to reserve a sample (such as a MSU) before instituting antibiotic therapy, not necessarily in all cases but particularly in those with recurrent illness.*

Antibacterial treatment

Choice of drug should be guided by a local formulary, as sensitivities and local policies may vary. Table 2 is a summary of typical first line drugs that might be used to treat specific infections while awaiting culture and sensitivity results.

Penicillins

The penicillins contain a β-lactam ring and inhibit the formation of peptidoglycan cross-links in bacterial cell walls (especially in Gram-positive organisms). This weakens the cell wall and water enters the cell by osmosis, causing cells to burst. Penicillins are bactericidal but can act only on dividing cells and are not toxic to animal cells, which have no cell wall.

Pharmacokinetics

The penicillins:

- are poorly lipid soluble and do not cross the blood–brain barrier in appreciable concentrations unless it is inflamed (so they are effective in meningitis)
- are actively excreted unchanged by tubular secretion in the kidney: this can be blocked by probenecid to potentiate penicillin's action, and will require dose reduction in severe renal failure
- may be acid labile (i.e. broken down by the stomach acid and so inactive when given orally) or acid stable.

Resistance

Usually resistance is the result of production of β-lactamase in the bacteria, which destroys the β-lactam ring. It occurs in organisms such as *Staphylococcus aureus* (90% of strains), *Haemophilus influenzae* (15%), *S. pneumoniae* and *Neisseria gonorrhoeae* (about 5–10%).

Examples

Benzylpenicillin (penicillin G) is acid labile and β-lactamase sensitive and is only given parenterally. It is the most potent penicillin but has a relatively narrow spectrum covering *Streptococcus pyogenes*, *S. pneumoniae*, *Neisseria meningitidis* or *N. gonorrhoeae*, treponemes, *Listeria*, *Actinomyces* and many anaerobic organisms, e.g. *Clostridium* sp.

Phenoxymethylpenicillin (penicillin V) is acid stable but not well absorbed. It is given orally for minor infections; it is otherwise similar to benzylpenicillin.

Ampicillin is less active than benzylpenicillin against Gram-positive bacteria but has a broader spectrum including (in addition to those above) *Streptococcus faecalis*, *H. influenzae*, and some *Escherichia coli*, *Klebsiella* and *Proteus* strains. It is acid stable and is given orally or parenterally; it is β-lactamase sensitive.

Amoxicillin is similar to ampicillin but better absorbed orally. Amoxicillin is sometimes combined with *clavulanic acid*, which is a β-lactam with little antibacterial effect but which binds strongly to β-lactamase. It therefore blocks the action of β-lactamase and extends the spectrum of amoxicillin. The combination is called co-amoxiclav.

Flucloxacillin is acid stable and is given orally or parenterally. It is β-lactamase resistant and is used as a narrow spectrum drug for *S. aureus* infections.

Table 2 Typical first line drug therapy for infections while awaiting laboratory tests

Infection	First line therapy
Respiratory tract	
Sore throat	Antibiotic not usually necessary
Tonsilitis	Phenoxymethylpenicillin or erythromycin
Sinusitis	Amoxicillin or erythromycin or doxycycline
Acute-on-chronic bronchitis	Amoxicillin or erythromycin
Community acquired pneumonia (healthy chest)	Amoxicillin and/or erythromycin
Community acquired pneumonia (COPD)	First line amoxicillin and/or erythromycin; second line co-amoxiclav or oral cephalosporin or fluoroquinolone
Severe pneumonia or hospital acquired pneumonia	Injectable third generation cephalosporin ± macrolide
Suspected 'atypical' pneumonia	Erythromycin
Tuberculosis	Rifampicin/isoniazid/pyrazinamide
Urinary tract	
Cystitis	Trimethoprim, nitrofurantoin
Pyelonephritis	Co-amoxiclav or ciprofloxacin
Pelvic inflammatory disease	Metronidazole and doxycycline, or co-amoxiclav
Skin	
Erysipelas	Amoxicillin
Cellulitis	Flucloxacillin (perhaps with amoxicillin)
CNS	
Meningitis	Initial blind therapy benzylpenicillin or ceftriaxone
Abdominal sepsis	
Biliary tree	Injectable cephalosporin or ciprofloxacin
Pseudomembranous colitis	Metronidazole or vancomycin orally
Peritonitis	Injectable cephalosporin and metronidazole
Endocarditis	
Streptococcus viridans	Benzylpenicillin with gentamicin
Streptococcus faecalis	Amoxicillin and gentamicin
Staphylococcus aureus or *S. epidermidis*	Flucloxacillin and gentamicin
Septicaemia	Injected cephalosporin or amoxicillin with gentamicin
Osteomyelitis	Flucloxacillin and fusidic acid

Piperacillin is not acid stable and is only used parenterally. It is β-lactamase sensitive and has a broad spectrum, which includes *Pseudomonas aeruginosa* and *Proteus* species. It is used i.v. for life-threatening infections, especially in immunocompromised patients, usually in combination with a tazobactam (which is similar to clavulanic acid) to extend its spectrum.

Adverse effects

Adverse effects are relatively unusual:

- Allergy occurs in 1–10% of patients, ranging from urticaria to potentially fatal anaphylaxis (this occurs in around 0.05% of patients); patients should always be asked about a history of previous exposure and adverse effects.

Rashes are common with ampicillin or amoxicillin (almost invariable if they are given in error to patients with infectious mononucleosis) and do not necessarily represent a true allergy.

About 10% of patients have been told that they are allergic to penicillin. Allergy is generally overdiagnosed because of the potential serious effects of readministration and because usually there are alternative antibiotics – many patients with so called 'allergy' have had minor non-allergic adverse effects, e.g. vomiting and diarrhoea. Patients with a history of anaphylaxis, urticaria or rash occurring early after administration of a penicillin should not receive a penicillin or other β-lactam antibiotic. If the patient has a minor rash 72 hours after

administration, this is probably not truly allergic: such patients might be given a penicillin if there is no reasonable alternative (but a true allergy is still possible)
- superinfections (e.g. oral thrush caused by *Candida*)
- diarrhoea: especially with ampicillin (20%), less common with amoxicillin, as it is better absorbed
- rare: blood dyscrasia or haemolysis; nephritis (ampicillin), hepatitis (co-amoxiclav, flucloxacillin), encephalopathy.

Drug interactions

The use of ampicillin (or other broad spectrum antibiotics) may decrease the effectiveness of oral contraceptives by diminishing enterohepatic circulation.

Cephalosporins

The cephalosporins also contain a β-lactam ring and are bactericidal. They are broad spectrum antibiotics.

There are many different cephalosporins with varying side chains; these side chains alter the pharmacokinetics, spectrum of activity and β-lactamase resistance. Cephalosporins are relatively expensive and, although good alternatives to penicillins when a broad spectrum drug is required, should not be used as first choice unless the organism is known to be sensitive. Some cephalosporins (e.g. cefotaxime) may be indicated for empirical use to treat life-threatening infections where the organism is probably sensitive.

Examples

Cefradine and cefalexin are well absorbed orally; cefradine can also be given parenterally. They are suitable for mostly Gram-positive organisms, e.g. *S. pyogenes, S. pneumoniae* and *S. aureus*, as well as some Gram-negative bacteria, although they are less effective in this than later cephalosporins. They are excreted by the kidney (reduce dose in renal failure).

Cefuroxime can be given parenterally or as an oral prodrug. It has a broader spectrum, including many Gram-negative bacilli.

Cefotaxime is given parenterally. It has an even broader spectrum, including many *Enterobacter, E. coli* and *Proteus* strains. *Ceftriaxone* is similar but has a long half-life and can be given only once per day.

Adverse effects
- allergy (10–20% of patients with penicillin allergy are also allergic to cephalosporins)
- nephritis and acute renal failure
- superinfections
- gastrointestinal upsets when given orally.

Aminoglycosides

The aminoglycosides are bactericidal. They cause misreading of mRNA by the ribosome, leading to abnormal protein production. To enter the bacterium, aminoglycosides need to be actively transported across the cell membrane; this does not occur in anaerobic organisms, which are, therefore, resistant.

Clinical pharmacokinetics

The aminoglycosides are:

- poorly lipid soluble and therefore not absorbed orally: parenteral administration is required for systemic effect
- unable to enter the CNS even when the meninges are inflamed
- not metabolised
- excreted unchanged by the kidney (where very high concentrations may occur, perhaps causing toxic tubular damage) by glomerular filtration (no active secretion); their clearance is markedly reduced in renal impairment and toxic concentrations are more likely.

Resistance

Resistance can develop through acquisition of plasmid-determined inactivating enzymes and through changes resulting in decreased transport of aminoglycosides into the cells.

Examples

Gentamicin is the most commonly used, covering Gram-negative aerobes, e.g. enteric organisms (*E. coli, Klebsiella, S. faecalis, Pseudomonas* and *Proteus* spp.), and is also used in antibiotic combinations against *S. aureus*. It is not active against aerobic streptococci. Gentamicin is often used blindly with other antibiotics in severe infections of unknown cause.

Streptomycin was formerly the mainstay of antituberculous therapy but is now rarely used in the developed world.

Tobramycin or *amikacin* are used for *Pseudomonas* and for some gentamicin-resistant organisms.

Topical use

Some aminoglycosides, e.g. gentamicin, may also be applied topically for local effect, for example in ear and eye ointments.

Adverse effects

The aminoglycosides have a narrow therapeutic window and toxicity is often related to plasma concentration. It is essential to *monitor plasma concentrations* (usually trough and peak, i.e. shortly before and after administration of a dose) to ensure adequate concentrations for bactericidal effect while minimising adverse effects, every 2–3 days during treatment:

- nephrotoxicity: may cause renal failure
- toxic to the 8th cranial nerve (ototoxic), especially the vestibular division
- other adverse effects are not dose related and are relatively rare, e.g. allergies, eosinophilia.

Macrolides

The macrolides are broad spectrum antibiotics to which resistance develops rapidly. They inhibit protein synthesis by binding to the ribosome and are bacteriostatic at usual doses but bactericidal in high doses.

Examples

Erythromycin is acid labile but is given as an enterically coated tablet; however, absorption is erratic and poor. It is given orally or parenterally. It is widely distributed in the body except to the brain and cerebrospinal fluid. Erythromycin is excreted unchanged in bile and is reabsorbed lower down the gastrointestinal tract (enterohepatic circulation). Its spectrum of activity includes *S. aureus*, *S. pyogenes* and *S. pneumoniae*. It is especially useful in these infections as an alternative to penicillins in allergic patients. In addition, it is specifically indicated in *Legionella pneumoniae*, *Mycoplasma pneumoniae* and *Chlamydia* infections.

Clarithromycin and *azithromycin* are newer macrolides that may have fewer adverse effects. Their use is similar to that of erythromycin. In addition, clarithromycin is used to treat *Helicobacter pylori* (see Ch. 11).

Adverse effects

- gastrointestinal upsets (common with erythromycin)
- rarely hypersensitivity, or cholestatic jaundice.

Drug interactions

Erythromycin (and to a lesser extent clarithromycin) inhibits cytochrome P450 enzymes. This can increase the effect of a wide range of other drugs such as warfarin, ciclosporin, some antiepileptics, etc. (see Ch. 21.)

Clinical sketch

A patient with epilepsy takes carbamazepine. The patient is allegedly allergic to penicillin and when she develops a respiratory tract infection with fever and sputum, she is prescribed erythromycin. Two days later the patient is drowsy and ataxic.

Comment: erythromycin is a good choice for respiratory tract infections in patients who are allergic to amoxicillin or patients in whom atypical organisms such as Legionella *or* Mycoplasma *are suspected. However, it does inhibit liver enzymes and they reduce metabolism of other drugs, such as carbamazepine, leading to toxic plasma concentrations of this drug. A better choice might have been to explore the details of the supposed allergy. If it seemed serious, then erythromycin might be used cautiously, or possibly another antibiotic entirely such as trimethoprim or tetracycline.*

Lincosamides; clindamycin

Clindamycin is chemically distinct to erythromycin but is similar in its mode of action and spectrum. It is rapidly absorbed and penetrates most tissues well, except the CNS. It is particularly useful systemically for *S. aureus* (especially osteomyelitis as it penetrates bone well) and anaerobic infections. It is also used in endocarditis prophylaxis.

Adverse effects

Diarrhoea is common. *Pseudomembranous colitis* is a serious inflammation of the large bowel caused by a superinfection with a strain of *Clostridium difficile*, which secretes a toxin that damages the mucosal lining; this may occur after any antibiotic but is especially common after clindamycin, which severely limits its use.

Sulphonamides and trimethoprim

Sulphonamides are rarely used alone today. Trimethoprim is not chemically related but is considered here because their modes of action are complementary.

Sulphonamides

Sulphonamides are competitive antagonists of para-aminobenzoic acid (PABA), a precursor of folic acid that is essential for the synthesis of purine nucleotides for DNA and RNA. Animals do not manufacture folate, depending on absorbed folate, and so are unaffected. The sulphonamides are bacteriostatic and effective against Gram-positive and many Gram-negative organisms.

Trimethoprim

Folate is activated by the enzyme dihydrofolate reductase to tetrahydrofolic acid. Trimethoprim inhibits this enzyme in bacteria and to a lesser degree in animals. It is bacteriostatic. Trimethoprim is well absorbed and excreted by the kidneys. It has a similar spectrum to the sulphonamides. It is widely used, especially for urinary tract infections and also for respiratory tract infections.

Co-trimoxazole

Co-trimoxazole is a combination of a sulphonamide (*sulfamethoxazole*) and trimethoprim. It blocks the same pathway at two different positions and is bactericidal. This combination is widely used in Europe and the USA, but in the UK is considered to have no advantage over trimethoprim alone in most indications, while being more toxic.

Co-trimoxazole is, however, the drug of choice for the treatment and prevention of pneumonia caused by *Pneumocystis carinii* in immunosuppressed patients.

Adverse effects

Gastrointestinal upsets can result from both components of co-trimoxazole.

Less common but more serious are effects of the components individually and as a combination:

- sulphonamides
  — allergy, rash, fever
  — agranulocytosis
  — Stevens–Johnson syndrome (a severe skin reaction)
  — haemolysis in patients with glucose 6-phosphatase deficiency
  — renal toxicity: sulphonamides may form crystals in an acid urine leading to tubular damage and severe renal impairment
  — inhibition of metabolism of other drugs
- trimethoprim:
  — macrocytic anaemia
  — thrombocytopenia

- co-trimoxazole:
  — aplastic anaemia (especially in the elderly).

Quinolones

The quinolones are effective antibiotics, but other less expensive drugs are often equally effective, especially for minor infections. Resistance to quinolones is becoming more common and, in general, their use as first line drugs should be limited.

Quinolones inhibit DNA gyrase and prevent recoiling of DNA after replication. This is bactericidal to dividing cells.

Examples

Nalidixic acid, the first quinolone, is used as a urinary antiseptic and for lower urinary tract infections as it has no systemic antibacterial effect.

Ciprofloxacin is a fluoroquinolone with a broad spectrum against Gram-positive and Gram-negative bacilli and *Pseudomonas* spp. It is given orally or i.v. to treat a wide range of infections, including urinary tract and respiratory infections (*Haemophilus*, *Branhamella*) as well as peritonitis (Gram-negative bacilli) and salmonella infection. It is used as prophylaxis for the contacts of patients with meningococcal meningitis.

Levofloxacin, an isomer of ofloxacin, has good activity against pneumococcus and is a second line drug for community acquired pneumonia. It hence may be useful in penicillin hypersensitivity.

Adverse effects

- gastrointestinal upsets
- fluoroquinolones may block the inhibitory neurotransmitter GABA, and this may cause confusion in the elderly and lower the fitting threshold; they should be used with caution in patients with epilepsy
- allergy and anaphylaxis
- tendinitis and rupture, e.g. of Achilles tendon; possibly damage to growing cartilage. Not recommended, therefore, for children or pregnant women.

Drug interactions

Ciprofloxacin is a liver enzyme inhibitor and may cause life-threatening interactions with drugs such as theophylline. Levofloxacin is less likely to cause these.

Tetracyclines

The tetracyclines are bacteriostatic and act by binding to the bacterial ribosome and interfering with protein synthesis.

Examples

Tetracycline, oxytetracycline have short half-lives, while *doxycycline* has a longer half-life and can be given once per day. These drugs:

- are not well absorbed
- bind avidly to heavy metal ions and so absorption is greatly reduced if taken with food, milk, antacids or iron tablets; they should be taken at least half an hour before food
- concentrate in bones and teeth
- are excreted mostly in urine, partly in bile
- are broad spectrum, active against most bacteria except *proteus* or *pseudomonas*; resistance is frequent
- are specifically indicated for *Mycoplasma, Rickettsia, Chlamydia* and *Brucella* infections
- are widely used to treat acne, given either orally or topically.

Adverse effects

- gastrointestinal upset
- superinfection: candidiasis
- discolouration and deformity in growing teeth and bones (contraindicated in pregnancy and in children under 12 years)
- renal impairment (should also be avoided in renal disease).

Metronidazole

Metronidazole binds to DNA and blocks replication. It is well absorbed after oral or rectal administration and can also be given i.v. It is widely distributed in the body (including into abscess cavities) and is metabolised by the liver.

Use

Metronidazole is:

- active against anaerobic organisms (e.g. *Bacteroides, Clostridia*), which are encountered particularly in abdominal surgery
- used to treat pseudomembranous colitis or severe antibiotic related diarrhoea (*Cl. difficile*)
- used against protozoa such as *Trichomonas, Giardia* and *Entamoeba* infections (Ch. 14)
- often part of the treatment of *Helicobacter pylori* (Ch. 11)

- used also to treat a variety of dental infections, particularly dental abscess.

Adverse effects

- nausea, anorexia and a metallic taste
- ataxia, caused by peripheral neuropathy
- disulfiram-like reaction (Ch. 18): metronidazole inhibits alcohol dehydrogenase (an enzyme in the pathway metabolising alcohol) and patients receiving it who drink alcohol may experience unpleasant reactions (flushing, abdominal pain, hypotension) as acetaldehyde accumulates; patients taking metronidazole should be advised not to drink alcohol
- possibly teratogenic if taken in the first trimester of pregnancy.

Drug interactions

Metronidazole may inhibit the metabolism of warfarin.

Nitrofurantoin

Nitrofurantoin is used as a urinary antiseptic and to treat Gram-negative infections in the lower urinary tract. It is taken orally and is well absorbed. It is excreted unchanged in the urine and is only antimicrobial when concentrated in the urine and so has no systemic antibacterial effect. It is ineffective in renal failure because of failure to concentrate. Resistance develops relatively quickly.

Adverse effects

- gastrointestinal upsets
- allergy (including pulmonary fibrosis)
- polyneuritis.

Fusidic acid

Fusidic acid is active only against *S. aureus* (by inhibiting bacterial protein synthesis). It is not affected by β-lactamase. It is given orally or parenterally and can be used alone or with flucloxacillin to reduce the development of resistance. It is well absorbed and widely distributed, including to bone (useful in osteomyelitis). It is metabolised in the liver.

Adverse effects

- gastrointestinal upsets
- hepatitis and jaundice.

Vancomycin and teicoplanin

The glycopeptide antibiotics vancomycin and teicoplanin interfere with bacterial cell wall formation and are only effective against Gram-positive organisms. They are not absorbed after oral administration and must be given parenterally. Both are excreted by the kidney. Vancomycin and teicoplanin are used i.v. to treat serious or resistant *S. aureus* infections and for prophylaxis of endocarditis in penicillin-allergic patients.

Vancomycin is given orally to treat pseudomembranous colitis (see above).

Teicoplanin is similar.

Adverse effects

Although not an aminoglycoside, vancomycin has similar plasma concentration-dependent toxicity and monitoring of plasma concentrations is essential. This is not necessary for teicoplanin, which is much less toxic. Effects include:

- nephrotoxicity
- ototoxicity
- allergy
- histamine release (after rapid injection of vancomycin: 'red man syndrome').

Linezolid

This is an antibiotic specifically used to treat MRSA and vancomycin resistant *S. aureus* infections. It is given intravenously or orally. It is a monoamine oxidase inhibitor with potential for serious interactions (see Ch. 21). It can also cause blood disorders.

13.3 Antibiotics for mycobacterial infections

> **Learning objectives**
>
> At the end of this section you should:
> - understand the significance of the increasing incidence of tuberculosis and the development of resistance
> - be aware of the current drug regimens for tuberculosis and leprosy
> - be aware of infections with atypical mycobacteria.

Mycobacteria spp. are intracellular pathogens that are resistant to host defences.

Tuberculosis

Tuberculosis (TB) is a major cause of death in many parts of the world (8 million new cases and 3 million deaths in 1996). In the developed world, TB is currently undergoing a resurgence, partly because of infection in immunosuppressed patients. *Mycobacterium tuberculosis* is an intracellular organism surviving inside phagocytes in a dormant form for many months. Consequently, therapy needs to be prolonged.

Drug-resistant mutants are often present and will proliferate if only single drug therapy is used; hence several drugs are used simultaneously to avoid resistance.

Failure of therapy is more often the result of poor compliance with the drugs rather than drug resistance. Supervision may be important to avoid this.

Regimens for treating pulmonary TB

Drug regimens will differ around the world, determined partly by bacterial resistance but mainly by economic factors. Currently recommended treatment in the UK is:

1. Initial phase: rifampicin, isoniazid, pyrazinamide and ethambutol for 2 months
2. Continuation phase: rifampicin and isoniazid for a further 4 months.

Some doubt the value of ethambutol and omit it. Several of these drugs are associated with liver toxicity and hepatic function should be checked pretreatment and again if the patient shows any signs of illness.

Isoniazid

Isoniazid is bactericidal but its mode of action is unknown. It is the most active of the anti-TB drugs. It is well absorbed after oral administration and widely distributed, including into the CNS.

Isoniazid is acetylated by the liver before excretion; this shows *genetic polymorphism* (i.e. variation in metabolism owing to genetic differences producing enzymes of different activity) giving rise to fast and slow acetylators, which occur with different frequencies in different populations (see Ch. 1). Acetylation ability may affect efficiency and toxicity in an individual.

Adverse effects

- peripheral neuropathy (occurs particularly in slow acetylators and is preventable by giving pyridoxine)
- hepatitis
- rashes
- drug-induced lupus syndrome: a syndrome resembling systemic lupus erythematosus.

Drug interactions

Isoniazid is a liver enzyme inhibitor (caution with phenytoin and warfarin).

Rifampicin

Rifampicin inhibits RNA synthesis in bacteria but not in humans and is bactericidal. It is also a valuable broad spectrum antibiotic but its use is restricted mainly to tuberculosis and to a small number of other uses: prophylaxis for the contacts of patients with meningococcal meningitis, and the treatment of *Legionella pneumoniae* and resistant *S. aureus*.

Rifampicin is well absorbed after oral administration (best taken on an empty stomach) and is widely distributed. It is metabolised in the liver and excreted in bile.

Adverse effects

- malaise, headache
- fever, rashes
- hepatitis
- invariably, all body secretions (urine, tears, etc.) become an orange–red colour.

Drug interactions

Rifampicin is a potent liver enzyme inducer and may cause interactions with anticonvulsants, warfarin, oral contraceptives, etc.

Pyrazinamide

Pyrazinamide is bactericidal. It is well absorbed and widely distributed, in particular achieving good penetration of the CNS.

Adverse effects

- hepatitis, especially if given at high doses; liver function tests should be monitored
- hyperuricaemia.

Ethambutol

Ethambutol is bacteriostatic but its mode of action is unknown. It is excreted by the kidneys.

Adverse effects

Optic neuritis, which is dose related and rare. Check visual acuity before starting therapy.

Reserve drugs

Reserve drugs in TB include para-*aminosalicylate, capreomycin, cycloserine, and streptomycin* which are also used in the treatment of atypical mycobacteria.

Leprosy

Leprosy is caused by infection with *Mycobacterium leprae*. A mixture of drugs are used to treat leprosy, depending on the type and severity of the infection and the local resistance patterns, e.g. *rifampicin* and *dapsone*. Dapsone is related to the sulphonamides and also inhibits folate metabolism (also used to treat dermatitis herpetiformis; see Ch. 16).

Adverse effects include haemolysis, gastrointestinal upsets and rashes.

Atypical mycobacteria

The atypical mycobacteria are environmental species that do not normally infect humans. They infect immunocompromised individuals causing pulmonary, skin, soft tissue infections and systemic infections. *M. avium intracellulare* (MAI) infection is a serious problem in HIV-positive patients. Treatment is difficult because they are often drug resistant but includes the reserve drugs listed for TB.

Thirteen

Self-assessment on Chapter 13: questions

Multiple choice questions

1. The following antimicrobials should be avoided in pregnant women:
   a. Gentamicin
   b. Tetracycline
   c. Amoxicillin
   d. Nitrofurantoin
   e. Trimethoprim

2. In treating any infection:
   a. Cultures must always be taken first
   b. The clinical picture is of no help in deciding appropriate antibiotic therapy
   c. Superinfection implies infection with an organism resistant to antibiotics
   d. Antibiotic therapy may be standardised for all patients with each infection
   e. Combinations of antibiotics are sometimes useful

3. Failure to respond to an antibiotic may result from:
   a. Microbial resistance to the antibiotics used
   b. Inappropriate selection of antibiotics
   c. Immunosuppression of the patient
   d. Inappropriate route of administration
   e. Good blood supply to the area infected

4. Penicillins:
   a. Are highly lipid soluble
   b. Are excreted by glomerular filtration
   c. Can all be destroyed by β-lactamase-producing bacteria
   d. Some may be given orally
   e. Are usually highly effective against streptococcal infection

5. Anaphylaxis:
   a. Should be treated with adrenaline (epinephrine)
   b. Is life-threatening
   c. May occur within seconds or minutes of administration of a drug
   d. Usually occurs on first exposure to the drug
   e. Is caused by endotoxin release

6. Aminoglycosides:
   a. Cross the blood–brain barrier
   b. Are metabolised by the liver
   c. May cause ototoxicity
   d. Require plasma concentration measurement
   e. Are effective against anaerobic organisms such as bacteroides

7. Erythromycin:
   a. May interact with phenytoin
   b. Is well absorbed after oral administration
   c. May cause nausea and vomiting
   d. May be used to treat *Legionella pneumoniae*
   e. Cross-allergy to penicillin may occur

8. Sulphonamides:
   a. May cause drug interactions by displacement from plasma proteins
   b. Inhibit nucleic acid formation in humans
   c. Co-trimoxazole may cause blood dyscrasias
   d. Co-trimoxazole may be used in the treatment of patients with AIDS
   e. Trimethoprim is more likely to cause adverse drug reactions than co-trimoxazole

9. Ciprofloxacin:
   a. Blocks protein synthesis
   b. Is the first choice drug for pneumonia
   c. May cause drug hypersensitivity
   d. Is effective against Gram-negative bacilli
   e. May cause interactions with theophylline

10. Tetracyclines:
    a. Are used to treat acne
    b. Should be taken with meals
    c. Should not be given to young children
    d. Bacterial resistance is rare
    e. Superinfection is common

11. Metronidazole:
    a. Is well absorbed
    b. Is effective in some protozoal infections
    c. Can be used to treat peptic ulcer disease
    d. May cause cerebellar damage
    e. May interact with ethanol

12. The antibiotic:
    a. Vancomycin is an aminoglycoside
    b. Vancomycin may be given orally to treat pseudomembranous colitis
    c. Fusidic acid and vancomycin are both effective against *Staphylococcus aureus*
    d. Linezolid is widely used for Gram-positive respiratory tract infections
    e. Nitrofurantoin is used for Gram-negative septicaemia

13. In treating tuberculosis:
    a. Multiple drug therapy is usual
    b. Treatment for 1 month is considered adequate
    c. Isoniazid is metabolised at different rates in different races
    d. Isoniazid may cause hepatic failure
    e. Isoniazid may cause liver enzyme induction

14. In treating tuberculosis (TB):
    a. Rifampicin is only used against TB
    b. Rifampicin inhibits the metabolism of warfarin
    c. Rifampicin may cause the urine to change colour
    d. Pyrazinamide may cause hepatitis
    e. Patients about to start taking ethambutol should have their eyes checked first

Case history questions

Case history 1

A 23-year-old woman presents with a urinary tract infection causing cystitis.

1. What general advice should be given to her?
2. What antibiotics should be considered?
3. If the woman was pregnant, how would this alter your choice of antibiotic?

Case history 2

A 54-year-old alcoholic man with no fixed address is found to have tuberculosis with acid- and alcohol-fast bacilli seen in the sputum.

1. Is he infectious?
2. What drugs should be administered and in what regimen?

3. Do his social circumstances pose any problems?

Case history 3

A 65-year-old man with a long history of chronic obstructive airway disease develops acute bronchitis: his doctor decides to prescribe an antibiotic.

1. What antibiotics would be appropriate first choices?

A week later, the patient returns to the doctor complaining of severe diarrhoea.

2. What diagnosis should be considered?
3. If this diagnosis is confirmed, how should it be treated?

Short note questions

Write short notes on:
1. Drugs used in the treatment of tuberculosis.
2. Adverse effects of antibiotics.

Essay question

List some strategies that can be adopted to reduce the risks of bacterial resistance to antibiotics developing.

Extended matching items questions

Theme: Antibiotics in primary care

Options
A. Flucloxacillin
B. Ciprofloxacin
C. Trimethoprim
D. Phenoxymethylpenicillin
E. Co-amoxiclav
F. Amoxicillin
G. Cefaclor
H. Erythromycin
I. Clindamycin
J. Levofloxacin

Which of the antibiotics options listed above would be the best choice in the following patients seen by their GP? There may be more than one reasonable option. Each option can be used once, more than once, or not at all.

1. A 67-year-old man with an exacerbation of his chronic obstructive pulmonary disease who is coughing increased volumes of purulent sputum. He has just recovered from an exacerbation during which he was treated with amoxicillin without any adverse effects.

2. A 26-year-old pregnant woman with dysuria, frequency and a temperature of 38.5°C. The urine dipstick is positive for nitrites and leucocytes.

3. A 60-year-old man, previously well, with a lobar pneumonia. There is a significant history of allergy to penicillin.

4. A 65-year-old diabetic woman with redness, swelling and pain in her ankle. The clinical diagnosis is cellulitis.

5. An otherwise healthy 20-year-old girl with a sore throat.

Theme: Choice of antibiotic and route of administration

Options

A. Oral gentamicin
B. Intravenous flucloxacillin
C. Intravenous ceftriaxone
D. Oral erythromycin
E. Oral trimethoprim
F. Oral ciprofloxacin
G. Oral metronidazole
H. Intravenous vancomycin
I. Intravenous benzylpenicillin
J. Intravenous metronidazole

Choose the most appropriate antibiotic and its route of administration from the list of options above to treat the following conditions. Each option can be used once, more than once, or not at all.

1. An intravenous drug user who presents with fever and an abscess in his left groin. Blood cultures have grown *Staphylococcus aureus*.

2. A 54-year-old man with no significant past medical history who presents with community-acquired pneumonia of mild/ moderate severity. He is probably allergic to penicillin.

3. A 70-year-old woman with chronic bilateral leg ulcers who presents with fever, cellulitis of the right leg and diarrhoea. Blood cultures have grown *Streptococcus pyogenes.*

4. A 20-year-old office worker who has been on holiday in Spain and, on returning to the UK, presents 2 days later with clinical features suggestive of acute bacterial meningitis.

5. An 80-year-old woman presents to her GP with a 4-day history of pain when passing urine and low abdominal pain. She suffers from recurrent urinary tract infections and *E. coli* has previously been cultured from the urine.

Theme: Serious infections in hospitals

Options

A. Ceftriaxone
B. Gentamicin
C. Co-amoxiclav
D. Teicoplanin
E. Clarithromycin
F. Flucloxacillin
G. Piperacillin
H. Metronidazole
I. Rifampicin
J. Ciprofloxacin

Choose the most appropriate antibiotic from the list above to treat the following conditions. Each option can be used once, more than once, or not at all.

1. Community acquired pneumonia with pyrexia, dyspnoea and a low oxygen saturation in an otherwise fit elderly man.

2. Staphylococcal cellulitis in the foot of a diabetic with peripheral vascular disease.

3. Methicillin-resistant *Staphylococcus aureus* (MRSA) septicaemia.

4. Severe diarrhoea and dehydration in a patient recently admitted and treated with intravenous cephalosporins for a respiratory tract infection.

5. Pneumonia in a patient recently admitted with a stroke.

Theme: Mechanisms of action and adverse effects

Options

A. Inhibits protein synthesis
B. Inhibits folate synthesis
C. Inhibits DNA synthesis
D. Inhibits plasma membrane synthesis
E. Inhibits cell wall synthesis
F. Diarrhoea
G. Impaired renal function
H. Anaphylaxis
 I. Marrow suppression
J. Drug interactions due to interference with liver enzymes

From the above list of options choose the most appropriate mode of action and a likely possible adverse effect of the following antibiotics. Each option can be used once, more than once, or not at all.

1. A patient with community-acquired pneumonia who is treated with an oral β-lactam antibiotic.

2. Trimethoprim used to treat urinary tract infection in an elderly female patient.

3. A patient with cystic fibrosis who is treated with a quinolone for chest infection.

4. A patient with high gentamicin trough concentrations.

5. Erythromycin given to a patient with penicillin allergy.

Self-assessment on Chapter 13: answers

Multiple choice answers

1. a. **True.** Aminoglycosides and vancomycin may cause 8th nerve damage in the fetus.
   b. **True.** Teeth and bone deformities may occur in the fetus.
   c. **False.** Widely used.
   d. **False.** May be used but should be avoided in late pregnancy or breastfeeding mothers.
   e. **True.** Folate antagonist and possibly teratogenic.

2. a. **False.** This is an ideal but not always possible, e.g. in severely ill patients.
   b. **False.** The clinical picture often gives clues, e.g. a lobar pneumonia is most often caused by *Streptococcus pneumoniae* and a penicillin is appropriate.
   c. **True.** At least to the antibiotic which has led to the superinfection.
   d. **False.** Although broad guidelines may be given, each case must be judged on its own merits (as occurs elsewhere in medicine).
   e. **True.** For example in treating tuberculosis.

3. a. **True.** For example, penicillinase-producing *Staphylococcus aureus* will not respond to amoxicillin.
   b. **True.** For example, use of benzylpenicillin to treat a Gram-negative infection would be inappropriate.
   c. **True.** If the patient is known to be immunosuppressed, antibiotic regimens will need to be more sophisticated and aggressive to achieve cure.
   d. **True.** For example, oral antibiotics to treat a septicaemia.
   e. **False.** Poor blood supply to an infected area may prevent antibiotic transport to the site, and importantly will also lead to poor tissue inflammatory responses and healing.

4. a. **False.** They are preferentially water soluble.
   b. **False.** They are excreted actively in the renal tubule.
   c. **False.** For example, flucloxacillin.
   d. **True.** For example, amoxicillin, etc.

e. **True.** Usually the drugs of first choice for this.

5. a. **True.** This is a physiological antagonist to histamine.
   b. **True.** If not treated promptly.
   c. **True.** Particularly after parenteral administration.
   d. **False.** The patient must have been sensitised to the drug previously, but a history of exposure may be difficult to find; patients have unwittingly been sensitised to penicillin by penicillin in milk.
   e. **False.** Endotoxin release by bacteria is important in septicaemic shock. Anaphylaxis is caused by histamine and other inflammatory mediators.

6. a. **False.** Since they are poorly lipid soluble.
   b. **False.** They are excreted by the kidney: this is a general feature of drugs that are not lipid soluble.
   c. **True.** A major adverse effect.
   d. **True.** To avoid some of the dose-related adverse effects.
   e. **False.** Only effective against aerobic organisms.

7. a. **True.** Erythromycin is a liver enzyme inhibitor.
   b. **False.** Absorption is erratic.
   c. **True.** The most common adverse effect.
   d. **True.**
   e. **False.** Widely used to treat patients thought to be allergic to penicillin.

8. a. **True.** Although enzyme inhibition may also occur.
   b. **False.** Humans cannot manufacture folate and so are not affected.
   c. **True.** Especially in the elderly.
   d. **True.** To treat *Pneumocystis pneumoniae* infection.
   e. **False.** Trimethoprim is part of co-trimoxazole and is far less likely to cause adverse effects than the sulphonamide component.

9. a. **False.** Interferes with nucleic acid coiling.
   b. **False.** Not as effective against *Streptococcus pneumoniae* as penicillins for instance.
   c. **True.** Anaphylaxis and other reactions are recorded.
   d. **True.** This is its main use.
   e. **True.** By liver enzyme inhibition.

10. a. **True.** And probably its most common use.
   b. **False.** Tetracycline will bind to heavy metal ions in the food and not be absorbed.
   c. **True.** Damage to teeth.
   d. **False.** Increasingly common.
   e. **True.**

11. a. **True.** And penetrates most tissues well.
   b. **True.** For example, amoebiasis.
   c. **True.** When peptic ulcer disease is associated with *Helicobacter* infection.
   d. **False.** May cause ataxia, but this is caused by peripheral neuropathy.
   e. **True.** The disulfiram reaction.

12. a. **False.** Although similar in its toxicity.
   b. **True.** But metronidazole is usually first choice on grounds of cost.
   c. **True.** Also flucloxacillin (the most widely used) and rifampicin.
   d. **False.** Considered too toxic for anything other than serious infections with MRSA or vancomycin resistant *S. aureus.*
   e. **False.** Nitrofurantoin is only effective after concentration in the urine.

13. a. **True.** To reduce resistance.
   b. **False.** Treatment for 6 months is usually the minimum for pulmonary tuberculosis.
   c. **True.** An example of genetic polymorphism.
   d. **True.** Especially in patients who are fast acetylators or who have their enzymes induced.
   e. **False.** Liver enzyme inhibitor.

14. a. **False.** Also used for *Staphylococcus aureus* and *Legionella pneumoniae*.
   b. **False.** Rifampicin is a liver enzyme inducer.
   c. **True.** Orange.
   d. **True.** This is rare at currently used doses.
   e. **True.** Since optic neuritis is a major adverse effect.

Case history answers

Case history 1

1. Copious fluid intake, rest and antipyretics as necessary.
2. Antibiotic choice will ideally be based on urine culture. Trimethoprim or nitrofurantoin would all be reasonable choices. Ciprofloxacin should be a reserve drug.
3. Treating minor urinary tract infections is more important in pregnant women because of the increased risk of progression to pyelonephritis. Neither trimethoprim nor ciprofloxacin would be appropriate.

Case history 2

1. Yes: he should be isolated if possible for the first 2 weeks of treatment.
2. Rifampicin and isoniazid for 6 months: pyrazinamide and possibly ethambutol for the first 2 months also.
3. This patient's compliance with long-term medication might be poor. It might be appropriate to admit him to hospital for the duration of his treatment or to ensure in some other way that he takes his medication under observation.

Case history 3

1. Amoxicillin or erythromycin, trimethoprim or levofloxacin would all be appropriate (in that order).
2. The patient may have pseudomembranous colitis as a result of the use of broad spectrum antibiotic. A stool sample should be sent for detection of the toxin, and a sigmoidoscopy performed.
3. Metronidazole is first choice, with vancomycin for resistant cases.

Short note answers

1. When asked to write a short note on any drug consider:
   a. its indications
   b. its mechanism of action
   c. its therapeutic use
   d. its adverse effects.

In this case, therefore, one would start by naming the major drugs (rifampicin, isoniazid, ethambutol and pyrazinamide) and for each include a mechanism of action where it is known. Discuss (in combination in this case) how all of the drugs are used together (rifampicin and isoniazid for 6 months, ethambutol and pyrazinamide for the first 2 months also) and why. And finally consider the drugs' adverse effects, listing the major adverse reactions for each one and their possible interactions. Here one would spend most time talking about rifampicin and isoniazid since they are the drugs used for the longest period and, therefore, the ones most likely to cause adverse reactions and interactions.

2. This is a very general question, but one should consider the patterns of adverse reactions to antibiotics which should include:

   a. hypersensitivity reactions, e.g. anaphylaxis to penicillin, drug fevers, fixed drug skin reactions, etc. These constitute the type B or bizarre adverse drug reactions (see Ch. 10). They are rare but potentially serious, and worrisome because of their unpredictable nature

   b. reactions which might arise as a result of the augmented effect of antibiotics, i.e. antimicrobial killing leading to superinfection with *Candida* or *Clostridium difficile*; drug-induced diarrhoea, etc.

   c. the long-term environmental hazards of these drugs, for instance in promoting antibiotic resistance.

Essay answer

Make the following points:

1. Restricting drug use to confirmed indications and sensitive bacteria
2. Using drug combinations if treatment is to be prolonged
3. Avoiding unnecessarily prolonged treatment
4. Establishing a hierarchy of drug usage, with more potent drugs reserved for resistant cases.

Extended matching items answers

Theme: Antibiotics in primary care

1. J best but B or E also reasonable. The likely organisms are *Streptococcus pneumoniae*, *Haemophilus influenzae* or *Branhamella* sp., or even all three. The last two in particular are showing increasing rates of resistance to amoxicillin. Amoxicillin is a reasonable first line choice but this infection has occurred immediately after such treatment and is likely to be with a resistant organism. The options then are to use a cephalosporin with increased activity against Gram-negative organisms such as *Haemophilus* (e.g. cefaclor) or a fluoroquinolone such as ciprofloxacin or trimethoprim. The last two would not be good first line choices since they do not have reliable effectiveness against *Streptococcus* spp. Since amoxicillin with its greater effectiveness against *Streptococcus* spp. has been used already in this case, we can assume that it is the *Haemophilus* or *Branhamella* sp. which is the culprit. Another alternative, not given here, is the combination of amoxicillin and clavulanic acid, co-amoxiclav.

2. G is the best choice. The concern in a pregnant woman is always about teratogenesis, i.e. causing fetal defects as a result of medication. Trimethoprim, ciprofloxacin and nitrofurantoin are, therefore, generally avoided. The safest option would be cefaclor. Co-amoxiclav would be a reasonable alternative; the resistance of the commonest organism causing urinary tract infection (*Escherichia coli*) to amoxicillin is too great to allow this to be used alone.

3. H. is best; J would be a reasonable choice also. The organism in lobar pneumonia is usually *Streptococcus pneumoniae*. This is usually very sensitive to penicillin and, therefore, one might think that either phenoxymethylpenicillin or amoxicillin (because of its better absorption) would be favoured drugs. However, as this patient has a history of allergy to penicillin, it is safest to avoid these. About 10% of the population has some vague history of allergy to penicillin, although true incidence is much lower. Often this history of 'allergy' arises from non-allergic adverse effects, such as stomach upsets. However, it is safer to avoid these drugs completely. As there is a 10% cross-reactivity between penicillins and cephalosporins, it is probably better to avoid cefaclor also. This would normally have very good activity against *S. pneumoniae*. Some authorities would argue that in a life-threatening situation and where there is anything less than a clear history of full-blown

anaphylaxis, it is reasonable to use a cephalosporin. However, this does not apply in this case when there are reasonable alternatives available.

4. Best answer is A. The likely organisms in cellulitis are *Staphylococcus aureus* and/or *Streptococcus pyogenes*. Treatment for these should be with flucloxacillin, possibly with amoxicillin in addition. Depending on the severity of the infection, it may be reasonable to treat these at home or it may be advisable to refer the patient to hospital for i.v. treatment. If the patient were allergic to penicillin, then erythromycin or clindamycin would be reasonable.

5. D. But the best answer here is not to use any antibiotic at all. Most sore throats are viral and will not benefit from antibiotics, so you are exposing the patient to the hazards of the drug needlessly. One could send a swab but the patient will probably be better by the time the result comes back. However, if there is a need for an antibiotic (patient pyrexial, swollen tonsillar glands, exudates), then phenoxymethylpenicillin is probably the best choice. The organism is likely to be *Strep. pyogenes*. Amoxicillin might be better absorbed but another cause of sore throat in a 20-year-old is infectious mononucleosis; giving amoxicillin to such a patient will probably produce a florid and unpleasant rash, whereas phenoxymethylpenicillin will not.

Theme: Choice of antibiotic and route of administration

1. B Intravenous flucloxacillin would be best but if you cannot get intravenous access (not uncommon in such patients) large oral doses may have to suffice. Do not forget to drain the abscess! A prolonged course of antibiotics would be wise, since *Staph. aureus* can seed itself in other tissues and only become apparent later – at least 10–14 days; i.v. vancomycin might be used if the organism was MRSA.

2. D Oral erythromycin should be adequate in most such cases.

3. I is best but there is a possibility of a mixed infection even if only one organism has been cultured. Many would use B as well.

4. C is best. I is an option but resistance to benzylpenicillin is growing and a third generation cephalosporin would be better.

5. E is best but F would be a reasonable alternative; however, beware of confusion in the elderly.

Theme: Serious infections in hospitals

1. A and probably E also. This patient is very ill. The most likely organism is *S. pneumonia* but atypicals such as *Mycoplasma* are also possible.

2. F is best first choice but other antibiotics such as D or I may be necessary if this does not respond quickly clinically. This patient is in danger of losing their foot. Seek advice from a vascular surgeon also.

3. D or I would be good choices here, in that order.

4. H This is likely to be *Clostridium difficile* related diarrhoea and maybe (depending on the clinical picture) a full blown pseudomembranous colitis.

5. A and probably H also. Hospital-acquired pneumonias are far more likely than community-acquired to have Gram-negative organisms and less likely to have atypical organisms involved so we need to cover these with a broad spectrum cephalosporin. In a patient with a recent stroke, the possibility of aspiration should be considered and metronidazole would often be used also to cover bacteroides.

Theme: Mechanisms of action and adverse effects

1. E for mechanism of action, F or H for the adverse effect.

2. B for mechanism of action and I for the adverse effect (though this is rare).

3. C for mechanism of action, and H or J for the adverse effect.

4. A for mechanism of action, G for the adverse effect (H also possible).

5. A for mechanism of action, D and J as adverse effects.

Chemotherapy for fungi, viruses and protozoa

14.1	Antifungal drugs	211
14.2	Antiviral drugs	213
14.3	Antiprotozoal drugs	216
	Self-assessment on Chapter 14: questions	218
	Self-assessment on Chapter 14: answers	220

Overview

Fungal infections are usually confined to the skin, mucous membranes and nails but, in immunocompromised patients, can give rise to systemic disease. Topical antifungal agents are largely without toxicity but systemic agents can also damage the host.

Viruses cannot grow or propagate outside living cells and use host cell mechanisms to reproduce. Although they are most vulnerable at this stage, the antiviral drugs are often toxic to the host.

The protozoa have life cycles outside the human and most protozoan pathogens multiply in the human having been acquired by ingestion, inhalation or an insect bite. Protozoan infections are unusual in general medical practice.

14.1 Antifungal drugs

Learning objectives

At the end of this section you should:
- be able to describe the main 'syndromes' caused by fungal skin infections
- know the appropriate treatment for common fungal skin infections
- be aware that systemic fungal infections are mainly a problem in immunosuppressed patients
- know the main adverse effects of amphotericin, systemic imidazoles and flucytosine.

Fungal infections are usually confined to the skin, mucous membranes and nails: these conditions are frequent and the general physician should have a working knowledge of the drugs used. Most of these drugs are used topically and are largely without major toxicity. In contrast, systemic fungal disease is unusual in the immunocompetent patient. Systemic antifungal drugs are a specialist area: these drugs are quite toxic and difficult to use.

Superficial cutaneous and mucous membrane infections

Superficial fungal infections can be classified as *dermatomycoses* and *candidiasis*.

Ringworm (tinea). There are various types of dermatomycosis; the commonest are tinea corporalis (which affects the trunk), tinea pedis ('athlete's foot') and tinea cruris (the groin). *All are equally common and easily treated. Identification of the fungus and drug sensitivity testing are neither practical nor necessary in the majority of cases.*

Candidiasis. Candida albicans causes opportunist infections when the skin is damaged, when antibiotic treatment alters normal flora or when the immune system is compromised.

Onychia. Infections of the nails can be hard to treat with topical agents and a long course of oral terbinafine may be required.

Clinical sketch

A woman brings her little boy to surgery because he has developed several raised, itchy red lesions on his arms. They have a red raised edge. The doctor diagnoses *tinea corporis* and prescribes clotrimazole cream.

Comment: these infections are common and usually respond to topical treatment.

A woman brings her 6-month-old baby to surgery with 'nappy rash'. The red area is mainly in the skin folds and is probably caused by wet nappies left on too long, but there are 'satellite' lesions over convex surfaces. The GP feels that there is an element of candidal infection; she advises more frequent changes of nappy, and gives clotrimazole cream.

Comment: nappy rash may be caused entirely by infrequent nappy changes, leading to wet, ammonia-exposed skin. However Candida albicans *frequently superinfects such areas.*

Clinical sketch

A woman has been on systemic antibiotics for life-threatening pneumonia. She develops an itchy vulva and a white vaginal discharge; in addition, her mouth is sore. Speculum examination reveals white 'plaques' on the vaginal mucosa; similar white plaques are seen in the mouth.

Comment: long courses of antibiotics encourage the growth of opportunists such as the yeast Candida albicans. *Topical treatment is indicated for both mouth and genitals.*

Clinical sketch

A man develops painless discoloration of his big toenails. They are yellow and thickened.

Comment: such fungal infections can be hard to treat with topical agents. A course of oral terbinafine is usually effective, but this might need to continue for up to 3 months.

Clinical sketch

A 20-week pregnant woman presents with painless discoloration of her big toenails. They are yellow and thickened.

Comment: this illustrates the need for 'benefit versus risk' assessment. Whereas a 3-month course of terbinafine is appropriate in the non-pregnant patient, the risks in this case are not warranted by the benefits. The woman should be advised of this, and treatment postponed.

Drugs for fungal skin infections

Topical nystatin

Nystatin is too toxic for systemic use and is not absorbed from the gut. Nystatin is used topically for cutaneous, oral, oesophageal and vaginal infections with C. *albicans* and various dermatophytes. Nystatin is not beneficial against fungal nail infections. Because it is mainly used topically, adverse effects are unusual: very high oral doses can cause gastrointestinal upset.

Topical imidazoles

Miconazole and *clotrimazole* are relatively toxic compounds. However, they are used topically for infections such as tinea and vaginal candidiasis. Under these circumstances, little drug is absorbed, and such topical use is usually safe. Allergic reactions are occasionally seen.

Systemic terbinafine

Terbinafine is used systemically, mainly for onychia, and might need to be used for up to 3 months to achieve improvement. Severe rashes have been reported and patients should be advised to stop the drug if they notice a rash. It can also cause hepatitis.

Systemic griseofulvin

Systemic griseofulvin is an alternative drug for onychia; treatment must last for several months. Griseofulvin is relatively non-toxic but can occasionally produce *adverse reactions* including rashes, agranulocytosis, systemic lupus erythematosus-like syndromes and peripheral neuropathy. Griseofulvin induces hepatic drug-metabolising enzymes and can affect warfarin therapy. A course of griseofulvin may last for several months to achieve cure.

Systemic fungal infections

The use of broad spectrum antibiotics, which decrease the normal non-pathogenic bacterial flora on the body, and the increase in the population with reduced immune responses (from AIDS, immuno-suppressant drugs, cancer chemotherapy) has led to an increase in systemic fungal disease. In the UK, the most common is systemic candidiasis, followed by cryptococciasis (meningitis or endocarditis), and aspergillosis (pulmonary).

Clinical sketch

A 40-year-old man was diagnosed HIV-positive 6 years ago and now has a very low CD4$^+$ lymphocyte count. He presents to hospital as an emergency with a 7 day history of malaise and fever. He is confused and has detectable neck rigidity. Lumbar puncture reveals yeasts when a special examination ('India ink examination') is done. He is treated with amphotericin and flucytosine.

Comment: such systemic fungal infections are rare, other than in immunosuppressed patients. If this man survives, he will need long-term maintenance treatment with fluconazole.

Drugs for systemic infections

Imidazoles

Ketoconazole and *fluconazole*, though structurally similar to clotrimazole and miconazole, are less toxic. They may be given orally or parenterally for systemic infection. Both are well absorbed, but ketoconazole does not readily cross the blood–brain barrier, and fluconazole is preferred for fungal CNS infection. All are hepatotoxic and are hepatic enzyme inhibitors (and, therefore, prone to drug interactions).

Amphotericin

Amphotericin is not absorbed from the gut; its oral formulations (such as amphotericin lozenges) are, therefore, for topical use only and are relatively free from adverse effects. It is given i.v. for life-threatening systemic fungal infections and then has frequent and severe toxicity. Rigors, fever and malaise are usual; renal failure, hepatic dysfunction and anaemia are common.

Flucytosine

Flucytosine is another toxic drug used for life-threatening systemic fungal infections. Bone marrow toxicity can be a major problem.

14.2 Antiviral drugs

Learning objectives

At the end of this section you should:
* know the main ways in which antiviral drugs work
* be able to describe some common syndromes caused by herpes simplex, herpes zoster, influenza and hepatitis viruses
* understand the concept of risk versus benefit in relation to the use of antivirus drugs
* know the principles of highly active antiretroviral therapy (HAART) for patients with HIV.

Most viral infections, although unpleasant, are self-limiting and require no treatment. Few of the vast number of viral infections are susceptible to drugs, and many of the available compounds suffer from variable efficacy, unacceptable toxicity or both. Viruses are more difficult 'targets' than bacteria: they are most vulnerable during reproduction, but all use host cell organelles and enzymes to do this; consequently, antiviral compounds are often as toxic to host cells as to the virus. Viruses have assumed increasing importance in the setting of immunosuppression – both drug-induced and AIDS. For the most part, the use of antiviral drugs, particularly in patients with AIDS, is a specialist area, but the general physician needs a basic grounding.

Modes of action of antiviral drugs

Antiviral drugs act in a number of ways:
* inhibition of viral 'uncoating' shortly after penetration into the cell; such drugs are best used prophylactically, or very early in the disease course (e.g. amantadine)
* interference with viral RNA synthesis and function (e.g. ribavirin)
* interference with DNA synthesis by acting as analogues of pyrimidine or purine bases (e.g. idoxuridine, cytarabine and vidarabine)
* inhibition of viral DNA polymerase (e.g. aciclovir and ganciclovir)
* inhibition of reverse transcriptase (relevant only to retroviruses such as HIV, e.g. zidovudine)
* inhibition of virus-derived enzymes (such as the protease inhibitors used for HIV, e.g. indinavir)
* use of complex 'natural' antiviral defences (e.g. the interferons).

Influenza virus. Although influenza is often acute and self-limiting, it can give rise to high mortality rates. Antigenic shift allows the virus to 'escape' previous immunity or vaccine cover.

The hepatitis viruses. Viruses of different groups can cause hepatocellular damage. Hepatitis A is spread by the faecal–oral route and is common where sewage disposal is inadequate. Hepatitis B and C are spread in blood and body secretions (e.g. during sexual intercourse), and are quite common in i.v. drug-abusers. Hepatitis B and C can lead to chronic liver disease and hepatocellular carcinoma.

Human immunodeficiency virus (HIV). Infection with HIV leads eventually to a depletion of $CD4^+$ T cells and impaired immune responses. HIV-positive individuals are then at risk for a number of secondary infections; these form the acquired immunodeficiency syndrome (AIDS).

Clinical sketch

A man is troubled with frequent and debilitating cold sores: they make his lips split and are embarrassing. The GP gives him aciclovir cream.

Comment: herpes simplex (cold sores) is a frequent indication for aciclovir. The drug should be applied as early after the onset of local discomfort as possible. Once ulceration has occurred its benefits are minimal. Sometimes cold sores may be a problem on exposure to bright sunlight (e.g. on holiday): in such cases, UV blocking creams may be helpful.

Drugs used in viral infections

Influenza

Zanamivir and oseltamivir

Zanamivir and oseltamivir can be used within 48 hours of close contact with either influenza A or influenza B in patients who are at increased risk of serious consequences (including chronic respiratory and cardiovascular disease). Zanamivir is taken by inhalation of powder, using an 'inhaler device', while oseltamivir is an oral formulation. Although patients with chronic lung disease are at grave risk from influenza (and would be among the patients who need protection), *zanamivir* can worsen bronchospasm and should be used with caution; the main caution for *oseltamivir* is in patients with renal impairment.

Amantadine

Amantadine has been used in the past for post-exposure prevention of influenza A, but it does not feature highly in current prescribing guidelines.

Herpes simplex and herpes zoster infections

Aciclovir

Aciclovir is active against herpes simplex; it also has activity against herpes zoster, but less so. Aciclovir is metabolised to its active form by a viral enzyme and, therefore, targets virus-infected cells quite specifically. The drug may be used topically, orally and i.v. Little drug is absorbed from topical formulations, and the bioavailability of the oral drug is low (about 20%). Once in the body, aciclovir crosses the blood–brain barrier. It is mainly excreted in the urine as the unchanged drug; this renal excretion is impaired by probenecid (see Ch. 8). *Adverse effects* include:

- renal impairment: mainly with high i.v. doses in dehydrated patients
- local inflammation following extravascular administration
- encephalopathy: mainly at high i.v. doses.

Other drugs

Famciclovir and *valaciclovir* are mainly used for herpes zoster.

Viral hepatitis

Acute uncomplicated viral hepatitis is usually managed with supportive care. However, both hepatitis B and C can cause chronic hepatitis. Chronic hepatitis B may be treated with *interferon-alfa* or *lamivudine*. Chronic hepatitis C may be treated with *ribavirin*, in combination with *interferon-alfa*.

Interferons

Interferons are a natural part of the body's defence system. They have protective effects against human viral infections and have been studied in hepatitis B and C infections. Interferon-alfa is not indicated for patients with acute hepatitis B but has proven beneficial in chronic hepatitis B, where around 40% of patients show benefit. Only a few studies have evaluated the use of interferon in acute hepatitis C infection but treatment may decrease the likelihood of chronicity and should be considered. In chronic hepatitis C infection, treatment has been effective in achieving sustained viral eradication in up to 20% of patients. *Adverse effects* include fever, alopecia, anaemia and gastrointestinal upset.

Lamivudine

Lamivudine is a nucleoside reverse transcriptase inhibitor (NRTI) used in HIV disease. It can also be used for chronic hepatitis B infection. Its use tends to be limited by adverse effects such as:

- gastrointestinal upsets
- alopecia
- peripheral neuropathy.

Ribavirin

Ribavirin is effective against a wide range of DNA and RNA viruses. It probably works by interference with the 'capping' of viral mRNA. Ribavirin may be given by inhalation, orally or i.v. It is eliminated both by metabolism and by renal excretion, with a terminal half-life of about 2 weeks. Other than hepatitis C, ribavirin may be used for severe respiratory syncytial virus (RSV) infections in young children (usually employed as an aerosol). Adverse effects include:

- dose-dependent bone marrow suppression
- gastrointestinal adverse effects.

HIV infection

There is no cure for HIV at present. Combinations of antiretroviral drugs are toxic but increase life expectancy. They should be used by experienced specialists.

Clinical sketch

A 30-year-old homosexual man is diagnosed HIV-positive after presenting with *Pneumocystis carinii* pneumonia (PCP). The PCP is treated with high-dose co-trimoxazole and he makes a slow recovery. His CD4$^+$ cell count is about 100×10^6 cells/L and his viral load is high. His physician starts highly active antiretroviral therapy (HAART) once he is better from the PCP.

Comment: HAART comprises a combination of antiretroviral drugs that work by different mechanisms: it is designed to avoid drug resistance (as in the case with tuberculosis). HAART has greatly increased life expectancy in AIDS but the drugs cause adverse effects.

- Treatment aims to reduce viral load (determined by blood test) and maintain this for as long as possible.
- Anti-HIV drugs should be started before the immune system is irreversibly damaged.
- Drug resistance is a major problem with monotherapy: standard treatment is now with drug combinations, so-called highly active antiretroviral therapy (HAART).

- HAART typically comprises two nucleoside reverse transcriptase inhibitors (NRTIs) with either a non-nucleoside reverse transcriptase inhibitor (NNRTI) or a protease inhibitor.
- HAART is usually started when the patient is clinically well (i.e. after they have recovered from the presenting infection).
- HAART may be limited by toxicity, treatment failure or both.
- In addition to efforts to reduce HIV loads, management relies on the prevention and prompt treatment of superimposed infections such as tuberculosis and infections with *Streptococcus pneumoniae* and cytomegalovirus.
- The management of HIV is expensive: most HIV sufferers worldwide do not have access to such treatment.

Nucleoside reverse transcriptase inhibitors (NRTIs)

HIV is an RNA virus capable of inducing the synthesis of a DNA transcript of its genome, which can then become integrated into the host cell's DNA, thereby allowing viral replication. Synthesis of the initial DNA transcript involves the enzyme reverse transcriptase. NRTIs resemble natural nucleoside substrates for the enzyme. These drugs are given by mouth. They are rapidly eliminated and must be taken more than once daily. Examples of these drugs, and their main adverse effects are:

Zidovudine (AZT): adverse effects include:

- bone marrow toxicity: about one-third of patients develop severe anaemia or neutropenia
- polymyositis: muscle pain and tenderness
- headache and insomnia.

Didanosine (ddI): adverse effects include:

- pancreatitis
- peripheral neuropathy.

Zalcitabine (ddC): adverse effects include:

- peripheral neuropathy
- myalgia
- bone marrow toxicity.

Non-nucleoside reverse transcriptase inhibitors (NNRTIs)

Drugs such as *nevirapine* also inhibit reverse transcriptase but by a different mechanism to that of the NRTIs. This difference in mechanism of action is crucial in the avoidance of drug resistance. Adverse effects of nevirapine include:

Fourteen

- severe rashes
- hepatitis.

Protease inhibitors (PIs)

Virus replication relies on the manufacture of new viral proteins, which are assembled into virus particles. The protease inhibitors interfere with this process. Again, this difference in mechanism of action is critical: HAART relies on the combination of differing drugs, and this reduces the risk of drug resistance. *Indinavir* and *ritonavir* are examples of this drug class. The main *adverse effects* are metabolic and include:

- hyperlipidaemia
- insulin resistance and hyperglycaemia
- lipodystrophy.

Cytomegalovirus (CMV) infection

CMV mainly causes disease in immunosuppressed patients. CMV retinitis is a common problem in people with AIDS.

Ganciclovir. This drug inhibits the DNA polymerase of CMV. Ganciclovir is used i.v. It causes severe adverse effects including neutropenia, thrombocytopenia and renal impairment.

Foscarnet. This drug has a wide spectrum of antiviral activity, working by inhibition of DNA polymerase. The drug is poorly absorbed from the gut and is usually given i.v. Elimination is mainly as unchanged drug in the urine. Foscarnet is indicated for life-threatening CMV infection. Adverse effects include renal impairment.

14.3 Antiprotozoal drugs

Learning objectives

At the end of this section you should:
- be aware of the protozoal infections likely to be seen in clinical practice
- be able to list the drugs used to prevent and treat malaria.

Clinical sketch

A woman comes to the surgery asking for malaria prophylaxis for her 2-week visit to Kenya. The GP consults current guidelines on malaria prevention and stresses that: (i) these drugs do not provide 100% protection; (ii) the patient needs to protect herself against mosquito bites (ideally by sleeping under an insecticide-dipped bed net); and (iii) she should seek medical advice for any influenza-like symptoms upon her return to Britain.

Comment: falciparum malaria is common in sub-Saharan Africa and can kill a non-immune patient within 24 hours of the onset of symptoms. Personal protection against bites and the use of chemoprophylaxis reduce risk.

The same woman develops fever, rigors and myalgia 2 weeks after her return from holiday. She is slightly confused. A blood film confirms *Plasmodium falciparum* infection. She is admitted to the local infectious diseases hospital and treated with i.v. quinine.

Comment: this is a medical emergency. Intravenous quinine is the drug of choice: resistance to quinine is unusual in Africa.

Clinical sketch

A homosexual man presents with severe breathlessness. His chest radiograph shows mid-zone shadowing and *Pneumocystis carinii* pneumonia (PCP) is suspected; he is found to be HIV-positive with a low CD4 cell count. He is treated with high-dose co-trimoxazole and recovers.

Comment: PCP is a common AIDS-defining illness. Upon recovery he will need lifelong secondary prophylaxis with either co-trimoxazole or pentamidine.

Common protozoal infections

Common protozoal infections include:

- falciparum malaria: a major cause of death in developing countries
- amoebiasis: causes dysentery and hepatic abscesses
- *Giardia lamblia*: causes diarrhoea and malabsorption
- *Pneumocystis carinii*: causes pneumonia mainly in immunosuppressed individuals
- toxoplasmosis: affects brain and eyes particularly; most common in immunosuppressed subjects.

Drugs

There is a wide range of antiprotozoal drugs, the most important of which are summarised below. Some antibacterial drugs, such as metronidazole, are also used against some protozoa (e.g. in amoebiasis).

Atovaquone. This is a well-tolerated drug that can be used for *Toxoplasma gondii* infections (seen in AIDS) and for the treatment and prevention of malaria.

Quinine. Quinine is mostly used parenterally for severe malaria. At high dose, adverse effects are common but rarely serious if standard regimens are used: deafness, vertigo and nausea are common, and ECG abnormalities may occur. In overdose quinine is very dangerous.

Mefloquine. This is used for the treatment and prevention of malaria. Psychosis and seizures are well-reported adverse effects.

Chloroquine. Malaria parasites resistant to chloroquine are now so widespread that its use cannot be recommended.

Pyrimethamine. This is usually combined with a sulphonamide for the treatment of uncomplicated malaria or for toxoplasmic encephalitis in AIDS patients. The doses used for malaria are usually without severe toxicity but the high doses used for toxoplasmosis cause bone marrow suppression. This can be reversed using folinic acid.

Co-trimoxazole. This combination of trimethoprim and sulfamethoxazole is used at high dose for the treatment of PCP. Toxicity is quite common at such high doses.

Pentamidine. This drug has many effects on *P. carinii* and is mainly used as an aerosol in the treatment and prevention of PCP. The main adverse effect is hypoglycaemia, which is common at high dose.

Fourteen

Self-assessment on Chapter 14: questions

Multiple choice questions

1. The following drugs reach high CNS concentrations when they are given by mouth:
   a. Nystatin
   b. Amphotericin
   c. Ketoconazole
   d. Aciclovir
   e. Fluconazole

2. Aciclovir:
   a. Is as effective for herpes zoster as it is for herpes simplex infections
   b. Is effective for all herpes virus infections
   c. Must be metabolised before it becomes active
   d. Interacts with allopurinol
   e. Interacts with probenecid

3. In the management of an influenza A outbreak:
   a. Oseltamivir should be given prophylactically to whoever requests it
   b. Oseltamivir and zanamivir have clinical benefit, even if started late in the illness
   c. The available influenza vaccines are of little use
   d. Zanamivir is safe in patients with chronic obstructive pulmonary disease
   e. Amantidine is contraindicated in pregnancy

Case history questions

Case history 1

A 40-year-old man with a renal transplant takes ciclosporin as an immunosuppressant. He develops a painful rash on his trunk and thinks it might be shingles (herpes zoster). His doctor agrees and starts oral aciclovir. A week later the patient is very unwell with fever and breathlessness: he is admitted to hospital as an emergency.

1. What may have happened?
2. Were the doctor's actions appropriate and adequate?

Case history 2

A 30-year-old man presents with life-threatening pneumococcal pneumonia. He has oral candidiasis, retinal features of cytomegalovirus infection and a low CD4$^+$ cell count. After counselling, an HIV test is done: unfortunately this is positive.

1. How would you manage this man?

Case history 3

An 18-year-old man has been backpacking in Kenya for 2 months. He took mefloquine every week while he was away but stopped it when he got back home. Two weeks after his return he presents with headache, fever, myalgia and sweats.

1. What should be done?

Extended matching items questions

Theme: Managing patients at high risk of influenza

Options

A. He should start oral zanamivir
B. He should start oral oseltamivir
C. He should start inhaled zanamivir
D. He should start inhaled oseltamivir
E. He should start oral amantidine
F. No drugs should be offered: the likelihood of influenza is too low
G. Bronchospasm
H. Gastrointestinal upset
I. Hepatic impairment
J. Renal impairment
K. Agranulocytosis
L. Hypotension

For each of the questions below choose the best response from the list of options above. Each option may be used once, more than once, or not at all.

1. A 65-year-old cigarette smoker with chronic obstructive pulmonary disease is cared for by his daughter. The daughter develops a febrile illness with severe rigors and myalgia, at the height of a 'flu epidemic, and the family is very concerned about her father. His chest is always pretty bad, despite home oxygen, nebulised bronchodilators and oral aminophylline. His peak expiratory flow rate is around 100 L/min at best. He is also known to have mild renal impairment (his last creatinine clearance was 50 ml/min). What should be done?

2. What particular adverse drug reaction should be looked for?

Master Medicine: Self-assessment on Chapter 14: answers

Multiple choice answers

1. a. **False.** Nystatin is not absorbed from the gut.
   b. **False.** Amphotericin is not absorbed from the gut.
   c. **False.** Ketoconazole undergoes extensive first pass metabolism and does not readily cross the blood–brain barrier.
   d. **False.** Aciclovir is poorly absorbed.
   e. **True.**

2. a. **False.**
   b. **False.** Aciclovir is very effective against herpes simplex, less so against herpes zoster and ineffective against Epstein–Barr virus and cytomegalovirus.
   c. **True.** Must be metabolised by thymidine kinase.
   d. **False.** Allopurinol (Ch. 9) inhibits xanthine oxidase and potentiates 6-mercaptopurine, an anticancer drug.
   e. **True.** Probenecid inhibits the renal tubular transport of some drugs including penicillin and aciclovir.

3. a. **False.** There are clear guidelines on the patient categories to whom oseltamivir may be offered (see the British National Formulary; BNF).
   b. **False.** Both drugs have demonstrable effects if started within 48 hours of the onset of symptoms. Beyond then they are not of proven use.
   c. **False.** At risk patients should be offered vaccination annually.
   d. **False.** Zanamivir may worsen bronchospasm. However, patients with chronic airways disease are at particular risk from influenza and zanamivir has proven benefit against influenza.
   e. **True.** Amantadine is teratogenic.

Case history answers

Case history 1

1. Immunosuppressed patients are at risk of disseminated herpes, which can cause pneumonia and other systemic illnesses. Aciclovir is the drug of first choice, but its bioavailability is very low. The drug may be given i.v. (which would require hospital admission) to particularly high-risk patients.

2. The doctor should have known all of this, and he has failed to act vigorously enough in the circumstances.

Case history 2

The life-threatening pneumococcal pneumonia is the first and most pressing problem. It will require the full range of supportive care as well as appropriate antibiotics (guided by assessment of drug sensitivity) and oxygen therapy. The oral candidiasis will often not respond to topical drugs such as nystatin in AIDS patients: fluconazole is probably the first choice drug. CMV retinitis is very serious and threatens sight: ophthalmologic advice is mandatory. Ganciclovir is the drug of first choice, but it must be given into a central vein as it causes phlebitis when given peripherally. HAART will be needed but should be postponed until the patient has recovered from his acute presentation.

Case history 3

This patient took weekly mefloquine, which probably has a protective efficacy of greater than 75%. Even so, there remains a risk of malaria transmission, and this diagnosis needs to be excluded *as an emergency*: non-immune patients may die within 24 hours of the onset of symptoms from falciparum malaria. If he does have parasites in his blood then he needs:

- emergency admission
- close monitoring of parasitaemia, blood sugar (hypoglycaemia is a complication), level of consciousness and haemoglobin
- oral treatment with quinine, three times daily for 7 days; there are concerns of additive cardiac toxicity when quinine is given to people with therapeutic mefloquine levels, and so daily ECGs would be wise.

Extended matching items answers

1. B. The main worry here is the father's chest. On the one hand there is the desire to protect against 'flu, while on the other hand there is the desire to avoid drugs that can cause bronchospasm. Guidelines issued by the National Institute for Health and Clinical Excellence (NICE) currently suggest treatment of high-risk patients like this within 48 hours of exposure. Oral oseltamivir is the best choice, since zanamivir can worsen bronchospasm. (Oseltamivir is not given by inhalation and zanamivir **must** be given by this topical route). Amantidine, although used in the recent past, is no longer included in NICE guidelines.

2. H. The father's creatinine clearance is not low enough for dose reduction of oseltamivir to be required; had it been below 30 ml/min then dose reduction guidelines are given in the BNF. The likeliest adverse events are nausea, vomiting and abdominal discomfort.

Anticancer chemotherapy

15.1	Principles of cancer treatment	223
15.2	Anticancer drugs	224
15.3	Palliative care	227
	Self-assessment on Chapter 15: questions	229
	Self-assessment on Chapter 15: answers	231

Overview

Malignant disease accounts for a high proportion of deaths in industrialised countries. Chemotherapy is one of several treatment options. Treatment aims to give palliation, induce remission and, if possible, cure. Because chemotherapeutic drugs will also affect normal healthy cells, drug regimens form an important part of prescription, using courses of drugs with gaps to allow normal cells to recover and drug combinations. The latter approach also contributes to avoidance of drug resistance.

15.1 Principles of cancer treatment

Learning objectives

At the end of this section you should:
- understand the differences between curative and palliative care
- understand the guiding principles underlying the use of anticancer drugs
- appreciate the benefit versus risk relationship with these drugs.

Prevention of malignant neoplasms continues to elude us because, despite strong epidemiological data linking certain high-risk activities (such as smoking) to cancer, changing the habits of a population is extremely difficult. Treatment options comprise *surgery*, *radiotherapy* and *chemotherapy*; the first two are outside the scope of this book.

Cancers may kill through the local effects of the primary lesion, such as compression of vital struc-

tures or invasion of major blood vessels, but more usually do so through organ 'failure' (e.g. liver, marrow, lung and brain) caused by metastases. The treatment of a patient with cancer may aim to:

- give palliation, for example prompt relief of unpleasant symptoms such as superior vena cava obstruction from a mediastinal tumour
- induce 'remission' so that all macroscopic and microscopic features of the cancer disappear, though disease is known to persist
- cure, for which all the cells of the clone must be destroyed.

The above options are ranked in increasing order of difficulty, and cure is often impossible with current drugs.

Unfortunately healthy cells, particularly those undergoing replication (e.g. those in the marrow, mucosa, skin and gonads), are also very susceptible to chemotherapeutic drugs, but *less* so than the malignant clone. A basic principle of anticancer therapy is that chemotherapy is given in *courses*, interspersed with gaps of varying duration to allow recovery of normal cells (Fig. 50). Another principle of chemotherapy is the use of *drug combinations*: though different drugs have additive (sometimes synergistic) therapeutic effects, aspects of their toxicity need not be additive. This approach has the further benefit of reducing the risk of tumour cell resistance to a particular drug. Rather like tuberculosis (Ch. 13), malignant clones contain cells with inherent drug resistance, and use of one drug may allow this population to flourish.

The drug treatment of malignancy is a specialist area. Solid tumours are usually managed by multidisciplinary teams of surgeons and oncologists. Haematological malignancies are the province of haematologists. The general physician consequently needs no more than an overview of the use of cancer chemotherapy. This is a rapidly changing field and

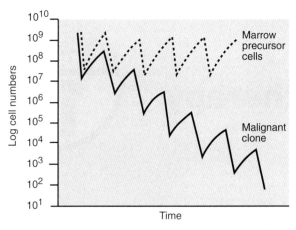

Fig. 50 Giving chemotherapy in courses allows recovery of normal cells.

practice is evolving all the time; consequently current prescribing guidelines should always be consulted.

15.2 Anticancer drugs

Learning objectives

At the end of this section you should:
- appreciate the different classes of drugs used to treat malignancy
- be able to list the main mechanisms of action of drugs used for malignancy
- be able to describe the therapeutic use of these drugs for a few common malignancies
- know the main adverse effects of the main drug groups

The clinical sketches in this chapter illustrate a few common malignancies – acute leukaemia, Hodgkin's disease, breast, prostate and lung cancer – and their chemotherapy.

Mechanisms of action of anticancer drugs

Alkylating agents

These drugs 'transfer' their alkyl groups to cell components, damaging the DNA and interfering with cell replication. They are the most widely used class of drugs in the treatment of cancer.

Examples include *cyclophosphamide, chlorambucil,* and *busulfan.*

Toxicity is mainly dose related and affects rapidly growing cell types such as bone marrow, skin and mucous membranes and the gastrointestinal tract. Gametogenesis is also severely affected.

Fig. 51 The folate pathway. dUMP, uridylate; dTMP, thymidylate.

An example of the alkylating agents: cyclophosphamide

Cyclophosphamide is well absorbed from the gut and widely distributed. It is metabolised in the liver to its active forms, which include a metabolite responsible for bladder toxicity. Most of a dose of cyclophosphamide is excreted as metabolites in the urine. Adverse effects include:

- marrow suppression: severe, dose related and often of long duration
- gonadal failure
- pulmonary fibrosis
- cystitis is a common problem caused by drug metabolites; this is usually avoided by co-administration of *mesna*, which protects the bladder epithelium
- carcinogenesis
- gastrointestinal upset is common and nausea may be severe
- cardiac toxicity, manifesting as arrhythmias and/or heart failure, may be seen at high doses.

Antimetabolites

These drugs 'mimic' a natural metabolite, thus impairing the efficiency of an essential biochemical path. For example *methotrexate* mimics dihydrofolic acid and binds strongly to the enzyme dihydrofolate reductase (Fig. 51), a mechanism that it shares with the antimicrobial drug trimethoprim. However, whereas trimethoprim does not bind strongly to the human enzyme, methotrexate does. It thereby interferes with DNA synthesis.

Examples include methotrexate, fluorouracil and mercaptopurine.

Toxicity is mainly dose related and affects rapidly proliferating tissues.

An example of the antimetabolites: methotrexate

Methotrexate is also used in low dose as an immunosuppressive in rheumatoid arthritis (Ch. 9).

Methotrexate may be given orally (it is well absorbed by an active uptake mechanism), i.v. or intrathecally. The drug is cleared unchanged, by renal excretion. Caution is needed in patients with renal impairment. Adverse effects include:

- marrow suppression, which manifests as agranulocytosis, thrombocytopenia and (to a lesser extent) anaemia; folinic acid has a useful therapeutic role
- mucositis, comprising ulceration and impaired function of the oral and intestinal mucosa; symptoms include stomatitis, nausea, diarrhoea and weight loss
- hepatitis, which varies between mild and life-threatening
- neurotoxicity, particularly with the high local concentrations achieved with repeated intrathecal administration.

Drug interactions. Methotrexate increases the toxicity of fluorouracil, cytarabine, 6-mercaptopurine and 6-thioguanine.

Clinical sketch: acute leukaemia

A 6-year-old girl presents with a short history of malaise, fever, bleeding gums and anaemia. She looks pale and has a temperature of 40°C but is otherwise normal: there is no organomegaly and no lymphadenopathy. Her haemoglobin is 9.0 g% (90 g/L), and she is both leucopenic and thrombocytopenic. Large numbers of primitive blasts are seen in the blood film; special staining reveals these to be lymphoblasts. She is given a blood transfusion and platelets, started on antibiotics and nursed in 'reversed barrier conditions'. Her haematologist starts cycles of combination chemotherapy including *vincristine*. After a stormy course, marked by many infections, she recovers. Five years later she is still in remission.

Comment: acute lymphoblastic leukaemia is the commonest childhood malignancy and responds well to chemotherapy. The prognosis is relatively good. Chemotherapy 'cocktails' vary, and their use is based on clinical trial data.

Clinical sketch: Hodgkin's disease

A 30-year-old man presents with fever and weight loss. Examination reveals cervical and axillary lymphadenopathy, and there is hilar adenopathy on his chest radiograph. Lymph node biopsy confirms Hodgkin's lymphoma. 'Staging computed tomographic (CT) scans' fail to show evidence of the disease below the diaphragm. After semen has been obtained and stored, his oncologist treats him with combination chemotherapy (including both *methotrexate* and *vincristine*) and radiotherapy. Five years later he is still disease free.

Comment: this young man did quite well considering that there were bad prognostic features including fever and weight loss. The prognosis of Hodgkin's disease very much depends on the stage at which it is caught. This man may well want a family in due course, and the treatment has left him infertile: the stored semen samples are important.

Plant alkaloids

These are naturally occurring plant molecules. Mechanisms of action are variable but include effects on the cytoskeleton and on the enzyme topoisomerase.

Examples include *vincristine* and *vinblastine*.

Adverse effects include bone marrow depression and neurotoxicity.

Example of the plant alkaloids: vincristine

Vincristine must be given i.v. and causes necrosis if it extravasates. Vincristine readily crosses the blood–brain barrier, whereas vinblastine does not. It is cleared by hepatic metabolism. Adverse effects include:

- neurotoxicity: this is more severe and frequent with vincristine than vinblastine; the effects may comprise peripheral neuropathy, cranial nerve lesions, autonomic dysfunction and seizures
- gastrointestinal problems are common but usually mild; however, paralytic ileus may occur
- marrow suppression is not usually marked.

Clinical sketch: breast cancer

A 55-year-old postmenopausal woman notices a breast lump and self-refers to the emergency breast assessment clinic. A fine needle aspiration is done the same day and breast cancer is confirmed. She is managed by a multidisciplinary surgical and oncological team. A segmental mastectomy is done and her axillary nodes are biopsied. Unfortunately, a metastasis is found in one of these local nodes. Postoperatively she is treated with cycles of chemotherapy (including *cyclophosphamide*, *methotrexate* and *doxorubicin*); she loses her hair and needs a wig. Thereafter, when she has recovered from initial treatment, she is started on *tamoxifen*. Unfortunately, 12 months later she presents with a pathological fracture and hypercalcaemia.

Comment: breast cancer affects around 10% of British women. It is treated with a combination of surgery, radiotherapy and chemotherapy. The prognosis is relatively poor if there is lymph node disease, since distant metastases are quite common.

Fifteen

Cytotoxic antibiotics

These are products of microorganisms, just like the drugs used to combat infection. Their mechanisms of action are variable but generally involve binding to host DNA.

Examples include *daunorubicin*, *doxorubicin* and *bleomycin*.

Adverse effects vary between drugs.

Examples of the cytotoxic antibiotics: doxorubicin and bleomycin

Doxorubicin is not absorbed from the gut and must be given i.v. It is extensively metabolised (some metabolites retain activity) and mainly excreted in the bile. Enterohepatic circulation occurs (see Ch. 1). It should be used with caution in patients with liver function impairment.

Bleomycin may be given i.v., i.m. or may be instilled into cavities (such as pleura or peritoneum). Bleomycin does not cross the blood–brain barrier but is otherwise widely distributed. It is mainly excreted unchanged, and renal impairment prolongs the half-life.

Adverse effects of doxorubicin include:

- marrow suppression, usually of short duration
- severe or total hair loss
- cumulative cardiac toxicity; this manifests as congestive cardiac failure and is usually avoided by careful recording of the cumulative dose given.

Adverse effects of bleomycin include:

- pulmonary fibrosis, which may affect 10% of patients; this is dose related and is more common in older patients
- anaphylactoid reactions
- mucositis, which may be severe
- marrow suppression: unlike most other anticancer drugs, bleomycin causes little myelosuppression, though it may be seen in patients with renal failure and drug accumulation.

Hormonal agents

Many common malignancies are hormone responsive (for example breast and prostate). These agents exploit this hormone-dependency.

Examples include *tamoxifen*.

Adverse effects vary between drugs.

Example of hormone therapy: tamoxifen

Tamoxifen is an oestrogen receptor modulator used for breast cancer. It is an oestrogen antagonist in breast tissue (see Ch. 12). It is taken orally in divided daily doses. Unlike the drugs described above, tamoxifen is well tolerated. Adverse effects include:

- hot flushes
- nausea
- fluid retention.

Other antineoplastic drugs

This is a diverse group of drugs used in the management of a wide range of different malignancies, including:

Imantinib. A protein tyrosine kinase inhibitor for chronic myeloid leukaemia. The most common adverse effects are nausea, myalgia and skin rash.

Cisplatin and **carboplatin** are platinum-based compounds used in the treatment of various solid-organ tumours. Cisplatin is very toxic, especially to the kidneys. Both cause nausea and vomiting.

Paclitaxel. This is a member of the taxane group of drugs, and is available for the treatment of ovarian cancer, metastatic breast cancer and non-small cell lung cancer. Hypersensitivity reactions are common.

Irinotecan. Irinotecan is an inhibitor of the enzyme topoisomerase I, one of the key enzymes involved in the replication of DNA. It can be used in colorectal cancer.

Trastuzumab. This is a treatment option in metastatic breast cancer as well as in early-stage disease. It is used in patients overexpressing the human epidermal growth factor receptor 2 (HER2) protein. It is given by intravenous infusion. Hypersensitivity reactions are of concern, as is potential cardiotoxicity.

Immunomodulating agents

There are a number of different drugs that will affect the immune response and are used in the treatment of haematological malignancy. *Prednisolone* is widely used in acute lymphoblastic leukaemia as well as in lymphoma. Monoclonal antibodies (of human origin) such as *rituximab* and *alemtuzumab* are also used in haematological malignancy. They are used with caution. A severe cytokine release syndrome can be seen with these immunomodulating monoclonal antibodies, and this can sometimes be fatal.

Supportive care

Synergistic drug combinations and gaps between courses of drugs minimises drug toxicity, but even so, cancer chemotherapy cannot be used without extensive supportive care, which is as important to the patient's survival as the chemotherapy itself. Key components of such care are described in Box 8.

15.3 Palliative care

Palliative care is an important part of the management of cancer. It encompasses methods of controlling debilitating or unpleasant symptoms, as well as the care of terminally ill and dying. The aim is to provide the best quality of life to the patient and their family. Patients may be managed in their own homes, hospitals or hospices. There is typically multidisciplinary involvement, with teams of specialist nurses working in hospitals and in the community. The emphasis is on symptom control and psychosocial support. Inevitably drugs feature as an important part of this care, although they are by no means the only part.

Pain. This is one of the most important symptoms to control. Analgesia will be determined by the nature and origin of the pain as well as its severity. Regular pain killers are typically more effective than those given when pain is felt most severely. Simple pain killers such as paracetamol and NSAIDs may be given alone or with opioid analgesia of varying strength (codeine, oxycodone and morphine). The route by which this will be given will depend on the patient's condition. Opioids can be orally, rectally, transdermally via skin patches, or parenterally via subcutaneous injection (sometimes through a syringe driver providing a continuous release of opioid into the circulation). Neuropathic pain may benefit from treatment with a tricyclic antidepressant (amitriptyline) or anticonvulsant (gabapentin or pregabalin). Bone pain may be amenable to radiotherapy.

Nausea and vomiting. These are unpleasant symptoms that can be quite common is patients with

Box 8 Components of supportive care

1. **Control of infection**. Predictable periods of agranulocytosis from marrow failure may cause life-threatening infection. Patients are routinely placed in *reversed barrier nursing* conditions. They are usually given *broad spectrum antibiotic* combinations at the first sign of infection. Granulocyte infusions are of limited use (colony-stimulating factors may be used; see Ch. 5).

2. **Awareness of thrombocytopenia**. Marrow failure predictably causes thrombocytopenia and a risk of severe bleeding. Intramuscular injections are absolutely contraindicated. Intravenous injections are safe (pressure can be placed on the bleeding). Platelet infusions may be valuable.

3. **Correction of anaemia**. Anaemia is often less of a problem because of the long half-life of red cells compared with platelets or white cells. However, transfusions are often needed. In the case of irreversible marrow failure induced by drugs and radiotherapy (e.g. in an attempt to cure certain leukaemias) bone marrow *transplantation* is often needed (usually from a related donor).

4. **Nausea**. This is often the worst symptom and requires aggressive management. Antiemetics are discussed in Chapter 11.

5. **Hair loss**. Though seemingly 'trivial' this may have a profound effect on morale. Patients must be warned if depilation is anticipated, and wigs should be made available.

6. **Palliative care**. This is dealt with in more detail in Section 15.3. Terminal care requires great medical and nursing skill, together with the appropriate use of drugs including analgesics (Ch. 7), antiemetics (Ch. 11) and laxatives (Ch. 11).

advanced malignancy. Opioid analgesia certainly does not help, and the underlying cause should be treated wherever possible. A range of different antiemetic therapies are available depending on the underlying aetiology but metoclopramide, haloperidol, cyclizine and levomepromazine are the most commonly used.

Constipation. This can be common, especially after opioid analgesia. The regular administration of a faecal softener and/or laxative may be beneficial.

Dyspnoea. Breathlessness through whatever cause is a distressing symptom. Morphine, starting in very small doses, can be helpful for this.

Excessive respiratory tract secretion. Antimuscarinic drugs such as hyoscine may help reduce excessive respiratory tract secretions.

Restlessness. Dopamine receptor antagonist such as haloperidol, chlorpromazine or levomepromazine may be used.

Anorexia. A poor appetite can be the result of many conditions, including malignancy. In palliative care, it can be a symptom that affects general wellbeing and can be relieved by steroids such as prednisolone or dexamethasone.

Self-assessment on Chapter 15: questions

Multiple choice questions

1. Methotrexate:
   a. Is antagonised by folic acid
   b. Is antagonised by folinic acid
   c. Enters cells by an active uptake mechanism
   d. Is potentiated by intracellular metabolism
   e. Is potentiated by hepatic disease

2. At standard dosage, the following drugs commonly cause the adverse effects to which they are linked in the question:
   a. Bleomycin and bone marrow suppression
   b. Cyclophosphamide and bladder carcinoma
   c. Doxorubicin and cardiac failure
   d. Methotrexate and macrocytosis
   e. Vincristine and peripheral neuropathy

3. The following statements concerning anticancer chemotherapy are true:
   a. Normal cells are usually more sensitive to the effects of the drugs than is the malignant clone
   b. The drugs are best given continuously for as long as possible
   c. Resistance to anticancer drugs is a major problem
   d. Most patients manage chemotherapy without the need for complicated supportive care
   e. Anticancer drugs cannot be given orally

Case history questions

A postmenopausal woman undergoes needle aspiration of a 3 cm lump in her breast. The aspirated cells are malignant, and she is admitted for segmental mastectomy and axillary lymph node sampling.

1. What are the two major roles of surgery here?

Thereafter she is offered six cycles of chemotherapy with fluorouracil–doxorubicin–cyclophosphamide.

2. By what mechanism might the tumour develop resistance to all these drugs?

She responds well to this cytotoxic regimen and is then started on tamoxifen, which is to continue for the next 5 years.

3. What is the most common adverse effect of tamoxifen that she should be warned about?

Short note question

Describe, giving examples, the mechanisms by which drugs used for cancer chemotherapy work. What adverse effects do the named drugs cause?

Extended matching items questions

Theme: Drug classes/mechanism of action in chemotherapy

Options
A. Alkaloid (plant)
B. Alkylating agent
C. Antimetabolite
D. Cytotoxic antibiotic
E. Hormonal agent
F. Monoclonal antibody
G. Platinum-based compound
H. Taxane
I. Topoisomerase I inhibitor

From the list of options above, select the single best term which describes the mechanism of action of the drugs listed below.

1. Goserelin
2. Paclitaxel
3. Cyclophosphamide
4. Methotrexate
5. Tamoxifen
6. Irinotecan
7. Busulfan

Questions

8. Doxorubicin

9. Bleomycin

10. Vincristine

11. Carboplatin

12. Rituximab

13. Cisplatin

14. Mercaptopurine

Self-assessment on Chapter 15: answers

Multiple choice answers

1. a. **False.**

   b. **True.** Methotrexate is a competitive inhibitor of dihydrofolate reductase (Fig. 51), the enzyme that reduces dihydrofolate back to tetrahydrofolate. The latter is a cofactor in the conversion of uridylate to thymidylate. Folic acid therefore 'precedes' the inhibited step. Folinic acid can 'bypass' this by conversion to methylene tetrahydrofolate (Fig. 51).

   c. **True.** Methotrexate is taken up by the same system that imports preformed folate into the cell; the lack of this system in microorganisms explains the lack of antimicrobial effect of the drug.

   d. **True.** Within the cell methotrexate becomes attached to glutamic acid residues: the polyglutamated form of the drug has activity against thymidylate synthetase (Fig. 51).

   e. **False.** Methotrexate is cleared unchanged: it is potentiated by renal disease.

2. a. **False.**

   b. **True.** Transitional cell carcinoma, resulting from chronic inflammation of the mucosa, is a problem unless mesna is used.

   c. **True.** This is an avoidable cumulative effect.

   d. **True.** Inhibition of DNA synthesis in red cell precursors results in fewer divisions and larger circulating cells.

   e. **True.**

3. a. **False.** Normal cells recover more rapidly than the malignant clones.

   b. **False.** It is usual to give courses of treatment interspersed with gaps to allow tissues (such as marrow, mucosal surfaces and skin) to recover.

   c. **True.** Especially if drugs are given as monotherapy. The mechanisms of resistance lie outside the scope of this book but include 'pumping' mechanisms that remove drug from the cancer cell.

   d. **False.** Almost everyone on cytotoxic treatment requires support in the areas of infection, blood products and nutrition.

   e. **False.** There are many drugs that are routinely given by mouth.

Case history answers

1. a. To reduce the size of the malignant clone by many log-orders.

   b. To permit microscopic examination of axillary lymph nodes, thereby clarifying prognosis and permitting decisions about further treatment to be made.

2. Multidrug resistance (or MDR) is usually caused by expression of P-glycoprotein pumps on cell surfaces. These pumps permit drug efflux from the malignant cell. These pumps can be opposed by such drugs as the calcium antagonist verapamil (which is more commonly used for its cardiac and hypotensive actions).

3. Tamoxifen is usually well tolerated, but hot flushes are quite common.

Short note answers

Modes of action

The major groups for discussion are:

Alkylating agents (e.g. cyclophosphamide and chlorambucil) transfer alkyl groups to nucleotide components of the DNA molecule. This results in misreading of the code, fragmentation of DNA and cross-linkage of DNA. Because alkylating agents interfere with transcription, their effects are not confined to rapidly dividing cells: any cell group may be affected.

Antimetabolites (e.g. methotrexate, mercaptopurine) compete with the substrate for the enzyme and inhibit enzyme function. Methotrexate resembles dihydrofolate, the substrate for the enzyme dihydrofolate reductase. Methotrexate also binds to, and inhibits, thymidylate synthetase, another enzyme important in the synthesis of pyrimidine nucleotides. The net effect is inhibition of DNA synthesis. 6-Mercaptopurine is an analogue of the purine bases adenine and guanine; it inhibits the enzymes responsible for interconversion of purines and is probably also incorporated into DNA. Antimetabolite drugs are mainly effective against rapidly dividing cells.

Vinca alkaloids (e.g. vincristine and vinblastine) bind to, and disrupt, the cytoskeleton (tubulin molecules). They produce arrest of mitosis and are effective mainly against rapidly dividing cells.

Cytotoxic antibiotics (e.g. daunorubicin) have been isolated from microbes (often fungi). They bind to DNA and block transcription and new DNA synthesis. They therefore have their effects on any cell, not just those which divide frequently.

Adverse effects

Suppression of bone marrow and mention the clinical consequences of this. All the above drugs, except the vinca alkaloids, produce marked marrow suppression.

Mucositis is produced by all the drugs to some extent, except the vinca drugs.

Nausea is produced by all the drugs (the vinca drugs to a lesser degree); mention its management briefly.

Alopecia occurs particularly with the antibiotics.

Specific organ toxicity can occur:

- pneumonitis: 6-mercaptopurine, bleomycin, methotrexate, antibiotics

- heart muscle damage: doxorubicin

- cystitis: cyclophosphamide (mention mesna)

- neurotoxicity: vinca drugs in particular

- hepatitis: any of these drugs, but particularly methotrexate and 6-mercaptopurine

- gametogenesis and fertility.

Extended matching items answers

1. E. Goserelin is a gonadotrophin releasing hormone analogue used in the treatment of prostate cancer.

2. H. Paclitaxel is a member of the taxane group of drugs, and is given by intravenous infusion along with a platinum based compound for the treatment of ovarian and breast cancer. Hypersensitivity reactions are quite common.

3. B. Cyclophosphamide is used in the treatment of some leukaemias, lymphomas as well as in solid tumours. There is a metabolite of cyclophosphamide which is excreted in the urine and can cause a haemorrhagic cystitis.

4. C. Methotrexate inhibits dihydrofolate reductase, an enzyme essential for the synthesis of purines and pyrimidines. Methotrexate can cause suppression of bone-marrow, and rarely, a pneumonitis.

5. E. Tamoxifen is used in breast cancer.

6. I. Irinotecan is an inhibitor of the enzyme topoisomerase I, one of the key enzymes involved in DNA replication. It is given by intravenous infusion.

7. B. Busulfan is an alkylating agent like cyclophosphamide. It is used to treat chronic myeloid leukaemia. Pulmonary fibrosis is a rare complication of treatment.

8. D. Doxorubicin is a cytotoxic used to treat the acute leukaemias, lymphomas and a variety of solid tumours.

9. D. Bleomycin can cause bone-marrow suppression and pulmonary fibrosis.

10. A. Vincristine is a vinca alkaloid drug like vinblastine. Neurotoxicity is a problem. It should *never* be given intrathecally.

11. G. Carboplatin is used in the treatment of advanced ovarian and lung cancer.

12. F. Rituximab is a monoclonal antibody which causes lysis of B lymphocytes and is licensed for aggressive types of lymphoma. Infusion-related side-effects are common.

13. G. Cisplatin is a platinum-based compound.

14. C. Mercaptopurine is an antimetabolite. It can be used in acute leukaemias but can also be used in inflammatory bowel disease. Azathioprine is metabolised to mercaptopurine and is used as an immunosuppressant for a whole variety of inflammatory conditions.

Drugs and the skin

16.1 Skin disorders	**233**
16.2 Skin and adverse drug reactions	**235**
Self-assessment on Chapter 16: questions	**237**
Self-assessment on Chapter 16: answers	**239**

Overview

Skin conditions are common; they may be confined to the skin, part of a wider systematic illness or caused by an adverse drug reaction. Many treatments for skin infections can be applied topically. Common conditions include eczema, psoriasis and acne. Common treatments are emollients to help rehydrate the skin, topical corticosteroids for inflammatory conditions and antibiotics for acne.

16.1 Skin disorders

Learning objectives

At the end of this section you should:
- be able to list the major common skin diseases
- be able to describe appropriate treatments for each of these conditions
- know the major adverse effects of these drugs.

The skin normally forms a water-resistant barrier and prevents loss of fluid. It also generally prevents entry of drugs, although certain drugs are now specifically formulated to enter through the skin; this avoids first pass metabolism and achieves direct entry into the systemic circulation. Sustained-release preparations are usually used with the drug contained in a reservoir held in place by an adhesive. Examples include glyceryl trinitrate, estradiol and progesterone, and nicotine (Chs 4 and 12).

The skin may suffer from a variety of conditions, usually not life-threatening but perhaps disfiguring. The skin may also be secondarily involved as part of a systemic illness.

Emollients

In the treatment of skin diseases, simple emollients are very important and are generally underused. These are bland substances that sooth and hydrate the skin and reduce irritation; they are very useful in conditions where the skin is dry and scaly. They may also be used as vehicles for drugs.

Examples include *aqueous cream* which is an oil in water emulsion. *Emulsifying ointment* is a water emulsion in oil and is more greasy and less pleasant to use but more effective for chronic dry skin lesions. It can be used as a skin cleansing agent instead of soap.

Topical antiinfectives

For many bacterial skin infections, such as cellulitis or erysipelas, systemic antibiotics are more appropriate as the infection is deep seated. Topical antibacterials are generally avoided: they may promote colonisation with resistant organisms and cause sensitisation. Simple cleaning of a wound is often adequate. Exceptions are a staphylococcal infection of the skin (impetigo) or in the treatment of skin colonisation with methicillin resistant *Staphylococcus aureus* in health care professionals. *Mupirocin* is a suitable topical treatment here.

There are specific preparations of some topical antibiotics for use on the conjunctiva (most often chloramphenicol eye drops, or in the ear for otitis externa (e.g. gentamicin or neomycin, often used with hydrocortisone).

Antiviral: aciclovir cream is widely used topically to treat labial herpes simplex.

Antifungals: skin fungal infections are common. Clotrimazole or itraconazole, or terbinafine are used topically (see Chapter 14).

Primary skin disorders

Eczema

> ### Clinical sketch
>
> A 21-year-old woman, who suffers from hay fever, reports that her skin is dry and irritated. This particularly bothers her on her face. She has had similar problems in the past, with no clear precipitant. She is particularly bothered now because the skin on her face is dry and flaking. She has had topical steroids in the past and wants them again now.
>
> *Comment: this is probably simple eczema. Short term use of 1% hydrocortisone to get control of the eczema would be reasonable. But longer term use of topical glucocorticoids or any use of more powerful glucocorticoids can cause skin thinning and atrophy. Long-term or very potent topical steroids should not be used on the face at all and elsewhere only intermittently. Use an emollient for the dryness and possibly oral antihistamines for the itching (if she is not already taking one).*

Eczema is an inflammatory response of the skin to either external or internal factors, acting either singly or in combination. These factors may be simple irritants, or there may be immunological mechanisms involved (there is an association of some forms of eczema with atopy). It may vary greatly in severity from dryness, scaling and itching, to severe itching with redness, formation of vesicles and perhaps exudation with crusting.

Treatment

An attempt should be made to identify and remove any causative irritants. If simple dryness of the skin and itching are present, an emollient to preserve the moisture of the skin may be adequate. In more severe cases, topical *glucocorticoid* creams and ointments are used in addition; a variety of such creams are available, of varying potency and strength (see Ch. 12 for their mode of action). The weakest preparation compatible with successful treatment should be used because of the adverse effects of topical glucocorticoids, including cutaneous atrophy and striae (it is particularly important to use topical glucocorticoids very sparingly on the face where such skin changes would be quite disfiguring). When they are withdrawn, a rebound exacerbation of the condition may occur. Rarely, systemic absorption of high-dose or high-potency topical glucocorticoids leads to systemic adverse effects and hypothalamic–pituitary–adrenal axis suppression.

Examples. Hydrocortisone is a low potency steroid, *betamethasone* medium potency and fluorinated steroids such as *clobetasol* high potency. These are available as creams or ointments.

In acute severe eczema with extensive exudate, *potassium permanganate* soaks are used initially. Oral sedating antihistamines are sometimes useful to reduce the itching.

Psoriasis

Psoriasis is a chronic inflammatory reaction of the skin of unknown aetiology, although there is often a family history. A form of psoriasis can arise after a streptococcal infection. The affected skin appears as thickened scaling plaques, often on the elbows, knees and scalp, although any area may be involved.

> ### Clinical sketch
>
> A 30-year-old man presents with red scaly lesions, most marked at his elbows and knees but also affecting his scalp and with some lesions on his trunk. The scalp is very itchy and the skin flakes readily. There is a family history of psoriasis, and he has had similar lesions for many years.
>
> *Comment: this sounds like plaque psoriasis. Topical treatment would be the first line, with emollients and maybe calcipotriol or dithranol. If unsuccessful and the psoriasis is severe, powerful immune suppressants may be needed.*

Treatment

In mild cases, simple emollients may be adequate. Topical keratolytic preparations containing *coal tar* (e.g. coal tar shampoo) or salicylic acid are effective but not pleasant to use. They act by softening and removing hardened skin and also have an anti-inflammatory effect. *Dithranol* acts in a similar manner and can be used for more severe disease; it is, however, irritant and can stain normal skin, so care must be taken to apply it only to the affected plaque. It is covered with a dressing for an hour and then washed off.

It was observed coincidentally that psoriasis improved in patients taking vitamin D. *Calcipotriol* and other vitamin D derivatives have been developed for topical use in psoriasis. It usually has no effect on systemic Ca^{2+} balance, unless large amounts are applied to very severe psoriasis where there may be systemic absorption; it should be avoided in patients with disordered Ca^{2+} metabolism. It is irritant, and local or generalised skin reactions can occur.

Specialist treatment. Ultraviolet light can improve psoriasis, and patients having this treatment may take a *psoralen* (a drug that increases the sensitivity of the skin) beforehand. This treatment needs careful supervision and is available in specialist centres only. Topical glucocorticoids are also used, but rebound of disease is a problem and they should be used only by specialists. Retinoids (see below) can be used. In severe cases, systemic immune suppression may be necessary: methotrexate (Ch. 15) or other systemic immune suppressants may be used. This is clearly associated with increased risks, but in some patients there may be no alternative.

Acne

Acne is a chronic inflammatory condition that particularly affects the face and back, characterised by the presence of comedones (blackheads), papules, pustules and cysts. In severe cases it may cause permanent scarring. It arises with the activation of the sebaceous glands at puberty, causing increased greasiness of the skin, and tends to clear with age. There may also be colonisation of the skin and sebaceous glands by *Propionibacterium acnes*, a bacterium that breaks down fats in the sebum to form irritant fatty acids.

Clinical sketch

An 20-year-old woman is distressed by the appearance of spots around her nose. She has blackheads and papules, and some pustules. She has been trying to hide these with cosmetics. She has some further lesions on her back.

Comment: acne is a common problem. This sounds moderately severe. Benzoyl peroxide should be used probably with a systemic antibiotic. If there is evidence of scarring or the acne does not respond quickly, she may need specialist referral. Isotretinoin could cause deformity of a fetus if she became pregnant and so would not be a safe option in a woman of this age unless there is rigorous use of contraception.

Treatment

Benzoyl peroxide kills the bacteria and peels the skin, unplugging the follicles: it can be irritant to the skin and a weak solution is applied to the face for a short period and then washed off; gradually, the duration of exposure and the strength of the preparation are increased. In moderate cases, long-term systemic or topical antibiotic treatment, usually with tetracycline or one of its derivatives or erythromycin is effective.

Co-cyprindiol consisting of cryproterone acetate and ethynylestradiol is a contraceptive with antiandrogen effects which may be useful in women who need both acne treatment and contraception. As with all oestrogenic compounds there is a risk of venous thromboembolism (see Ch. 12).

In very severe cases, vitamin A derivatives such as *isotretinoin* can be used. These may be used topically (*tretinoin, isotretinoin*) in mild to moderate acne, or orally (*isotretinoin*) in severe acne. Their adverse effects used topically include local irritation, redness and photosensitivity.

Isotretinoin's systemic adverse effects when given orally include hepatitis and altered serum lipids; most importantly, it is teratogenic and is usually given only to males, or to females who are using careful contraception (for at least a month before and after treatment: but longer afterwards is wise since isotretinoin concentrates in body fat and may take up to 2 years to be completely cleared). Isotretinoin may rarely cause severe depression. Because of these hazards, isotretinoin can only be prescribed by hospital specialists.

Topical retinoids do not usually have systemic adverse effects but must be avoided in pregnancy and used only in females with careful contraception.

16.2 Skin and adverse drug reactions

Learning objectives

At the end of this section you should be aware of:
- the potential for skin disorders associated with drug therapy
- the seriousness of the reaction.

The skin is also a common site for manifestation of adverse drug effects, often allergic in nature. Rashes or itching can occur shortly after the drug is first taken, but sometimes not until 2–3 weeks later. Almost any type of reaction may occur, and these can mimic many skin conditions, including rashes, itching, photosensitivity, hair loss, purpura, blistering and pigmentation. A fixed drug eruption is a drug reaction that occurs in the same place on each exposure. Some reactions are particularly associated with certain drugs:

- morbelliform (measles-like): ampicillin, amoxicillin
- lichen planus-like: gold, antimalarials
- exfoliative dermatitis: penicillin, gold.

Clinical sketch

A newly diagnosed epileptic is prescribed carbamazepine for the first time. Two weeks later, he has developed ulceration in his mouth such that he has difficulty drinking. He is feverish and feels very unwell.

Comment: the diagnosis is Stevens–Johnson syndrome, a severe and unusual form of skin reaction to carbamazepine. This is an example of a type B adverse drug reaction.

Most skin reactions are mild and self-limiting. Stevens–Johnson syndrome is a severe and usually fatal condition with skin blistering. It is associated with the use of some drugs such as fluconazole and carbamazepine.

Self-assessment on Chapter 16: questions

Multiple choice questions

1. The following statements are correct:
   a. The skin prevents the entry of all drugs
   b. Topical corticosteroids may cause systemic adverse effects
   c. Psoriasis is treated with keratolytic agents or vitamin D derivatives
   d. Acne is treated with topical corticosteroids
   e. Vitamin A derivatives are teratogenic

2. The following statements are correct:
   a. Isotretinoin is used to treat herpes simplex
   b. Adverse drug reactions often affect the skin
   c. Methotrexate is used topically in severe psoriasis
   d. Eczema of the face is treated with high-potency fluorinated glucocorticoids
   e. Topical treatment is adequate for all skin conditions

3. The following drugs may be applied directly to the skin for systematic therapeutic effect (i.e. can affect the whole body)
   a. Hydrocortisone
   b. Estradiol
   c. Aspirin
   d. Glyceryl trinitrate
   e. Fusidic acid

Case history questions

An 18-year-old man presents with acne. This is moderately severe and has failed to respond to simple peeling agents used for some weeks.

1. What would you consider is the next line of treatment?

There is some improvement on your second line treatment but the condition does not resolve and there are some large inflamed areas. There is concern that these may go on to scar, since they are on the face.

2. What drug treatment would you consider now?

3. What precautions would you take and which warning would you give before starting this treatment?

Extended matching items questions

Theme: Acne

Options
  A. Isotretinoin
  B. Hydrocortisone
  C. Tetracycline
  D. Emollient
  E. Coal tar
  F. Cyproterone
  G. Benzoyl peroxide
  H. Calcipotriol

Answer the questions below by choosing the most appropriate option from those listed above. Each option can be used once, more than once, or not at all.

1. A peeling agent, used as first line in mild to moderate acne
2. A drug which may have serious teratogenic effects if used in women
3. An antiandrogen
4. An antibiotic used systemically in acne
5. A drug used which may cause photosensitivity

Theme: Miscellaneous skin conditions

Options
  A. Isotretinoin
  B. Hydrocortisone
  C. Clobetasol
  D. Emollient
  E. Coal tar
  F. Amoxicillin
  G. Chlorpheniramine
  H. Calcipotriol

Answer the questions below by choosing the most appropriate option from those listed above. Each option can be used once, more than once, or not at all.

1. A sedating antihistamine useful in itchy conditions

2. A vitamin D derivative used in psoriasis

3. A high potency topical glucorticoid

4. Used in conditions with dry skin

5. A drug which may cause a measles-like rash

Self-assessment on Chapter 16: answers

Multiple choice answers

1. a. **False.** While true for most drugs, there are many preparations specifically designed to penetrate the skin.
   b. **True.** If used in very high dose.
   c. **True.** Keratolytics to reduce the scaling; calcipotriol's mode of action is unknown.
   d. **False.** Peeling agents and some antibiotics are used: corticosteroids would make things worse.
   e. **True.** So only given to women of child-bearing potential if they are using effective contraception.

2. a. **False.** Isotretinoin is used to treat acne and other skin disorders.
   b. **True.** A very common site of manifestation of adverse drug reactions.
   c. **False.** Used systemically.
   d. **False.** This would cause striae etc. on the face. Less potent steroids may be used with great care.
   e. **False.** For example, methotrexate, etc.

3. a. **False.** Commonly used in dermatology for local effect but will not have a systematic effect. More potent corticosteroids may if applied in sufficient quantity have a systematic effect, as proven by adrenocortical suppression.
   b. **True.** Used in oestrogen patches for systematic effect in the treatment of postmenopausal problems.
   c. **False.** Too irritant to use topically at all, although some salicylates are used in traditional rubefacients for relief of musculoskeletal pain, and salicylic acid can be used in psoriasis. These do not have a systematic effect.
   d. **True.** Used in patches or creams to treat angina.
   e. **False.** Although used topically to treat local infections, for instance in the eye.

Case history answers

1. Since topical peeling agents alone have been unsuccessful, it is time to consider systemic antibiotics. Topical antibiotics are generally less effective. Long-term oxytetracycline or erythromycin should be considered. It can take some weeks for this to have its maximum effect.

2. Since systemic antibiotics in addition to topical agents have failed to resolve the condition satisfactorily, it is time to consider vitamin A derivatives such as isotretinoin.

3. The potential adverse effects are hepatitis and altered serum lipids and teratogenicity. Fortunately, teratogenicity is not an issue in this male patient, but blood should be sent for serum lipids and for liver function tests before starting the therapy and intermittently during it. The patient should be warned of the major adverse effects. Because of these hazards and the need for careful monitoring, isotretinoin is usually only prescribed by hospital specialists.

Extended matching items answers

Theme: Acne

1. G. Benzoyl peroxide is widely used alone and with other treatments.

2. A. Isotretinoin can be teratogenic in women: it must only be used in women of childbearing age who are using effective contraception, and who will continue to use it after withdrawal of the retinoid.

3. F. Sometimes used with ethinylestradiol as a contraceptive in women with acne, but has a higher risk of thromboembolism than many low dose oestrogen preparations.

4. C. Tetracycline or its derivatives are used in this way.

5. A and C. Isotretinoin and tetracyclines may both cause photosensitivity.

Theme: Miscellaneous skin conditions

1. G. Chlorpheniramine. But remember to warn patient about driving, etc.

2. H. Avoid in patients with e.g. hyperparathyroidism or sarcoidosis.

3. C. Clobetasol. Hydrocortisone is a low potency glucocorticoid.

4. D. 'Emollient' is not a specific preparation but a description of what we expect such preparations to achieve, e.g. emulsifying ointment.

5. F. Amoxicillin is the most likely culprit.

Drug overdose and poisoning

17.1 The principles of supportive care   **241**

17.2 Specific drugs   **243**

    Self assessment on Chapter 17: questions   **246**

    Self assessment on Chapter 17: answers   **248**

Overview

Poisoning is one of the most common medical emergencies. In the majority of cases, it is deliberate, the result of social pressures or psychiatric illness, but accidental overdose by children remains common, despite 'child-proof' medicine containers. In an industrial setting, inadvertent acute poisoning can occur from a variety of non-therapeutic compounds, including heavy metals, insecticides and gases such as cyanide and carbon monoxide.

Management of drug overdose involves identifying the causative agent, assessing the dose involved, supportive care and minimising the adverse effects, with antidotes if possible.

17.1 The principles of supportive care

Learning objectives

At the end of this section you should:

* know the management of a poisoned patient, the principles of decontamination, acceleration of drug elimination, specific antidotes and supportive care
* understand the principles of supportive care
* know the main antidotes used and the drugs for which they are used
* be able to describe the principles underpinning the use of alkaline diuresis and haemodialysis/ haemoperfusion for enhancing drug elimination.

Initial resuscitation and an assessment of level of consciousness and vital signs should be followed by an attempt to discover:

* what drug(s) or toxin(s) were taken (bearing in mind, 'cocktails' of drugs may be taken)
* what dose(s) were taken (empty bottles can be very useful)
* approximately the time of ingestion (although the patient's assessment of time lapse can often be unreliable).

Management comprises:

* decontamination
* supportive care
* specific measures to reduce toxicity through the use of 'antidotes' or to enhance elimination.

The clinical sketches in this chapter illustrate the more frequently encountered overdose/poisoning situations and their likely presentation.

Supportive care

Detailed consideration of supportive care is beyond the scope of this book, but the student should be aware of the principal ways in which poisoning can cause problems, and ways in which these problems can be managed. In general, supportive care is the mainstay of treatment – oxygen and intravenous fluids may be all that is required. The National Poisons Information Service (NPIS) provides up-to-date expert advice on the management of any overdose: the lethality of the dose ingested, the clinical features to be vigilant for and the specific treatment required. NPIS is available 24 hours a day (either via an online database TOXBASE® www.spib.axl.co.uk or via the telephone) and should always be consulted for all but the most straightforward cases.

Coma. Death may result from obstruction of the airway by soft tissues, by aspiration of vomit or by depression of the respiratory centre. It is essential that level of consciousness be monitored (e.g. using tools such as the Glasgow Coma Scale). Protection of the airway is critical: nursing in the recovery position will usually be sufficient, but some patients may need endotracheal intubation. Monitoring of arterial gases is critical in such severely ill patients: respiratory failure necessitates mechanical ventilation.

Seizures. CNS excitation, resulting in seizures, can coexist with profound coma and can contribute to respiratory failure. Antiepileptic drugs may be needed, and resistant cases may need to be paralysed and ventilated on an intensive care unit.

Cardiovascular toxicity. Toxins may cause arrhythmias (fast or slow), reduced stroke volume, vasodilatation or a combination of these: the resulting shock may prove fatal. In many cases acid–base and electrolyte imbalance are major contributing factors. Electrolyte/pH correction, temporary cardiac pacing, inotropic drugs and antiarrhythmics may all be needed in supportive care.

Renal failure. This is another common life-threatening problem. Careful clinical assessment is required; treatment ranges from the administration of intravenous fluids to emergency haemodialysis/haemofiltration.

Clinical sketch: paracetamol

An 18-year-old girl takes an overdose of paracetamol following a row with her boyfriend. Thereafter, although she feels okay, she regrets her actions and is scared. She presents to hospital about 8 hours after drug ingestion. The doctors measure her plasma paracetamol concentration: it is above the 'treatment line', so an infusion of *N*-acetylcysteine is started. Her clotting parameters and liver function tests remain normal and she makes an uneventful recovery.

Comment: patients are relatively asymptomatic between ingestion of the drug and development of liver impairment between 48 and 72 hours thereafter. The insidious nature of this problem probably contributes to its mortality since patients can present too late for help. Prolonged prothrombin time and elevated transaminase levels are the first indication of impending illness; thereafter clinical features of acute liver damage develop. This young girl was caught before clinically apparent liver damage was done.

Clinical sketch: salicylate

A 22-year-old woman takes an impulsive overdose of aspirin. She feels unwell almost at once with nausea, vomiting and tinnitus. She presents to A&E where she is found to be ill, tachypnoeic and dehydrated. Her arterial pH is 7.05 and her salicylate level is very high. Rather than rely on alkaline diuresis, the clinical team decides that haemodialysis is needed: she is moved to ITU.

Comment: metabolic acidosis is the commonest acid–base disturbance seen in adults after significant salicylate overdose. There is no specific antidote; management hinges on accelerating elimination of the drug. Alkaline diuresis (see text) increases the rate of elimination but haemodialysis is required in the most serious cases.

Clinical sketch: opiates

A young i.v. drug abuser is found unconscious in the street by the police. He has pinpoint pupils and is deeply cyanosed; his blood pressure is unrecordable. His arterial gases are as follows: pH 7.15, PCO_2 10.5 kPa, PO_2 6.5 kPa. The doctors gain i.v. access and give him i.v. naloxone. This improves his clinical features but he remains very ill: he is intubated and ventilated. The naloxone is repeated periodically in ITU.

Comment: this man has pronounced CNS depression causing type 2 respiratory failure and respiratory acidosis. He may have inadvertently taken too much heroin (street supplies vary in their purity); alternatively he may have taken more than one drug. Naloxone is a specific opiate antagonist; it has a very short half-life necessitating repeated dosing, usually with an infusion. Patients normally respond rapidly and completely if their only intoxication is with an opiate. Supportive care on ITU is provided until the drug is eliminated from the body.

Clinical sketch: tricyclic antidepressants

A 50-year-old man lost his wife a year ago and has been depressed ever since. His GP has prescribed amitriptyline, and this may have helped (he has been sleeping better). However, after leaving a suicide note, he takes a massive overdose of amitriptyline and is found by his daughter late that afternoon. A&E doctors find an unconscious man who starts to fit soon after arrival. He is transferred to ITU, where he dies of cardiac arrhythmias despite best efforts.

Comment: tricyclic antidepressants cause profound CNS depression, seizures, arrhythmias and shock. There are no accepted means of enhancing elimination, and no specific antidote is available; management is supportive. Fortunately such scenarios are rare. More modern antidepressants such as serotonin-specific reuptake inhibitors are (relatively) safer in overdose, and are hence beneficial in a population of patients already at high risk of overdose and deliberate self-harm.

Decontamination

Decontamination includes both removal of toxin from the skin and clothes in industrial accidents (followed by copious washing) and removal of drug from the gastrointestinal tract. Most overdoses are taken orally, but the absorption of most drugs is pretty rapid and there is little to be gained by attempting to remove the drug – indeed this may be positively dangerous. Gastric lavage is very rarely indicated, and is only carried out if a life-threatening amount has been ingested within the previous hour, and only if the airway can be properly protected. The induction of vomiting (emesis) by potent emetic drugs such as ipecacuanha is not recommended. Emesis and gastric lavage are absolutely contraindicated where corrosive substances such as bleach have been ingested – these may do more damage, including exacerbating oesophageal damage, and increase the risk of a life-threatening aspiration pneumonitis.

Activated charcoal may be given orally following an overdose to bind the poison within the gastrointestinal tract to prevent absorption. The aim is to give it as soon as possible, although drugs which delay gastric emptying, or modified release preparations are particularly susceptible to the use of activated charcoal.

Specific antidotes

Specific antidotes are available for some drugs/ toxins (Table 3).

Methods of enhancing elimination

Manipulation of urinary pH

Some drugs become unionised at urinary pH and may be reabsorbed in the distal tubule. Relatively small changes in urinary pH produce relatively large changes in the fraction of drug unionised (see Ch. 1 for the Henderson–Hasselbach equation, which describes this relationship) and alter renal clearance. This is of practical value with overdoses of:

- salicylates
- phenobarbital.

Table 3 Specific antidotes

Drug/toxin	Antidote
Paracetamol	*N*-acetylcysteine is a specific antidote
Opiates	Naloxone is an antagonist
Benzodiazepines	Flumazenil is an antagonist
Iron	Desferrioxamine chelates
Copper	Penicillamine chelates
Lead	Edetate (EDTA) chelates
Mercury, arsenic	Dimercaprol chelates

In both cases, sodium bicarbonate is given as an intravenous infusion. This increases urinary pH. This is termed an alkaline diuresis. However, haemodialysis is the treatment of choice for severe salicylate poisoning.

Haemodialysis and haemoperfusion

Drugs with relatively small apparent volumes of distribution (VD) are largely restricted to the plasma, whereas those with large VD are extensively distributed to the tissues. Drugs with a small VD may be removable by haemodialysis (the extracorporeal pumping of blood across a large surface area of semipermeable membrane) or haemoperfusion (the pumping of blood through a column of adsorbent material, such as charcoal).

Factors influencing the utility of these measures for a particular drug include molecular weight, water solubility and protein binding.

Haemodialysis may be valuable for:

- salicylate
- aminophylline
- lithium.

Haemoperfusion may be valuable for:

- phenobarbital
- carbamazepine.

17.2 Specific drugs

> **Learning objectives**
>
> At the end of this section you should be able to:
> - describe the clinical syndromes that are commonly encountered after overdoses of paracetamol, salicylate, opiates, benzodiazepines, stimulants, tricyclic antidepressants, heavy metals and organophosphates.

Many patients overdose with more than one drug. It is important to establish the history as accurately as possible.

Paracetamol

In therapeutic doses, paracetamol is principally metabolised to non-toxic, water-soluble conjugates. However, in overdose, conjugation becomes saturated and 'excess' drug is oxidised to a toxic metabolite. The toxin forms covalent bonds with proteins, both structural and enzymic, thereby denaturing them. Cells employ glutathione as a defence against such toxins: it forms non-toxic conjugates with the

Seventeen

toxin. However, intracellular glutathione 'stores' are soon exhausted after a significant paracetamol overdose. Glutathione cannot be used as an antidote because of its inability to enter cells. N-acetylcysteine is a glutathione precursor. Although generally very safe, N-acetylcysteine is not without risk (hypersensitivity) and should not be used indiscriminately.

The risk of liver damage correlates well with plasma paracetamol concentration, and this measure is used to guide therapy. Because drug absorption may not be complete within the first 4 hours after ingestion, measurement of plasma paracetamol should not be done within this period. Thereafter, patients with a plasma concentration above the 'treatment line' (see the British National Formulary or TOXBASE) should be given N-acetylcysteine (as an i.v. loading dose, followed by i.v. infusion).

Beyond 14 hours after paracetamol overdose, the benefits of N-acetylcysteine are less clear, though most units would still try using it even in late presenters. Most physicians err on the side of caution when deciding to administer N-acetylcysteine in the presence of ambiguity. Established acute liver failure needs to be treated in specialist centres and carries a high mortality rate; transplantation may be required.

Methionine, an amino acid given orally, can also be used to regenerate glutathione stores but is less effective than N-acetylcysteine. It tastes particularly foul and is only effective if given within the first 10–12 hours. It can, however, be useful in remote areas where there may be a delay in seeking specialist medical help, provided the patient is not vomiting.

Salicylate

Aspirin has several metabolic effects: it stimulates the respiratory centre, interferes with carbohydrate and lipid metabolism and is itself a relatively strong acid. Stimulation of the respiratory centre, which causes hyperventilation, results in a *respiratory alkalosis*, typically seen early on. To compensate for this, there is renal loss of bicarbonate ions, which reduces buffering capacity; higher salicylate concentrations then induce a *metabolic acidosis* readily (both directly and by changes in carbohydrate and lipid metabolism).

Salicylate poisoning gives symptoms soon after drug ingestion: abdominal pain, nausea, tinnitus, deafness, vertigo and hyperpnoea. If the overdose is large, fever, dehydration, metabolic acidosis, renal impairment and cardiovascular collapse may follow.

The severity of poisoning can be assessed by measuring the plasma salicylate concentration: plasma salicylate over 700 mg/L (5.1 mmol/L) confirms severe poisoning (though better guidance may be given by serial measurements to establish whether concentrations are rising).

Rehydration is an important part of general care. Drug elimination can be enhanced by alkalinisation of the urine or, in severe cases, by haemodialysis.

Opiates

Sedation, cough suppression and respiratory depression occur as a direct consequence of stimulation of opioid μ-receptors. This results in deep coma with pinpoint pupils, hypotension and hypothermia.

Patients with *respiratory failure* should receive the specific antidote *naloxone* as an i.v. injection. This opioid receptor antagonist causes prompt improvement in the level of consciousness unless other sedative drugs have been taken. Naloxone's duration of action is very short, and it may need to be given frequently. Methadone has a particularly long duration of action. Naloxone induces a state of acute opiate withdrawal in those patients addicted to opiates and is not used unless respiratory failure is a problem. Buprenorphine, a synthetic opiate, may not be reversed by naloxone.

Benzodiazepines

The GABA agonist action of the benzodiazepines causes CNS depression. However, benzodiazepines have a relatively flat dose–response curve and do not induce surgical levels of anaesthesia even after overdose. They are consequently safer than the barbiturates in this setting. However, patients may still vomit and aspirate, and those with chronic pulmonary disease are still at risk of respiratory failure.

The use of *flumazenil* (a specific benzodiazepine antagonist) can be particularly hazardous in mixed overdoses involving tricyclic antidepressants or in those patients who are physically dependent on benzodiazepines. It can precipitate seizures; its use should therefore be with expert advice only. Flumazenil has a short duration of action and may need to be repeated frequently.

Tricyclic antidepressants

Tricyclic antidepressants have complex pharmacological effects (Ch. 6) including inhibition of reuptake of noradrenaline (norepinephrine) into neurones, anticholinergic actions and quinidine-like antiarrhythmic effects:

- combined effects on the CNS cause agitation at lower concentration but result in profound CNS depression and seizures at higher levels
- anticholinergic effects cause tachycardia
- quinidine-like action results in QT prolongation and ST changes in the ECG and reduced stroke volume (hence reduced cardiac output). Arrhythmias, such as torsades-de-pointes (a polymorphic form of ventricular tachycardia), can result and be very difficult to treat.

Early features may include blurred vision, retention of urine, dry mouth and agitation. Features of severe poisoning include coma, seizures, arrhythmias and shock. Because anticholinergic effects delay gastric emptying, activated charcoal can be indicated even beyond 12 hours after ingestion.

Tricylic antidepressants have very large volumes of distribution. Consequently, measures such as haemodyalisis are of no value (there is simply too little drug in the plasma for any impact to be made). With no accepted means of enhancing elimination, and no specific antidote, management hinges on supportive care. Sodium bicarbonate may be given intravenously to those with an abnormal ECG.

Stimulants (e.g. 'Ecstasy')

Ecstasy (see Ch. 18) is an amfetamine derivative, *methylenedioxymetamfetamine*. It is widely available to young people and taken orally. Its use is entirely illicit, i.e. it is not made by reputable manufacturers and therefore quality control is poor and tablet contents may vary.

Clinical effects include vomiting, tachycardia, hyperthermia and hypo/hypertension. Rhabdomyolysis (destruction of skeletal muscle), renal failure and disseminated intravascular coagulation (a blood clotting disorder) may be seen.

Death is usually caused by cardiac arrhythmias. There is no specific antidote and neither haemodialysis nor haemoperfusion is beneficial. Management is entirely supportive.

Heavy metals

Iron. Desferrioxamine chelates iron. The symptoms of iron poisoning evolve over several days:

phase 1 is characterised by gastrointestinal features and may involve severe ulceration; it evolves over about 6 hours
phase 2 between 6 and 24 hours, comprises resolution of symptoms – most patients have no further problems
phase 3 between 12 and 48 hours after serious poisoning: a minority of patients develop shock, acidosis and renal/hepatic failure
phase 4 comprises late complications (2–6 weeks after poisoning) from high intestinal or pyloric strictures.

Lead. Lead poisoning can present with encephalopathy and peripheral neuropathy. *Chelators* include EDTA, penicillamine and calcium edetate.
Mercury. Mercury poisoning can present with tremor, encephalopathy and renal impairment. *Chelators* include dimercaprol and penicillamine.

Organophosphates

These insecticides are widely used in farming. They are extensively absorbed from the skin and inhibit acetylcholinesterase.

The main acute effects of massive exposure are respiratory muscle paralysis and coma.

Atropine is used to oppose the excessive acetylcholinergic activity in the autonomic nervous system. Pralidoxime is used to help regenerate acetylcholinesterase.

Seventeen

Self-assessment on Chapter 17: questions

Multiple choice questions

1. Poisoning with benzodiazepines:
   a. Causes seizures
   b. Causes respiratory depression
   c. Should be reversed with flumazenil in all cases
   d. Is more severe in the presence of respiratory disease
   e. Can be reversed by haemodialysis

2. In the case of iron poisoning:
   a. Gastric lavage causes oesophageal damage
   b. Oral desferrioxamine is adequate to chelate the fraction of the dose that has been absorbed
   c. Oral desferrioxamine is useless
   d. Patients may be discharged within 24 hours of poisoning
   e. Serum iron concentrations give a good idea of prognosis

3. Following paracetamol poisoning:
   a. Symptoms and signs develop quickly
   b. Serum paracetamol levels should be estimated as soon as possible after poisoning
   c. Estimation of the International Normalised Ratio is the most useful guide to severity of poisoning in patients who present late
   d. N-acetylcysteine works by chelating paracetamol
   e. N-acetylcysteine should be given to all patients irrespective of their drug concentrations

Case history questions

Case history 1

A man takes a deliberate overdose of amitriptyline, but 4 hours later regrets this and presents to hospital.

1. How essential is it to measure drug concentrations?
2. Should he be given any prophylactic drugs?

He is given activated charcoal, and he is sent to the ward. His plasma potassium is 2.9 mmol/L (reference range 3.5–5.0 mmol/L). His heart rate is 140 beats/min, regular, and his blood pressure is 110/60 mmHg.

3. Should anything be done at this stage?

Later, he becomes unconscious, has a series of generalised fits and his pulse rate rises to 180 beats/min with blood pressure of 100/60 mmHg. The doctor gives him physostigmine for the coma and convulsions.

4. Why physostigmine?
5. Is this drug of first choice for convulsion in a tricyclic overdose?
6. Should an antiarrhythmic drug be given?

Case history 2

A 20-year-old i.v. drug abuser is admitted comatose after a probable opiate overdose. She is given naloxone i.v. and her level of consciousness improves. She is admitted and sent to the ward.

1. What else must be done?

Short note questions

1. Consider the following model illustrating volume of distribution (VD): 1 g each of two compounds, A and B, are added simultaneously to a small glass beaker, of unknown volume. The beaker is filled with water and has some black powder (looks like charcoal) in the bottom. We lack the means to measure the volume of the beaker directly but can measure the concentrations of A and B: that of A is about 1 g/L, that of B is about 0.001 g/L.
   a. What are the VD values of A and B?
   b. What is the probable explanation for the difference?
   c. What does the charcoal represent in this model?

d. If the relative VD values of two drugs are the same in vivo as A and B in this model, which is more amenable to removal by dialysis in the event of overdose?

2. Write short notes on the clinical features and management of severe aspirin poisoning.

Extended matching items questions

Theme: Clinical features of poisoning

Options

A. Alcohol

B. Amitriptyline

C. Aspirin

D. Ecstasy

E. Ferrous sulphate

F. Methadone

G. Nifedipine

H. Paracetamol

For each of the following clinical scenarios, select the most appropriate culprit drug explaining the presentation from the options listed above. Each option may be used once, more than once, or not at all.

1. Abdominal pain and vomiting 36 hours following ingestion. The liver function tests are all very abnormal and the prothrombin time is elevated.

2. Coma and respiratory depression. The blood pressure is low and the pupils are pinpoint.

3. Acute renal failure caused by rhabdomyolysis. There is hyperpyrexia.

4. Convulsions and metabolic acidosis. The pupils are dilated and the QRS interval is prolonged.

5. Initial tinnitus associated with hyperventilation and a respiratory alkalosis followed by a metabolic acidosis.

Theme: Specific antidotes

Options

A. Atropine

B. Desferrioxamine

C. Dimercaprol

D. Edetate (EDTA)

E. Flumazenil

F. *N*-acetylcysteine

G. Naloxone

H. Verapamil

For each of the drugs listed below, select the most appropriate antidote from the options listed above. Each option may be used once, more than once, or not at all.

1. Diazepam

2. Paracetamol

3. Dihydrocodeine

4. Lead

5. Mercury

Self-assessment on Chapter 17: answers

Multiple choice answers

1. a. **False.** Benzodiazepines cause sedation, and seizures are very uncommon.

   b. **True.** Respiratory depression is rarely severe enough to threaten life.

   c. **False.** Flumazenil should only be given with caution.

   d. **True.** Precipitation of respiratory failure is more likely in patients whose respiratory function and blood gases are usually poor.

   e. **False.** Benzodiazepines have very large volumes of distribution.

2. a. **False.** Gastric lavage is contraindicated for corrosive substances (such as bleach) but not iron.

   b. **False.** Desferrioxamine is not absorbed; it must be given parenterally to chelate absorbed iron.

   c. **False.** When desferrioxamine is given into the stomach, it chelates unabsorbed iron.

   d. **False.** The symptoms of serious iron poisoning evolve over several days.

   e. **True.** Serum iron >90 mmol/L indicates the need for parenteral desferrioxamine. Although desferrioxamine is generally safe, adverse reactions to it include anaphylaxis, hypotension and visual/hearing impairment.

3. a. **False.** Most patients remain asymptomatic until they develop hepatic necrosis (takes at least 24 hours to become apparent).

   b. **False.** Estimates made in the first 4 hours after ingestion are not reliable because drug absorption is still in progress.

   c. **True.** Clotting abnormality is a sensitive indicator of developing liver damage. The International Normalised Ratio (INR) is a standardized form of the prothrombin time (PT).

   d. **False.** *N*-acetylcysteine is a glutathione precursor that forms adducts with reactive paracetamol metabolites.

   e. **False.** *N*-acetylcysteine does cause anaphylaxis occasionally and should be reserved for those patients with drug concentration above the 'treatment line' on the standard graph.

Case history answers

Case history 1

1. There is no antidote for tricyclics, and no means of increasing their clearance, so knowing drug concentrations will not alter management. All cases of tricyclic poisoning should be admitted, and most physicians would want to observe for a period of at least 48 hours because of the tendency for late complications.

2. No. Vital signs should be observed, and electrolyte concentrations should be measured.

3. He is hypokalaemic: this predisposes to tachyarrhythmias and should be corrected using an i.v. infusion of potassium chloride diluted in 0.9% saline or 5% glucose. His tachycardia is currently insignificant, and his blood pressure is well maintained: antiarrhythmic drugs are not indicated. A cardiac monitor should be used, and the patient should be nursed in a high-dependency area (such as a coronary care unit).

4. Tricyclic drugs have marked antimuscarinic properties, which may cause coma and fits. Physostigmine is an anticholinesterase (Ch. 8) that potentiates acetylcholine; furthermore, it crosses the blood–brain barrier.

5. The effects of physostigmine are short lived, and it is not considered first-line therapy; i.v. diazepam is probably preferable to terminate fits, and if coma becomes a problem (through respiratory failure) ventilation is indicated.

6. His blood pressure is still well maintained, so the arrhythmia is unlikely to be life threatening at the moment. However, an ECG should be done and the arrhythmia should be identified. Acidosis, if present, needs to be corrected. Sodium bicarbonate may be given. Antiarrhythmic drugs should be reserved for life-threatening arrhythmias; their early use will often make the situation worse. Lidocaine,

beta-blockers and phenytoin are most often employed.

Case history 2

Naloxone has a very short duration of action, and repeated doses may be needed: ward doctors should be warned of this, and close observations made of the level of consciousness. Opiates like dihydrocodeine are formulated in compound tablets with paracetamol, and patients often take more than one type of pill: unless paracetamol concentrations are measured this poisoning may go unnoticed until liver failure ensues. Salicylate concentrations should also be measured, given the ready availability of this drug, to judge whether alkaline diuresis is required.

Short note answers

1. a. For compound A, VD = 1 g ÷ 1 g/L = 1.0 litres. For compound B, VD = 1 g ÷ 0.001 g/L = 1000 litres.
   b. The likeliest reason for the difference is that compound B binds avidly to the charcoal.
   c. In this model, charcoal represents the tissues.
   d. The drug with the smaller VD will be more readily removed from the body.

2. Make the following points:
   a. Discuss pertinent pharmacokinetics:
      — aspirin has a small volume of distribution
      — much of the drug is eliminated unchanged in the urine
      — aspirin is an acid, and tubular reabsorption of aspirin can be reduced if the urine is made alkaline
      Mention also that salicylate pharmacokinetics become zero order at high concentration and that the protein binding of the drug can be saturated at high plasma concentration (so the unbound drug fraction rises; explain the importance of this).
   b. State that management is heavily influenced by plasma salicylate concentrations. Mention that salicylate concentrations often need to be measured more than once (in case absorption is slow).

c. Activated charcoal may reduce drug absorption.
d. Supportive care is important and comprises:
   — rehydration
   — correction of hypokalaemia, hyperglycaemia and severe acidosis.
e. Drug clearance is increased by alkalinisation of the urine if plasma salicylate exceeds 750 mg/L:
   — 1.4% sodium bicarbonate is infused i.v. to achieve a urine pH between 7.5 and 8.5
   — input/output balance including central venous pressure should be measured.
f. In severe poisoning (plasma salicylate >700 mg/L), or poisoning complicated by renal failure, haemodialysis may be required.

Extended matching items answers

Theme: Clinical features of poisoning

1. H. This is typical of paracetamol poisoning. Clinical features are relatively late. The prothrombin time is a marker of synthetic liver function.
2. F. This is opiate poisoning and is common in intravenous drug users. Methadone may be either obtained illicitly or via a drug rehabilitation programme.
3. D. There are a number of very serious effects of ecstasy including convulsions, arrhythmias, rhabdomyolysis (which can cause renal failure) and intracerebral haemorrhage.
4. B. This patient needs supportive care on an intensive care unit. Sodium bicarbonate should be given with appropriate monitoring.
5. C. This pattern is very characteristic of salicylate poisoning.

Theme: Specific antidotes

1. E. However, flumazenil can cause problems when multiple drugs have been taken (including tricyclic antidepressants) or when the patient is benzodiazepine dependent.
2. F. *N*-acetylcysteine is the treatment of choice in paracetamol overdose. Hypersensitivity reactions can be a problem. Methionine is another donor of glutathione and is an alternative.

3. G. The half-life of the opiate compared to the half-life of naloxone needs to be considered.

4. D. Lead poisoning can present with encephalopathy and peripheral neuropathy.

Chelating agents include EDTA, penicillamine and calcium edentate.

5. C. Chelators for mercury include dimercaprol and penicillamine.

Substance dependency and abuse

18.1	Drug use	251
18.2	Substances abused	252
	Self-assessment on Chapter 18: questions	257
	Self-assessment on Chapter 18: answers	260

Overview

Substance use is very common. Depending on the substance used and the extent of its use, this may be very harmful. This chapter reviews some of the issues around substance abuse, the commonly abused substances, including alcohol and tobacco, and the treatments available. The success rate for maintaining abstinence in many forms of substance abuse is low but this should not discourage repeated attempts.

18.1 Drug use

Learning objectives

At the end of this section you should:
• be able to define key terms related to substance abuse
• be aware of general issues which apply across many forms of substance abuse.

A wide variety of legal and illegal drugs and substances can be used to create a sense of wellbeing or to escape from an unpleasant situation. Most societies have legal restrictions on the use of such drugs. There are a number of risks associated with drug use:

• overdose
• direct physical or mental damage from a drug, e.g. liver cirrhosis with alcohol abuse
• inappropriate behaviour and legal considerations, e.g. driving while drunk

• distortion of perception and response to environment: self-neglect, drift into criminal subculture (perhaps to finance illegal drug use)
• exposure to unknown substances: users of illicit drugs may not know what they are using; adulteration is common
• spread of disease, e.g. hepatitis B or C, or HIV disease, by sharing needles between injecting drug abusers
• drug dependency.

Definitions

Drug dependency (*addiction*) is a compulsion to continue taking a drug, either because of its pleasant effects or, more commonly, because of fear of drug withdrawal. Dependency is sometimes described as *physical* where there is a clear physical withdrawal syndrome, or *psychological* where the drug is used for pleasure or as support and there is no clear withdrawal syndrome. The distinction becomes less clear-cut as our understanding of the biochemistry of the brain improves. Drug dependency may be stable if the patient has an easily obtainable supply but may have severe detrimental effects on the individual and society if the supply is difficult, when the patient may resort to criminal behaviour to obtain the drug.

Tolerance occurs if the body adapts to the continual presence of a drug so that greater doses are required to achieve the same effect. This occurs with many drugs of abuse and may occur because of increased metabolism of the drug (alcohol, barbiturates) or because of altered receptor sensitivity (opioids).

The range of substances that can be used is wide. What is being used at any time and in any place is a matter of popular culture. Some of the more commonly used substances are described below. Relapse rates despite treatment are high for most forms of substance abuse. Simultaneous abuse of multiple drugs is also common.

18.2 Substances abused

Tobacco

Tobacco is usually smoked. One of its many components is nicotine, which is a CNS stimulant. The user may, therefore, feel more alert, more calm and more in control. Nicotine is addictive and there is a withdrawal syndrome that encourages continued use. Tolerance to its effects tends to occur. The kinetics of nicotine after smoking are almost the same as after intravenous use: very rapid absorption, leading to the desired CNS effects. Nicotine itself increases blood pressure and in larger doses can cause CNS toxicity, but much of the harm from smoking comes from the associated tars and gases inhaled from the burning tobacco. These cause cancers of the aerodigestive tract (particularly the lung) and are associated with bladder cancer. They cause chronic lung damage, and usually manifest as emphysema or chronic bronchitis. They are also a major risk factor for ischaemic heart disease. Smoking tobacco is, therefore, a major public health problem.

Treatment

Patients can be weaned off smoking onto nicotine replacement therapy. This can be taken as a spray, as a chewing gum or as a transdermal patch. The aim is to reduce the dose received gradually and withdraw the drug completely. This obviously does not avoid the harmful effects of nicotine but does avoid the other effects of smoking.

Buproprion (amfebutamone). This is an SSRI (selective serotonin reuptake inhibitor) antidepressant that is used for the treatment of smoking in reducing doses over 7 weeks. It reduces the compulsive behaviour involved in smoking and the urge to smoke. It can be used with nicotine replacement therapy. It is moderately effective. Adverse effects are those of other SSRIs (see Ch. 6). Bupropion can rarely include seizures.

Alcohol (ethanol)

Alcoholic drinks contain from 4% (weak beer) to 45% (whisky, brandy) ethanol in water. It is the most widely abused drug and a major cause of drug dependency (alcoholism). Its abuse is a major public health problem. A unit of alcohol is a crude measure of about 8 g of alcohol; a glass of wine or a pint of beer is about two units, a measure of spirits about one unit and an alcopop about one and a half units. Recommendations are that males should not exceed 21 units per week and females 14 units.

Clinical pharmacokinetics

Alcohol is rapidly absorbed after ingestion, although this may be slowed by food. It is metabolised in the liver to acetaldehyde by two pathways: a specific alcohol dehydrogenase and the less specific microsomal enzymes. These microsomal enzymes are inhibited by acute ethanol intake but induced by chronic intake; this is a possible source of drug interactions. The acetaldehyde is then broken down further by aldehyde dehydrogenase. Small amounts of ethanol are excreted unchanged in urine and in the breath. The metabolism is saturable, i.e. at high doses, alcohol exhibits zero-order metabolism and the clearance of alcohol is not exponential but is at a steady rate (see Ch. 1). Women are in general less tolerant of the acute and long-term effects of alcohol than men.

Psychological effects. Alcohol is a depressant and causes disinhibition and relaxation, with slowing of mental function. Aggression and confusion may occur. Tolerance and drug dependency may develop with prolonged use.

Physical effects. These can be considered in the short term, overdose, and over a longer term if taken at high dosage.

* short term (overdose)
  — incoordination
  — injury because of intoxication
  — unconsciousness
  — death in severe overdose.

* long term (high doses)
  — hypertension
  — peripheral neuropathy
  — damage to the cerebrum, partly caused by vitamin deficiencies, and the cerebellum
  — cirrhosis
  — nutritional deficiencies (especially vitamins)
  — cardiomyopathy
  — fetal alcohol syndrome.

Withdrawal. On withdrawal, the patient becomes tremulous, anxious and confused. In severe cases, delirium tremens (DTs) may occur with hallucinations, convulsions, coma and death.

Treatment

In the acute stage of alcohol withdrawal, sedatives such as *chlordiazepoxide* or other benzodiazepines are used over several (2–7) days in gradually decreasing doses to avoid convulsions and other withdrawal symptoms. (Clomethizole should *not* be used any more.) The patient may also have nutritional deficiencies, particularly vitamin B_1, and should receive supplements to prevent serious CNS or cardiac effects. This may be given intravenously as a vitamin complex preparation or orally.

Disulfiram inhibits aldehyde dehydrogenase; as a result, the acetaldehyde accumulates with toxic effects. It is used to dissuade alcoholics from taking alcohol, as if they drink while taking it, they will experience unpleasant adverse effects, with nausea and vomiting and flushing; severe cases may be fatal. It is useful in a small number of alcoholics who are determined to stop drinking.

Acamprosate reduces the compulsion to drink and so may be useful in maintaining abstinence in combination with counselling and other support.

Clinical sketch

A patient is brought to the A&E department by ambulance having been found collapsed in the street. On examination, the patient seems to be intoxicated; he is confused and uncoordinated. He smells of alcohol. The patient seems to be complaining of chest pain and a chest radiograph reveals several fractured ribs.

Comment: drunkenness is common and patients who have been injured while drunk occupy much of the time of staff in the A&E department. Fractured ribs are particularly common – often caused by falls where the patient has made little effort to protect himself.

The patient sobers up and gives a history of heavy alcohol abuse over some months. The patient agrees not to drink again and is allowed home. Two days later the patient is readmitted in a delirious state complaining of visual hallucinations.

Comment: alcohol is a CNS suppressant. As with any CNS suppressant that is withdrawn suddenly, the brain may, in effect, become overactive. This man's symptoms are due to cessation of alcohol use. In this severe case, it is manifest by confusion, delirium and hallucinations. In alcohol abuse, this state is an alcohol withdrawal syndrome, an extreme of which is

---

known as delirium tremens and can progress to fitting. It is potentially fatal and should be treated as a medical emergency with hospital admission and sedatives such as benzodiazepines. The patient probably also needs high-potency vitamin B_1 (thiamine) to avoid the development of Wernicke's encephalopathy. This deficiency of vitamins is the result of chronic malnutrition since the patient may have been deriving most of his calorie intake from alcohol. When recovered, he will need intense and sustained counselling and support to stop drinking. This is the first step in a long-term plan towards abstinence.

Clinical sketch

A 20-year-old man is brought to A&E unconscious and with minor facial injuries on a Saturday night. He smells of alcohol. He is observed while he recovers. When awake, he denies any problem with alcohol use as, he says, he only drinks at weekends when he consumes 30–40 units over Friday and Saturday. He shows no signs of alcohol withdrawal.

Comment: binge drinking is a common cultural phenomenon in some countries including the UK. It can be highly dangerous – patients can die with acute alcohol overdose, and are prone to injury or violence. The unconscious patient needs urgent investigation to exclude other causes (e.g. head injury, hypoglycaemia), and then careful observation until recovered. Although not alcohol 'dependent', this patient clearly has a drinking problem.

Sedatives/hypnotics

Benzodiazepines

The potential for benzodiazepines (see Ch. 6) to cause tolerance and dependence was not recognised by doctors for many years. As a result, doctors unwittingly caused many cases of dependence in otherwise well patients by overprescribing of these drugs.

These drugs are also abused illegally, either alone or in combination with other drugs. They may be taken orally, or the tablets may be crushed and dissolved in water or other solvents and then injected. Temazepam is a widely used hypnotic that is particularly favoured by injecting drug abusers.

The psychological effects are similar to those of alcohol. The physical dangers are less, although injury may occur. Overdose, accidental or deliberate, is not usually fatal unless there is underlying cardiac or respiratory disease or other drugs are abused simultaneously. The withdrawal syndrome consists of increased anxiety, insomnia and sometimes convulsions.

Barbiturates

Barbiturates (Ch. 6) were widely used as hypnotics and sedatives before the benzodiazepines were available. They are now rarely used for medical purposes and hence are not readily available as drugs of abuse. Their effects are similar to those of alcohol. Barbiturates are metabolised by the liver and are liver enzyme inducers. Tolerance, therefore, occurs in regular use. Barbiturates are particularly dangerous in overdose, when coma and cardiovascular collapse may occur. Withdrawal often causes severe confusion, agitation and convulsions.

Cannabis

Cannabis is widely used as a relaxant and mild intoxicant. The dried leaves of the cannabis plant may be smoked or eaten (marihuana). A more concentrated form is the resin from the plant, compressed into blocks (hashish). There are several active compounds in cannabis; Δ^9-tetrahydrocannabinol (THC) is thought to be the most important. There are specific cannabinoid receptors in the brain (CB1), although their physiological function is at present not clear, and in other organ systems (CB2). The endogenous ligands include anandamide and may be involved in memory and pain awareness.

Psychological effects. Relaxation, talkativeness and increased awareness of sensation occur. Concentration and coordination are impaired. Occasionally, a user will experience anxiety and paranoia, and even a toxic psychosis. The long-term effects of the drug are debated; many claim it has none; others point to evidence of brain damage in some users. Users of cannabis are more likely to use other drugs. A mild withdrawal syndrome is described in heavy users.

Some cannabis derivatives are used medically. Nabilone is used as an antiemetic (see Ch. 11), and a preparation of THC and cannabidiol is under investigation for possible use in multiple sclerosis and some other neurological conditions.

Amfetamines

Amfetamines are stimulants and indirect sympathomimetics, i.e. they stimulate the release of endogenous catecholamines and so activate the sympathetic nervous system. Initially, they were used for the treatment of depression and as appetite suppressants; now they are used very rarely in medicine to treat narcolepsy. Amfetamines are widely abused; most amfetamines are now made in illegal laboratories. They may be taken orally, sniffed or injected.

Effects. The physiological and psychological effects are similar to those of adrenaline (epinephrine): hypertension, tachycardia (sometimes reflex bradycardia) and mydriasis; in large doses, cardiac arrhythmias, angina or sudden death may occur. The user may become exhilarated, energetic, lose his appetite and feel that his physical and mental abilities have been expanded; with long-term use, anxiety and irritability may occur. In high doses, confusion and psychosis may be seen. The amfetamines postpone fatigue rather than prevent it and, after use, many users feel exhausted. On withdrawal, depression is common, and amfetamines are said to be psychologically but not physically addictive. Tolerance occurs with chronic use.

Methylenedioxymethamfetamine (MDMA, Ecstasy) is an amfetamine derivative that has, in addition to the effects of amfetamines, hallucinogenic properties (see below). It has become particularly widely used in recent years and has caused a number of deaths as a result of cardiac arrhythmias or as a result of myolysis and subsequent renal failure.

Clinical sketch

A 19-year-old woman is admitted to hospital from a nightclub. She is confused and hyperthermic. Her friends admit that they and she have taken Ecstasy. The patient rapidly develops rhabdomyolysis and renal failure. Despite the best supportive care, she goes on to develop multiple organ failure and dies.

Comment: Ecstasy (MDMA) is a widely used illicit amfetamine derivative. The reaction described is not common and it is not clear whether it is caused directly by the drug, by the circumstances in which it is used (e.g. with intense exercise, heat and dehydration) or by impurities in the illegal tablets.

Cocaine

Cocaine is derived from the coca leaf. It is an indirect sympathomimetic and a membrane stabiliser and is still used by ear, nose and throat surgeons as a local anaesthetic (see Ch. 8). Cocaine hydrochloride is a white powder that can be injected but more commonly is sniffed and absorbed through the nasal mucosa. In this form, cocaine is an expensive drug popular with wealthy users. Cocaine freebase is powder treated with alkali to form nuggets ('crack'), which can be smoked. It is said to give very rapid effects and has been sold relatively cheaply.

Effects. The effects are similar to amfetamines: exhilaration, loss of appetite and fatigue, occasionally anxiety, panic or psychosis. After inhalation, the effects last for about 15–30 minutes and repeated doses are usually used. After-effects include fatigue and depression. Physical effects include tachycardia and hypertension, and possibly angina, acute myocardial infarction, cardiac arrhythmia and sudden death. Cocaine sniffing will cause intense vasoconstriction of the nasal mucosa and may cause necrosis of the nasal septum. Cocaine is said to be psychologically rather than physically addictive.

Gamma-hydroxybutyrate

Gamma-hydroxybutyrate (GHB) is a naturally occurring substance, a precursor of the inhibitory neurotransmitter GABA. It is produced illegally as a liquid. It is a CNS depressant and may therefore cause loss of inhibition, euphoria and intoxication with drowsiness, impaired memory, unconsciousness, fitting and death, depending on dose and individual response. It has been implicated as a drug used in 'date rape'; it may be given to the victim in other drinks where it is difficult to detect, and the victim may subsequently have no memory of events.

Opioids

Opioids (see Ch. 7) can all be abused; the partial agonist drugs *(pentazocine, buprenorphine)* were developed in an unsuccessful attempt to produce an analgesic with agonist/antagonist effects and no abuse potential. Raw opium was widely smoked in the Far East. The refined alkaloids *morphine* and *codeine* are taken orally, injected or smoked. *Diamorphine (heroin)* is a potent morphine derivative that is particularly widely available and abused.

Effects. When injected, the user experiences a 'rush' or sensation of intense pleasure. The chronic user, in contrast, mainly uses it to avoid the unpleasant effects of withdrawal. In large doses, sedation is more prominent. Overdose can occur with respiratory depression and death. Tolerance occurs quickly, requiring larger doses, but can also be lost quickly (e.g. users sent to prison who have limited or no access to opioids). Physical dependence also occurs within a few weeks of regular use and a severe withdrawal syndrome occurs within a few hours of the last dose: muscle aches, sneezing and rhinorrhea, and yawning, progress on to chills and piloerection ('going cold turkey'). There is also psychological dependence. Abuse by injection is associated with the infectious hazard outlined above. Sniffing or inhaling the fumes of heroin ('chasing the dragon') is increasingly common, as is smoking. Chronic users of opioids often abuse them with other drugs in an attempt to regain the 'rush'.

Methadone is an opioid with a long half-life, active after oral administration. It is used to avoid the withdrawal symptoms in opioid users, its advantage being that it can be given once per day under supervision. The dose can be gradually reduced over a period of a few weeks or months until total withdrawal is achieved. Many patients are maintained indefinitely on it. *Buprenorphine* is also used as maintenance treatment: its partial agonist/antagonist effects may limit the effects of other opioids if taken in addition.

Naltrexone, an oral pure opioid antagonist, can also be used as a maintenance treatment to avoid relapse, in patients who have been off opioids for 7–10 days. Use in a patient recently using opioids may cause a withdrawal syndrome.

Clinical sketch

A doctor who regularly treats i.v. drug abusers muses about what the attraction of opiates is and wonders whether he should self-administer diamorphine to try to understand this better. He is not worried about addiction since he does not intend to use it more than once and is aware of the risks.

Comment: this kind of dangerous curiosity has led to many doctors becoming addicted to opiates and other drugs. Doctors are at relatively high risk of becoming drug abusers, in part because of their easy access to them. Knowledge of the dangers of the drugs and their effects are no protection against addiction and may even encourage some individuals to try these drugs, thinking that they cannot be affected.

Clinical sketch

A 26-year-old man is admitted with fever and feeling unwell with shortness of breath. He has obviously been neglecting himself. He has oral candidiasis, splinter haemorrhages and a murmur of aortic regurgitation. There are extensive needle tracks on his arms and a sinus in the groin. He admits to injecting heroin for several years.

Comment: this patient has some of the complications of intravenous heroin abuse. He may have infective endocarditis involving the aortic and other valves, due to the injection of infected and impure material. He has probably injected many times into his femoral vein (or even artery) due to difficulty of access to peripheral veins which are largely all thrombosed. He is likely to have hepatitis C and possibly hepatitis B. The oral candidiasis raises the possibility of systemic immune suppression due to HIV disease. All of these problems require investigation and treatment.

Eighteen

Hallucinogens

LSD (lysergic acid diethylamide) is a synthetic ergot derivative and a hallucinogen that is widely used. It acts largely by blocking 5-HT receptors. Users report intensification of all the senses and synaesthesia (merging of the senses, e.g. seeing music or feeling colours). Distortions of the senses occur and users may see pseudohallucinations (which they know to be false) or true hallucinations. Some users describe mystical experiences, others experience severe anxiety, disorientation or acute psychosis. Rarely LSD users may harm themselves or others during the 'trip'. Many users experience 'flashbacks' where they may re-experience the effects of LSD without having taken any. Occasionally long-term psychotic reactions may occur in LSD users. Physical effects do not occur, nor does classical physical dependence.

Other hallucinogens. Many other naturally occurring alkaloids can act as hallucinogens, including *atropine*, *muscarine* and *psilocybin* from fungi or *mescaline* (from a cactus).

Solvents

Many organic solvents can be inhaled to produce effects similar to those of alcohol: disinhibition, euphoria, disorientation and dizziness leading to stupor. These can be found in glues, dry cleaning fluids, paints, nail varnish remover and many other household substances. They are commonly put into a plastic bag from which the user inhales. Because organic solvents are lipid soluble, the acute effects clear quickly when the use is stopped. Solvents are particularly abused by children. The adverse effects in short-term use are injury and occasionally sudden death caused by sensitisation of the myocardium to catecholamines by the solvent. In the long term, the adverse effects include poor concentration, liver and kidney damage and possibly permanent brain damage.

Self-assessment on Chapter 18: questions

Multiple choice questions

1. The following statements are correct:
   a. Drug dependency describes a compulsion to continue taking a drug
   b. Tolerance means that an increased dose of the drug has no effect
   c. Alcohol is associated with a physical withdrawal syndrome
   d. Alcohol is mostly excreted unchanged in the urine
   e. Disulfiram is used to treat alcohol dependency

2. The following statements are correct:
   a. Benzodiazepine abuse is common
   b. Tolerance occurs to benzodiazepines
   c. Benzodiazepines may cause liver enzyme induction
   d. Barbiturates are safe in overdose
   e. Physical withdrawal syndromes are seen with benzodiazepines

3. Amfetamines:
   a. Cause catecholamine release from nerve endings
   b. May cause angina
   c. May cause weight gain
   d. Withdrawal may cause rebound depression
   e. Are usually diverted from legal medical use

4. The following statements are correct:
   a. Cocaine is a local anaesthetic
   b. Sniffing cocaine may destroy the nasal septum
   c. Opioid dependency only occurs after i.v. use
   d. Opioid withdrawal syndrome includes constipation, drowsiness and miosis
   e. Methadone is a long-acting opioid used to treat dependency

Case history questions

Case history 1

A 24-year-old man is found unconscious in a public toilet and is brought to an A&E department. There are no signs of injury and blood sugar is normal. He has needle track marks on his arms and is noted to have small pupils and slow, shallow respiration.

1. What is the likely diagnosis?
2. What treatment should be given immediately?

The patient recovers consciousness initially but an hour later becomes unconscious again.

3. What has happened?
4. What are the effects of sudden withdrawal of the drugs to which this patient is addicted?
5. What other drugs are commonly abused intravenously?

Case history 2

A 60-year-old man is found to have hepatomegaly. He admits to drinking a bottle of whisky a day.

1. What is the likely cause of the hepatomegaly?
2. What is considered a 'safe' maximum weekly intake of alcohol?
3. Will the patient's capacity to metabolise drugs be increased or decreased?
4. What drugs are synergistic with alcohol in affecting the CNS?
5. What antibiotic should be avoided in such a patient?

Case history 3

A 60-year-old man has ischaemic heart disease. He has smoked 40 cigarettes per day for 45 years and has attempted to stop on many occasions unsuccessfully. He has been put on a waiting list for coronary artery surgery but has been told that if he does not stop smoking, the operation will be worthless. He comes to you again to ask for help.

1. What pharmacological treatments are available?
2. Are there any concerns about their use in this case?
3. What other support should the patient be offered?

Short note questions

Write short notes on:

1. Treatment of alcoholism.
2. Treatment of opiate addiction.
3. Illicit misuse of prescribed drugs.

Extended matching items questions

Theme: Drugs of abuse

Options

A. Heroin
B. Cocaine
C. Pethidine
D. 'Cold turkey'
E. Barbiturates
F. Tolerance
G. Dependency
H. Ecstasy
I. Temazepam
J. Methadone
K. Naloxone

For each of the following questions, select the most appropriate option from the list above. Each option may be used once, more than once, or not at all.

1. A 24-year-old man is brought to the GP by his mother who requests treatment for him. He admits to using illicit drugs. He has very small pupils and seems very relaxed. The doctor notes marks on the patient's left forearm that the patient says were caused by a cat scratch. Choose one drug which this patient could be abusing.
2. Choose a drug which could reverse the effect of this.
3. Patients on such drugs often require escalating doses to achieve the desired effect. What is this phenomenon called?
4. What is the withdrawal syndrome commonly called?
5. What drug may be used to try to avoid a withdrawal syndrome and maintain withdrawal in such drug users?
6. Multiple drug use is common. Which other drugs might be commonly used in this patient, though not clinically obvious at present?

Theme: Effects of drugs of abuse

Options

A. Cirrhosis
B. Hepatitis A
C. HIV
D. Benzodiazepines
E. Hepatitis B
F. Acamprosate
G. Ecstasy
H. GHB
I. Thiamine
J. Delirium tremens
K. Disulfiram

For each of the following questions, select the most appropriate option from the list above. Each option may be used once, more than once, or not at all.

1. A 40-year-old man comes to his GP complaining of unsteadiness when he walks and is noted to have an enlarged liver. On questioning, he admits to drinking about half a bottle of whisky per day as well as wine and beer. Choose one liver complication caused by alcohol abuse.
2. What may happen to a heavy drinker who suddenly stops drinking?

3. What drug might be used to diminish the severity of the withdrawal syndrome?

4. What other drug treatments might be considered?

5. Pick an infectious disease likely to complicate intravenous drug abuse.

6. An 18-year-old girl is brought to A&E unconscious, having collapsed at a party. What drug or drugs are likely to be responsible?

Self-assessment on Chapter 18: answers

Multiple choice answers

1. a. **True.** A distinction is sometimes made between dependency and addiction but we consider this spurious.
   b. **False.** Tolerance means that an increased dose is needed to achieve the same effect.
   c. **True.** This may be very severe.
   d. **False.** Mostly metabolised.
   e. **True.** By inhibiting alcohol dehydrogenase, toxic metabolites of alcohol are formed, hopefully discouraging use of alcohol as it will cause a very unpleasant reaction.

2. a. **True.** Often iatrogenic.
   b. **True.** Tendency to increase the dose occurs, even in therapeutic use.
   c. **False.** No effect.
   d. **False.** On the contrary, one of the most dangerous of overdoses.
   e. **True.** Including insomnia, anxiety, etc.

3. a. **True.** The definition of an indirect sympathomimetic.
   b. **True.** May cause tachycardia and hypertension.
   c. **False.** May cause loss of appetite and weight loss.
   d. **True.** Hence a psychological compulsion to continue taking the drug.
   e. **False.** Amphetamines have few medical uses today.

4. a. **True.** Still used by ENT surgeons.
   b. **True.** Because of intense vasoconstriction.
   c. **False.** Although obvious, this is a common misunderstanding by opioid users.
   d. **False.** These are all opioid effects: the withdrawal syndrome is, therefore, the opposite of these.
   e. **True.** It has relatively little potential for abuse itself and avoids the withdrawal syndrome in well-motivated users. It may be used as a maintenance or in gradually decreasing doses to achieve complete withdrawal.

Case history answers

Case history 1

1. Opiate (probably heroin) toxicity.
2. Intravenous naloxone.
3. Naloxone has a short half-life, unlike many commonly abused opiates: the naloxone has probably been cleared, allowing the opiate effects to reappear.
4. Muscle aches, sneezing and rhinorrhoea, yawning, mydriasis, progressing on to chills and piloerection ('cold turkey').
5. Drug abusers may abuse many drugs intravenously and often use mixtures of drugs. Commonly used are a variety of opioids, benzodiazepines, amfetamines and cocaine.

Case history 2

1. Alcoholic hepatitis, fatty infiltration of the liver or cirrhosis (with regeneration). Patients with cirrhosis are at risk of hepatomas also.
2. Roughly 21 units per week for men and 14 for women.
3. Alcohol acutely inhibits liver enzyme drug metabolism but in the long term is a liver enzyme inducer; this is the likely condition in this patient when he is not acutely drinking.
4. Any CNS depressant, especially benzodiazepines.
5. Metronidazole; this can have a disulfiram-like effect.

Case history 3

1. This patient could be given nicotine replacement therapy (or could buy it over the counter himself) or buproprion (*amfebutamone*), or both.
2. Bupropion can cause a range of adverse effects including gastrointestinal upsets and anxiety. Nicotine may stimulate angina, by causing tachycardia and hypertension. So should he be given nicotine replacement therapy? This is, as in all prescribing decisions, a question of balancing risk and benefit: in general in such cases, the balance favours giving the nicotine replacement.

3. The effectiveness of both of these drugs is greatly enhanced if the patient is part of a well-defined support programme to monitor and encourage the patient. This should be part of the 'contract' made with the patient before prescribing either of these drugs. It would be worth defining why previous attempts have failed.

Short note answers

1. This should consider immediate detoxification with benzodiazepines and vitamins. Psychological treatments rather than pharmacological treatments have a major role to play in treating alcohol abuse. Acamprosate is used in selected patients to reduce the desire to drink. Clomethiazole should be avoided as a sedative in the early stages, since patients may substitute a clomethiazole addiction for their alcohol addiction.

2. Patients should be transferred from illicit opiates to oral methadone or buprenorphine. Only doctors with special licences may legally prescribe any other drug for the treatment of opioid addiction. The replacement could either be gradually reduced until the patient is weaned off the drug, which would be the ideal, or be used as maintenance treatment with no dose reduction. This is clearly less desirable than total withdrawal and might be considered damage limitation in that it will avoid the patient needing to seek illegal supplies of opioids with all of the attendant risks of injection, illegal activity, etc. Unfortunately, some patients continue to misuse illicit drugs in addition to their methadone. Naltrexone is under study as a treatment for opioid addiction in the hopes of reducing patients' craving for the drug.

3. This needs to consider the therapeutic drugs which have psychotropic effects and potential for abuse. The single largest group of these are the benzodiazepines. These are overused in medicine, especially in long-term treatment. Illicit benzodiazepines are almost all diverted from medical use and their abuse could be largely eliminated with better prescribing. Barbiturates are rarely used in medicine now and are rare as drugs of abuse. Opiates might also be abused, especially such drugs as dihydrocodeine or buprenorphine. Again, better prescribing is the key. Drugs such as diamorphine are almost never diverted from medical use. In addition to considering the potential drugs in this answer, it is also important to consider what we mean by better prescribing: this means only issuing these drugs for short-term use, explaining this carefully to the patient, and so avoiding the potential for abuse. Many patients are on such drugs long term already and may need to be weaned off them – changing this culture is very difficult but essential.

Extended matching items answers

Theme: Drugs of abuse

1. A or C. This patient is probably using an injected opioid – probably heroin (diamorphine), but pethidine is also possible.

2. K. Naloxone will reverse the effects of acute intoxication with opioids.

3. F. Users need to increase the dose to achieve the same effect as the number and sensitivity of opioid receptors is decreased (downregulation).

4. D. Because of the piloerection which is supposed to resemble a plucked turkey.

5. J. Methadone has a long half-life and can be given orally once per day under supervision. It is useful to avoid withdrawal symptoms in patients who are opioid dependent. Some argue against its use since some addicts will use methadone with other illicit opioids, or they may become addicted to the methadone. Buprenorphine is an alternative.

6. B and I. Benzodiazepine and cocaine are often co-used in these patients.

Theme: Effects of abuse

1. A. Cirrhosis is common. Alcoholic hepatitis may occur, but not hepatitis A or B, which are infections.

2. J. Confusion, agitation, and fitting in some cases. In severe cases, it may be fatal.

3. D. Chlordiazepoxide (or other benzodiazepines) are used to diminish the risks of sudden withdrawal.

4. I, F, K. Acutely, thiamine should be considered. If the patient wishes to maintain abstinence disulfiram or acamprosate as well as psychological support could be considered.

5. C or E. Hepatitis B and HIV are often spread between drug abusers who share needles and other injecting equipment. Medical and paramedical staff may be at risk because of their contact with blood and other body fluids.

6. D, G, H. All are possible but beyond the current list, the potential range is huge; do not forget alcohol alone or in combination, or opioids.

Drugs in pregnancy, breastfeeding, children and the elderly

19.1	**Pregnancy and breastfeeding**	**263**
19.2	**Children**	**266**
19.3	**The elderly**	**267**
	Self-assessment on Chapter 19: questions	269
	Self-assessment on Chapter 19: answers	271

Overview

Prescribing for certain groups of patients requires particular care. This is because, by virtue of a physiological state, their response to drugs and their vulnerability to adverse drug reactions are altered. The groups considered here are pregnant and breastfeeding women (where the major concerns are of harm to the fetus or the child), and children and the elderly (where the major concerns are around pharmacokinetic and pharmacodynamic differences in drug response compared to the young adult).

19.1 Pregnancy and breastfeeding

Learning objectives

At the end of this section you should:
- be aware of the hazards of prescribing to women at different stages of pregnancy
- understand which drugs can be safely given to breastfeeding mothers.

Drug use in pregnancy is now limited by doctors' and patients' awareness of the possible harm that may be done to the fetus. This was brought home by the thalidomide disaster of the 1960s, when thalidomide used as a treatment for morning sickness by pregnant women caused deformities of the limbs in the fetus. Despite the risks, some medical conditions require drug treatment during pregnancy and the benefits and risks of this need to be carefully

weighed. A broad principle, however, is to avoid drugs in pregnancy as much as possible. There are many drugs that have been used quite safely throughout pregnancy, and these are generally used in preference to new or untried drugs. This might also be considered to apply to women of childbearing age – who might after all be pregnant at the time you write a prescription or become pregnant while taking a drug prescribed by you.

Drugs and the fetus

Drugs may adversely affect development of the fetus and cause deformities (teratogenic), particularly during the first trimester of pregnancy when the major organs and limbs are being formed. This is a particularly sensitive time, and a time when the woman may not have even realised she is pregnant. The period of greatest risk is from the third to the eleventh week of pregnancy. The list of teratogenic drugs is long: some, such as cytotoxics, might be anticipated; others may be unexpected and found during animal testing (although this is not completely reliable – thalidomide had not been identified as a teratogen in animal studies, partly because it had been tried only in rodents) or found tragically by chance. It must be remembered that 1–2% of all births are of a child with a malformation of some kind, and it is important not to over- or underestimate the potential of a drug to cause deformity. Not all exposures to a teratogenic drug will cause a malformation, e.g. warfarin causes deformities in only about 5% of cases. A teratogenic drug may be taken by a woman before she realises that she is pregnant; in some cases, the risks of using a teratogenic drug may be outweighed by the benefits, e.g. warfarin in a patient with a prosthetic heart valve.

Some teratogenic drugs:

- phenytoin: craniofacial and limb abnormalities
- carbamazepine: craniofacial and limb abnormalities
- sodium valproate: neural tube abnormalities, spina bifida
- ACE inhibitors: abnormalities of the skull
- alcohol: growth retardation and cranial abnormalities
- diethylstilbestrol: adenocarcinoma of the vagina in the daughters of women exposed during pregnancy.

After the first trimester

The second and third trimesters are mainly stages of growth and development, and drugs taken by the mother may still affect the fetus. Antithyroid drugs may lead to goitre or hypothyroidism in the fetus. Tetracyclines may interfere with bone and tooth formation. There are many other drugs that may have adverse effects on the fetus; a full list should be consulted before prescribing for a pregnant woman. The British National Formulary (BNF) provides a table of drugs to be avoided or used with caution during pregnancy. It should also be appreciated that drugs given shortly before or during labour may adversely affect the health of the neonate.

Drugs in the pregnant mother

The pharmacokinetics of drugs may be altered in pregnant women.

Absorption. Gastrointestinal motility is slowed, which increases absorption of poorly soluble drugs such as digoxin.

Distribution. Plasma volume and extracellular fluid increase up to 50% and this will reduce the plasma concentration of drugs with a small volume of distribution for a given dose. Changes in albumin also occur: this falls by around 20% while α_1-acid glycoprotein, to which basic drugs bind, increases by about 40%. This will mean increased free drug for a given concentration for acidic drugs (phenytoin, valproate), while for basic drugs (propranolol, chlorpromazine), the free fraction will fall for a given plasma concentration. This may be of importance if therapeutic drug monitoring is undertaken.

Elimination. Renal plasma flow increases but this is important only for a few drugs, such as ampicillin, where larger doses may be needed. For most drugs, renal elimination is relatively unaltered. Liver metabolism is induced by progesterone in pregnancy and so the clearance of drugs metabolised by the liver may be enhanced.

Some common chronic conditions in pregnancy

Epilepsy

There is an increased incidence of congenital deformities in the children of pregnant epileptic women, probably largely because of the use of anticonvulsant drugs. Although most anticonvulsants are teratogenic, the risks to the mother and to the fetus of uncontrolled epilepsy usually outweigh any risks of teratogenesis, and so pregnant epileptic women are advised to continue their medication. *Carbamazepine* is probably the least likely to cause deformities, although little comparative evidence is available.

Altered pharmacokinetics may make drug treatment for epilepsy difficult in pregnancy; total anticonvulsant concentrations tend to fall because of increased volume of distribution and enhanced metabolism, although this may be slightly countered by decreased protein binding. Measurement of plasma concentrations at frequent intervals is advised during pregnancy for drugs such as *phenytoin*, with dosage adjustment as necessary. It is not usually possible to measure free drug, and so to compensate for this, it is common practice to keep the plasma concentration at the lower end of the therapeutic range; however, as in all therapeutic drug monitoring, the wellbeing of the patient and not the plasma concentration is the major measure.

Infections

Urinary tract infections in particular are common in pregnancy, and appropriate drug treatment must be determined by sensitivity testing. Suitable drugs include penicillins, cephalosporins and nitrofurantoin.

Antimicrobials to avoid in pregnant women:

- tetracyclines: teeth and bone deformities in the fetus; hepatitis is more common in pregnant women
- metronidazole: possibly teratogenic
- trimethoprim: folate antagonism, possibly teratogenic
- quinolones (such a ciprofloxacin): may damage growing cartilage
- isoniazid, rifampicin: use with great care because of the risk of hepatitis
- aminoglycosides: 8th nerve damage in the fetus.

Clinical sketch

A woman is 20 weeks pregnant. She develops frequency and dysuria and urine testing shows blood and leucocytes. The doctor thinks about what antibiotics might be prescribed.

Comment: urinary tract infections are common in pregnant women and should always be treated vigorously since they may give rise to pyelonephritis or premature delivery. At 20 weeks, the risk of developing fetal malformation is small, since we are now in the second trimester. However, the appropriate antibiotics need to be considered carefully. The best choice would be a cephalosporin or co-amoxiclav. Nitrofurantoin would also be safe for lower urinary tract infections.

Clinical sketch

A woman is 26 weeks pregnant. She develops pleuritic chest pain and shortness of breath, and the admitting team is concerned about the possibility of a pulmonary embolus.

Comment: this is a life-threatening condition and there is a significant risk to the mother (and therefore of course to the fetus). Anticoagulation with low molecular weight heparin is warranted under these circumstances. Although the first trimester is complete, it would probably be unwise to switch to oral anticoagulation with warfarin as this is slow to reverse and may cause problems with bleeding postpartum. It is likely that this patient would therefore remain on subcutaneous low molecular weight heparin throughout the rest of her pregnancy and in the postpartum period.

Diabetes mellitus

Diabetes mellitus may become unstable in pregnant women and some pregnant women may develop gestational diabetes for the first time. All such women need careful specialist monitoring and very tight control of the diabetes. Some diabetic women may be adequately controlled on diet, but many will require insulin. Oral antihyperglycaemic drugs should not be used.

Hypertension

Pregnant women may develop hypertension with proteinuria as part of toxaemia of pregnancy (pre-eclampsia), in which case fetal loss is high. Alternatively, they may have hypertension as an incidental problem. Few antihypertensive drugs have been evaluated in pregnancy. *Methyldopa* has been established by long usage to be safe, as has *labetalol* and *hydralazine*. Diuretics and ACE inhibitors are not

suitable. The role of other beta-blockers or calcium-channel blockers has been questioned as, although effective in treating hypertension, they do not seem to improve the fetal prognosis. Some, such as *atenolol*, seem to lead to low birth-weight. Bed rest is also important in the management of hypertension in pregnancy. Occasionally, hypertension is sufficiently severe to require early delivery of the fetus.

Hyperthyroidism

Carbimazole can cross the placenta and cause hypothyroidism and goitre in the fetus. The lowest possible dose of carbimazole should, therefore, be used, along with beta-blockers to control symptoms.

Breastfeeding

Although many drugs taken by the mother may be detectable in breast milk, in many cases the concentrations are low and the dose to the child is clinically unimportant.

Drugs that can be given safely to mothers who are breastfeeding:

- penicillins, cephalosporins
- theophylline or beta-agonists
- glucocorticoids (although high doses may affect the fetus and cause adrenal suppression)
- anticonvulsants
- tricyclic antidepressants
- neuroleptics such as chlorpromazine
- antihypertensives such as methyldopa, hydralazine
- warfarin or heparin.

Drugs to be avoided in mothers who are breastfeeding:

- aspirin
- ergotamine
- sulphonamides, ciprofloxacin, tetracyclines, chloramphenicol
- benzodiazepines
- lithium
- antithyroid drugs or iodine
- sulphonylureas
- antineoplastic drugs.

Drugs that inhibit lactation:

- bromocriptine
- oestrogens and progestogens (high doses)
- thiazides.

Clinical sketch

A 30-year-old woman gives birth to a normal child but develops a deep vein thrombosis (DVT) immediately afterwards. She is breastfeeding the child.

Comment: treatment of the DVT will require heparin (unfractionated or low molecular weight forms) followed by warfarin for a period of 6–12 weeks. Warfarin does appear in breast milk in very low concentrations but should not be harmful to the child. It is, therefore, reasonable for her to continue breastfeeding.

19.2 Children

Learning objectives

At the end of this section you should:
- be aware of the pharmacokinetic and pharmacodynamic factors that are distinct to children and will affect drug levels
- understand the issues in prescribing for children.

Half of all children visiting GPs' surgeries will be issued with a prescription, usually for short-term medication, especially antibiotics. Using drugs properly in children requires an understanding of the alterations in pharmacokinetics and pharmacodynamics that occur, especially in neonates (age up to 1 month) and infants (age up to 4 years). Very few drugs have been developed specifically with children in mind (with children as clinical trial subjects), and many drugs routinely prescribed are technically being used outside of their product license when they are used in children.

Pharmacokinetics

Distribution. Children and neonates have a higher body water/fat ratio than adults, which will result in relatively higher concentrations of water-soluble drugs. Lipid membranes may be more permeable in neonates: in particular, the blood–brain barrier will not be effective. Protein binding will be reduced in neonates.

Metabolism. In neonates, this will be reduced: in older children, it may be relatively greater than in adults. For instance, children may need relatively higher doses of theophylline or phenytoin than adults (based on a dose per unit body weight) to attain therapeutic concentrations.

Excretion. Neonates have diminished glomerular filtration rate and tubular excretion compared with adults: this decreases the clearance of such drugs as *penicillin*. Older children have renal function similar to that of adults.

Pharmacodynamics

Some drugs will demonstrate a reduced effect in neonates compared with adults or older children (e.g. *digoxin*), while some have an increased effect (e.g. CNS depressants). This is sometimes the result of altered pharmacokinetics (for instance, the volume of distribution of lipid-soluble CNS depressants); in other cases, there are alterations in tissue sensitivity.

Clinical sketch

A 7-year-old child with severe asthma is prescribed an inhaled corticosteroid. The mother is concerned that this may give rise to impaired growth.

Comment: systemic corticosteroids can give rise to impaired growth in children. High-dose inhaled corticosteroids may have a sufficient systemic effect also to impede growth. However, far more likely to impede growth is uncontrolled disease, such as asthma. As always, the benefits of therapy must be weighed against the risks and in severe childhood asthma the inhaled corticosteroid is appropriate.

Adverse effects

Adverse effects may differ slightly from those seen in adults; for instance, long-term *glucocorticoid* use may lead to impaired growth or even adrenocortical suppression (even when inhaled), while *theophylline* may lead to overactivity and learning difficulties. *Aspirin* may cause Reye's syndrome (hepatic failure).

Dosage in neonates and children

Altered pharmacokinetics and pharmacodynamics make determination of doses difficult in children. Doses are sometimes calculated on the basis of body weight; the use of square metre of body surface area is better, usually derived from nomograms of height and weight. However, effective doses with minimal adverse effects are often determined only by experience. It is vitally important to consult an appropriate source of doses related to age etc., before prescribing for young children.

Drug licensing and children

A common problem in prescribing for children (affecting about 40% of all drug use in children) is that the drug has not been adequately evaluated in children and so is not licensed in this age group. This requires 'off-label' prescribing, i.e. prescribing outside the terms of the product licence and labelling. A manufacturer may not seek a licence for use in children: the necessary trials would be expensive and difficult, and there would be little commercial return on this investment. Licensing agencies are increasingly aware of this problem and encourage or even require companies to submit data on children.

Where possible, a licensed product should be prescribed. Where not possible and where 'off-label' use is necessary, it is important that the prescribing should be as evidence based as possible, i.e. supported by randomised clinical trials and with good information on the pharmacokinetics and dynamics of the drug in children.

19.3 The elderly

Learning objectives

At the end of this section you should:
- be aware of the physiological and pathological factors common in elderly people that may influence drug effects
- be aware of the effect of coexisting medical problems on drug effects
- know the likely drug interactions that can occur in this group.

Drugs are widely used in the elderly: the elderly (over 65 years) account for about 15% of the general population but about 40–45% of prescriptions. The elderly are prone to many chronic degenerative diseases, which may influence drug effects and which promotes prescribing. They may have several medical problems that may lead to multiple drug therapy (polypharmacy) (Fig. 52).

Often there are difficulties of diagnosis in the elderly, and doctors may be excessively enthusiastic in their desire to treat symptoms. Some complaints may be inappropriately treated with drugs, e.g. dizziness caused by age-related loss of postural stability might be treated with *prochlorperazine*, which may lead to parkinsonism and further treatment. Many problems of the elderly are psychosocial and cannot be expected to respond to drugs. Often, drugs are started in the elderly and not discontinued although the original indication for the drug has long since resolved.

Adverse drug reactions

Adverse reactions are more common in the elderly and may result in one in 10 admissions of elderly

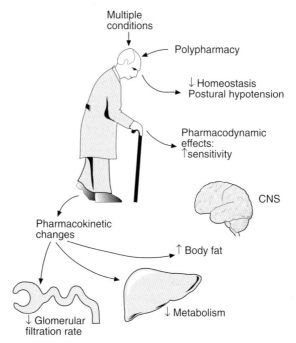

Fig. 52 Drugs in the elderly.

patients to hospital. The adverse drug reactions are largely related to increased drug action (type A, see Ch. 21), rather than the idiosyncratic adverse effect (type B). There are several reasons:

- *increased use* of drugs makes adverse reactions more likely, and *polypharmacy* increases the risks of drug interactions
- *altered pharmacokinetics*: many drugs have not been adequately studied in the elderly
  — absorption may be slower in the elderly
  — distribution may be altered because of decreased serum albumin concentrations and a relative increase in body fat and decrease in body water; lipid-soluble drugs may have an increased volume of distribution, which, coupled with reduced elimination, may prolong the duration of their effects
  — elimination of many drugs in the elderly is reduced: glomerular filtration rate and tubular secretion will be reduced, which may increase adverse reactions from drugs such as *cimetidine* or *digoxin*; liver size and hepatic blood flow and hence enzyme metabolism will also be reduced in the elderly – this is particularly important for drugs that undergo first pass metabolism, which will have greater bioavailability in the elderly, e.g. *propranolol* or *verapamil*
- *altered pharmacodynamics*, with increased organ or receptor sensitivity: this applies to many CNS

depressants, such as *benzodiazepines*, for reasons that are not entirely clear, and to other drugs such as antihypertensives

- *diminished homeostatic reserve*: as a result many drugs that affect homeostasis in vital organs have a disproportionate effect in elderly patients, e.g. antihypertensives may lead to postural hypotension because of reduction of the normal reflex responses
- *the disease state* may influence the response to drugs; for instance, patients with rheumatoid arthritis may be more prone to suffer gastrointestinal bleed after NSAIDs.

Clinical sketch

A 75-year-old woman comes to ask for a repeat prescription for her usual medicines: nifedipine 20 mg twice per day, bendroflumethiazide 5 mg, ranitidine 150 mg twice per day, Slow K tablets one three times per day, diclofenac 50 mg three times per day, and allopurinol 300 mg per day. The case notes contain the diagnoses of hypertension, dyspepsia and gout. She feels reasonably well but complains with a smile that she rattles as she walks! Her blood pressure is unsatisfactory at 180/100 mmHg.

Comment: this patient states that she has no complaints. But is there really no problem? She may suffer from hypertension, dyspepsia and gout, but she definitely has one other problem: **polypharmacy***! Careful analysis and monitoring will reveal whether the patient really needs all these drugs.*

How did she end up on all of these drugs? The sequence of events was that she was noted at a routine health check to have a blood pressure of 170/102 mmHg. Her doctor prescribed nifedipine 20 mg twice daily. A month later, her blood pressure was 120/60 mmHg and she complained of dizziness, dyspepsia and swollen ankles. Her doctor added in bendroflumethiazide 2.5 mg per day, and ranitidine 150 mg twice per day. Another month passed and her ankles remained swollen: her serum potassium was 3.2 mmol/L. Her doctor increased the dose of bendroflumethiazide to 5 mg per day and added in potassium supplements, two tablets twice per day. Two weeks later, she had her first ever attack of gout and was treated with diclofenac 50 mg three times per day. Allopurinol was later added in, while the diclofenac was continued. A month later her blood pressure was 180/100 mmHg.

If you look up the adverse effects of nifedipine (ankle swelling and dizziness), diuretics (hypokalaemia and gout) and non-steroidal anti-inflammatory drugs (worsening of antihypertensive control), it is possible to work out that much of this is iatrogenic. Drugs are best avoided wherever possible. Even then it is better to avoid further drugs to overcome adverse drug reactions.

Compliance

Compliance with prescribed drugs may be poor or sporadic in the elderly, especially where several drugs are prescribed together. This may be the result of poor understanding by the patient and poor explanation by the doctor of the purpose of the prescription.

Recommendations for prescribing in the elderly

1. Assess the clinical situation carefully, considering other drugs, previous history and the need to prescribe at all.
2. Keep the drug regimen as simple as possible and treat only major problems.
3. Start with the lowest effective dose (often 50% of the usual adult dose) and build up the dose gradually as necessary. Consider carefully the choice of drug in the elderly and work from a limited range of drugs with which the prescriber is very familiar.
4. Explain carefully to the patient the proposed therapy, its purposes, administration and its adverse effects. Verbal explanation may need to be supplemented with written material. Issue a clear prescription for the pharmacist.
5. Avoid inappropriate and overenergetic treatment: consider the patient as a whole and not as a collection of symptoms or diseases.
6. Review medication and compliance frequently and be alert for adverse drug reactions, which may mimic other disease or present in a nonspecific manner in the elderly.

Self-assessment on Chapter 19: questions

Multiple choice questions

1. The following drugs may be safely given to a pregnant woman in the first trimester:
   a. Carbamazepine
   b. Prednisolone
   c. Ciprofloxacin
   d. Co-trimoxazole
   e. Etretinate

2. In pregnant women:
   a. The plasma volume decreases
   b. The free portion of acid drugs rises
   c. Plasma drug concentration monitoring is accurate
   d. Carbimazole may cause fetal goitre
   e. Sulphonylureas may be used to manage gestational diabetes mellitus

3. In prescribing for children:
   a. Children are basically small adults
   b. Doses for children are best calculated on a simple body weight basis
   c. Adverse drug reactions may occur of a type that are not seen in adults
   d. In a child aged 5 years, the liver metabolism of drugs is proportionately less than that of an adult
   e. Children have relatively high water to fat ratios

4. In prescribing for the elderly:
   a. Pharmacokinetic alterations may occur compared with younger patients
   b. Increased sensitivity to doses of benzodiazepines is an example of pharmacodynamic changes
   c. Polypharmacy is common
   d. Homeostatic mechanisms are well maintained
   e. Compliance with prescribed drugs is variable

Case history questions

Case history 1

An epileptic woman becomes pregnant. She is taking phenytoin.

1. Is she at an increased risk of having a child with a congenital defect?
2. Concerned about the safety of her child, she wishes to discontinue her antiepileptic medication; what do you advise her?
3. If her dose remains unchanged, how will the pregnancy affect the total and free plasma phenytoin concentration?
4. Is this of clinical significance?
5. Can she breastfeed without risk to the infant?

Case history 2

A 75-year-old man is diagnosed as hypertensive and the doctor wishes to institute drug treatment with a water-soluble beta-blocker.

1. Is this patient in general more likely to suffer adverse drug reactions than a younger patient?
2. Will the clearance of the drug prescribed be affected by the patient's age?

The patient subsequently complains of falling episodes and is found to have postural hypotension.

3. What should the doctor do?
4. The patient later develops Parkinson's disease and is given levodopa and selegiline, and later still digoxin because of atrial fibrillation. What problems might the use of so many drugs pose?

Short note questions

Write short notes on:

1. Polypharmacy in the elderly.
2. Pharmacokinetic and other differences between children and adults.
3. Drug treatment of epilepsy in a pregnant woman.

Extended matching items questions

Theme: Drug selection in young women and pregnancy

Options

A. Aspirin
B. Carbamazepine
C. Cefalexin
D. Ciprofloxacin
E. Dalteparin
F. Paracetamol
G. Phenoxymethylpenicillin
H. Phenytoin
I. Streptokinase
J. Trimethoprim
K. Valproate
L. Warfarin

From each of the clinical scenarios given below, select the most appropriate drug from the list of options above.

1. A 25-year-old woman is pregnant and sees her GP with symptoms suggestive of a urinary tract infection.
2. A 25-year-old woman is pregnant, and complains of a sore throat. Her pharyngeal muscosa is inflamed.
3. A 25-year-old woman is pregnant. She is diagnosed with a deep venous thrombosis.
4. A 25-year-old woman is diagnosed with epilepsy. She has just got married and tells you that she wants to start a family.

Self-assessment on Chapter 19: answers

Multiple choice answers

1. a. **False.** It may cause fetal abnormalities but nevertheless it is the anticonvulsant of choice in pregnancy, as it seems to be the safest of the antiepileptic drugs.
   b. **True.** As generally used. Very high doses for long periods might be harmful.
   c. **False.** There is a theoretical risk of damage to fetal cartilage.
   d. **False.** Risk of teratogenesis as trimethoprim is a folate antagonist.
   e. **False.** A vitamin A derivative and highly teratogenic.

2. a. **False.** Substantially increased.
   b. **True.** As albumin binding is proportionately decreased.
   c. **False.** Although free drug levels remain much the same, total drug (which is what is measured in therapeutic drug monitoring) is altered because of changes in protein binding.
   d. **True.** Also neonatal hypothyroidism.
   e. **False.** Insulin therapy must be instituted.

3. a. **False.** This is a common but potentially dangerous mistake. Children should be considered quite separately from adults.
   b. **False.** The best way is probably on a dose per body surface area basis.
   c. **True.** For example, Reye's syndrome on aspirin, or stunted growth on glucocorticoids.
   d. **False.** Children have relatively well-developed liver drug-metabolising enzyme systems.
   e. **True.** Hence they may need lower doses than predicted of many water-soluble drugs.

4. a. **True.** For example reduced clearance, etc. If this were an essay question could you discuss it with examples?
   b. **True.** Again, a slight change to this question would make it suitable for an essay or short answer.

   c. **True.** Because of increased illness and perhaps poor prescribing. Around 75% of elderly patients have taken a therapeutic drug within the preceding 2 weeks compared with 33% of younger patients.
   d. **False.** These become increasingly impaired with time.
   e. **True.** Often poor, especially if the patient is required to take a complex drug regimen: occasionally too good, with the patient taking excessive drug.

Case history answers

Case history 1

1. Yes, probably from both the epilepsy and the drugs. Cleft lip deformities are associated with phenytoin.
2. It would have been desirable to have this patient on carbamazepine before she became pregnant. Now, however, the risks to her and to her child of stopping therapy outweigh those of continuing.
3. The total plasma phenytoin will fall because of the increased volume of distribution, and because of the reduction in serum albumin. However, the free phenytoin will remain roughly the same.
4. The free drug is active, and since this remains largely unchanged, the change in total drug is of little clinical consequence. However, if a doctor measures total plasma concentrations and finds them low, he may mistakenly increase the dose of the drug.
5. Yes.

Case history 2

1. In general yes, for many reasons: the most important of which is increased drug use in this age group.
2. Yes: water-soluble beta-blockers are cleared by the kidney through glomerular filtration and this will fall with advancing age. The dose of beta-blocker used should be low initially and titrated for effect. The use of a low starting dose is advisable for other reasons also, such as increased sensitivity to the effects of drugs.

3. There are many factors that need to be considered in causing postural hypotension in the elderly, but a reasonable first step would be to stop the beta-blocker. It might be worth trying another antihypertensive (e.g. a thiazide). However, if the patient shows a poor tolerance for such drugs, even if he is hypertensive off treatment, it may be best to leave the hypertension untreated.

4. There may be an increased risk of drug interactions and of poor drug compliance.

Short note answers

1. The issues to be considered are:
   - possible inappropriate responses to multiple symptoms
   - inappropriate treatment of adverse effects of some medications with other medication
   - increased risk of adverse reactions and interactions in the elderly
   - problems with poor patient concordance and adherence to prescribed medication
   - need to take holistic overview of the patient's condition to avoid polypharmacy.

2. A comparison of adults and children in pharmacology should cover:
   - need to consider different relative distributions of fat and water between adults, children and neonates
   - appropriate dosing regimens, based on milligrams or unit dose per body surface area
   - decreased renal function in neonates relative to adults and children
   - relatively well-preserved hepatic function in children compared with adults
   - different patterns of adverse reactions in children compared with adults, e.g. theophylline causing hyperactivity and attention deficit disorders, sedatives causing paradoxical excitation, etc.

3. Key elements are:
   - the need to maintain control of the epilepsy, which if uncontrolled would be more harmful to the fetus and the mother than any drug
   - choice of appropriate drug or least harmful drug before the woman becomes pregnant (most often carbamazepine)

- potential misleading plasma concentration levels in pregnancy because of changed body water and plasma protein levels
- possible prenatal diagnosis of such potential drug effects as spina bifida, which may allow the woman to decide to abort a malformed fetus if tested early enough.

Extended matching items answers

Theme: Drug selection in young women and pregnancy

1. C. It is likely that this woman will be treated with an antibiotic provided there is reasonable suspicion of a urinary tract infection, as untreated infections like this can develop into something more serious and can provoke pre-term labour. A dipstick of her urine will be needed at the very least, and this should be sent for microscopy, culture and sensitivity. It would be reasonable thereafter to treat her empirically with a cephalosporin antibiotic such as cefalexin.

2. F (or nothing at all). This is almost certainly going to be viral and would not therefore benefit from antibiotics anyway. Simple analgesia with paracetamol (and NOT aspirin) would be advisable. Good practice would generally suggest she returns to see you again if her symptoms are not self-limiting. The diagnosis and hence need for antibiotic therapy could thus be reviewed.

3. E. There is a risk of thromboembolism. Low molecular weight heparins are not known to be harmful in pregnancy. Warfarin is best avoided. Streptokinase would only be considered in a massive life-threatening pulmonary embolus when there is an immediate threat to the life of the mother.

4. B. There is probably most experience with carbamazepine under these circumstances. Women with epilepsy should also be given folate supplementation as part of pre-pregnancy counselling, and be offered closer medical supervision throughout pregnancy, including screening for fetal abnormalities.

Effects of disease state on drug response

Chapter
20

20.1	Pharmacokinetic factors	273
20.2	Pharmacodynamic factors	275
	Self-assessment on Chapter 20: questions	278
	Self-assessment on Chapter 20: answers	280

Overview

For the majority of drugs, clinically serious interindividual variation in response is not a frequent problem – most drugs have fairly reproducible effects. However, certain diseases alter drug response predictably, necessitating dose alteration to avoid either toxicity or therapeutic failure. Disease may affect either pharmacokinetic factors (absorption, distribution, metabolism or excretion) or pharmacodynamic factors (dose-concentration–response relationships).

You should be familiar with Appendices 2 and 3 of the British National Formulary (BNF). These give warnings and recommendations concerning dosing in hepatic and renal disease, which are the two most commonly encountered disease states of relevance. Individual hospital formularies or medicines information services also provide advice under these circumstances.

20.1 Pharmacokinetic factors

Learning objectives

At the end of this section you should:
- know the pharmacokinetic mechanisms whereby disease may alter drug response
- be able to give clinically relevant examples of disease-related changes to the processes of absorption, distribution, metabolism and excretion
- be able to describe the important features of drugs likely to be affected by changes in liver function (be aware of Appendix 2 in BNF)
- be able to describe the important features of drugs likely to be affected by changes in renal function (be aware of Appendix 3 in BNF).

Disease states can affect all four of the key pharmacokinetic parameters determining how the body handles a given drug:

- absorption
- distribution
- metabolism
- excretion.

Absorption

Absorption can be altered by *blood flow*:

- reduced blood flow to the gut: this rarely compromises drug absorption
- reduced muscle blood flow: the i.m. route of administration is prone to slow absorption if muscle blood flow is reduced, as it can be in shock.

Altered transit time. Acute gastrointestinal infections, both viral and bacterial, may increase motility, reducing transit and hence drug absorption. The severe chronic diarrhoea often seen in AIDS patients may reduce the absorption of anti-tuberculosis drugs.

Clinical sketch: drug absorption

The victim of a road traffic accident is in great pain from multiple injuries. His blood pressure is 80/30 mmHg. The emergency team's doctor is happy to use diamorphine, and gives it i.m. at the roadside, but it does not seem to work.

Comment: there are many reasons why diamorphine may be problematic in such circumstances (head injury, for example). However, in this hypothetical case, it has been given by the wrong route. Muscle blood flow is reduced in shock, and the drug will not be reliably absorbed.

Distribution

Plasma protein binding

Drugs are transported in the plasma bound to plasma proteins, mainly albumin and α_1-acid glycoprotein. Diseases that change plasma protein concentrations alter drug effect by increasing or decreasing the drug concentration unbound in the plasma water. The concentration of α_1-acid glycoprotein rises in acute infection, inflammation or infarction. Albumin concentrations may be markedly reduced by chronic liver disease and nephrotic syndrome.

Clinical sketch: protein binding and drug distribution

A 50-year-old man with type 1 diabetes mellitus has been on phenytoin for epilepsy for many years. He develops peripheral oedema and notices foamy urine. Shortly thereafter he develops severe ataxia, and presents acutely to hospital.

Comment: phenytoin has serious concentration-dependent adverse effects, including ataxia and sedation, which are dependent on its unbound fraction and so are potentiated by hypoalbuminaemia. It sounds like this man has developed nephrotic syndrome (probably a complication of his diabetes). He probably has hypoalbuminaemia, and this is the likeliest cause of his phenytoin toxicity.

Clinical sketch: protein binding and drug distribution

Patient A has cerebral malaria and is treated with quinine: the peak drug concentration is 20 µg/ml. *Patient A* recovers uneventfully. In contrast, *patient B*, who is healthy, takes an overdose of quinine (his mother's prescription – she was given it for night cramps). On admission, his peak drug concentration is also 20 µg/ml. *Patient B* develops bilateral blindness, which never fully recovers.

Comment: concentrations of α_1-acid glycoprotein are low in health but rise in some diseases, because it is an acute-phase reactant. Although the total quinine concentrations in patients A and B are identical, the free drug levels are markedly different because of the variation in the level of α_1-glycoprotein to bind drug: hence the marked difference in response.

Clinical sketch: tissue distribution

A patient with meningococcal meningitis is treated with high doses of i.v. benzylpenicillin. As he recovers, and can take drugs by mouth, ampicillin is started in place of benzylpenicillin. From this point, his improvement falters: repeat lumbar puncture suggests inadequate treatment.

Comment: this would be unusual management – it is produced here to illustrate a point. The penicillins are polar compounds that do not readily cross the blood–brain barrier. In meningitis, this barrier becomes inflamed, allowing a greater partition of the antibiotic into the CNS. The danger comes as meningitis resolves, because care must be taken that CNS drug concentrations are maintained to achieve full resolution.

Tissue distribution

Most drugs have their effects in specific tissues, diffusing out of the plasma to reach effective local concentrations. Inflammation of membrane barriers and changes in local pH may affect this process.

Metabolism

Alteration in drug metabolism is among the most commonly encountered causes of disease-induced changes in drug response. Predictably, the drugs concerned:

- are extensively metabolised to inactive derivatives
- have serious concentration-dependent toxicity
- have narrow therapeutic indices.

Most drugs are metabolised in the liver. This organ has tremendous reserve, and changes in drug effects may not be seen until there is loss of much of the parenchyma. Even so, caution is recommended in both acute and chronic liver disease. Both first pass metabolism and systemic metabolism may be reduced.

Clinical sketch: drug metabolism

An alcoholic patient develops decompensated liver failure as a result of pneumonia. He is given pethidine because of pleuritic chest pain.

Comment: this could be extremely dangerous. Even 'weak' analgesics such as codeine may precipitate coma.

Clinical sketch: drug metabolism

A man with known alcoholic cirrhosis is seen in clinic. He smokes, and complains of wheeze. He is already taking salbutamol, and the doctor starts aminophylline.

Comment: he is at risk from aminophylline toxicity. This drug has a narrow therapeutic range and is eliminated by hepatic metabolism.

Clinical sketch: drug metabolism

An alcoholic patient takes an overdose of paracetamol and presents to the A&E department about 6 hours thereafter. His paracetamol level is below the 'normal treatment line' but he is given N-acetylcysteine nevertheless.

Comment: alcohol is an inducer of the CYP450 enzymes that metabolise paracetamol to its toxic metabolite. Such patients are at increased risk of severe liver damage. Patients taking liver enzyme inducers should be treated at lower plasma concentrations of paracetamol.

Excretion

Drugs that cause concern in patients with renal impairment usually fulfil the following criteria:

- they are excreted unchanged
- they cause serious concentration-dependent toxicity
- their therapeutic indices are all narrow.

Both acute and chronic renal failure reduce drug excretion rate in proportion to the reduction in glomerular filtration rate. Major examples include:

- aminoglycosides
- digoxin
- sulphonylureas.

Appendix 3 of the British National Formulary lists many others.

Clinical sketch: drug elimination

An elderly woman with impaired renal function is treated with digoxin for new-onset atrial fibrillation. She presents to the A&E department 6 months later in complete heart block, and her digoxin level is found to be greatly above the therapeutic range.

Comment: digoxin concentrations ought to have been measured and the dose adjusted.

Clinical sketch: drug elimination

An obese 55-year-old man with type 2 diabetes mellitus has been treated with metformin for many years. During his annual diabetes review his GP notes that his renal function has become significantly abnormal. The metformin is stopped and he is transferred to insulin therapy.

Comment: metformin is almost exclusively eliminated from the body by renal excretion. Serious toxicity in the form of lactic acidosis can occur in the presence of renal failure, resulting from drug accumulation, and hence the drug is contraindicated in the presence of even relatively mild renal impairment. The cause of the deterioration in this man's renal function should be investigated – it is most likely a result of his diabetes.

Clinical sketch: drug elimination

A young man is admitted with extensive burns and develops Gram-negative septicaemia. He is treated with antibiotics, including gentamicin. His renal function has not been as closely monitored as it should have been. Gentamicin concentrations have been measured during the admission but towards the end of a bank holiday weekend he complains of tinnitus, deafness and vertigo.

Comment: this man was always at high risk of renal failure (through Gram-negative sepsis and hypovolaemia from the burns), and frequent monitoring of renal function and gentamicin concentrations is mandatory. Ototoxicity is not unusual with the aminoglycosides, which may also cause worsening renal function themselves.

20.2 Pharmacodynamic factors

Learning objectives

At the end of this section you should:
- be able to classify the influences of disease states on drug response
- understand the pharmacodynamic mechanisms that explain both reduced and increased drug responses
- be able to outline some clinical examples of such altered drug response.

Reduction in drug effect

Less responsive 'target'

Disease may compromise the function of target organs or alter their receptor status. For example, type 1 diabetes mellitus cannot be treated with sulphonylureas because the disease state results from the loss of pancreatic beta-cells. Since much of the response to sulphonylureas results from increased insulin secretion, their activity is much diminished. In contrast, of course, sulphonylureas are routinely used in the treatment of type 2 diabetes where peripheral insulin resistance is involved.

Clinical sketch: less responsive 'target'

An elderly man presents with pulmonary oedema caused by a myocardial infarction. The A&E doctor gives him 80 mg furosemide, puts in a catheter and waits for diuresis to reduce the pulmonary oedema. The patient's dyspnoea diminishes a little, but there is only a sluggish diuresis. Meanwhile, some blood results have come through: haemoglobin 8.6 g% (86 g/L; normochromic and normocytic), urea 90 mmol/L, creatinine 400 µmol/L.

Comment: this man probably has chronic renal impairment, judging by his haemoglobin. If so, the relative lack of response to the loop diuretic is understandable. The initial reduction in his breathlessness will have been the result of the vasodilatation caused by furosemide. Larger doses of furosemide might have to be used to achieve the same diuretic effect.

Clinical sketch: less responsive 'target'

An intravenous drug user is admitted with a fractured humerus. He is given diamorphine for his pain, but it does not seem to work well.

Comment: there is downregulation of opiate receptors in opiate addicts, and response to a given dose is lower than expected. However, common sense suggests other reasons why the patient may be asking for a larger dose: clinical judgement is required here.

The presence of endogenous ligands

If the disease allows the accumulation or increased synthesis of endogenous compounds with the opposite effect to that of the drug, the drug will be rendered less efficacious. For example, phaeochromocytomas are catecholamine-secreting tumours (usually benign; usually in the adrenal cortex). They present with hypertension (often accelerated hypertension). Use of beta-blockers in patients with phaeochromocytomas may cause a rise in blood pressure because the high concentration of circulating catecholamines binds readily to α-adrenoceptors, causing vasoconstriction (and hence an increase in peripheral resistance), while the beta-blockers may decrease the vasodilatation previously experienced by the patient.

Clinical sketch: endogenous ligands oppose drug action

A man with chronic renal failure is being treated for chronic duodenal ulcers. These seem remarkably 'resistant' to treatment with ranitidine.

Comment: the gastric hormone gastrin is normally metabolised in the kidneys and accumulates in patients with chronic renal failure, opposing the effects of H_2 blockers such as ranitidine.

Enhanced drug effect

More responsive 'target'

Disease may already mimic the desired drug effect, so that addition of the drug causes unexpectedly marked response. The interactions between chronic liver disease and anticoagulant/antiplatelet drugs are commonly encountered in this regard. Clotting factors are synthesised in the liver, and parenchymal liver disease often prolongs tests of intrinsic and extrinsic clotting cascades. Consequently, the effects of warfarin and aspirin are more pronounced than in health.

Clinical sketch: more responsive 'target'

A patient is admitted with pleuritic chest pain and a normal chest radiograph. Ventilation perfusion scanning suggests a 'moderate' probability of pulmonary embolism. D-dimers are raised. Warfarin is started using a standard dosing regimen. The first INR, performed 4 days later, is 8.0; liver function tests become available at the same time and suggest liver disease.

Comment: use of warfarin in patients with unrecognised liver disease may cause uncoagulable blood, and tests of coagulability should always be done before starting treatment.

Clinical sketch: more responsive 'target'

A man with chronic pancreatitis presents with atrial fibrillation and is put on warfarin. The first INR, performed 4 days later, shows an INR of 6.0.

Comment: clotting factors II, VII, IX and X are dependent upon vitamin K, a lipid-soluble vitamin, for their synthesis. Pancreatitis often manifests with maldigestion/malabsorption of fat. This man may well be vitamin K deficient.

Clinical sketch: more responsive target

An elderly woman, on longstanding diuretics for congestive cardiac failure, is started on an angiotensin converting enzyme (ACE) inhibitor. After the first dose, on rising from the seated position, she collapses and is found to be hypotensive.

Comment: homeostasis is often poorly maintained by the elderly. This problem is exacerbated here by the naturesis induced by her diuretic. Such patients should be started on extremely low ACE inhibitor doses.

Clinical sketch: more responsive target

An elderly woman suffers diarrhoea from villous adenomas of the large bowel: she has refused surgery. She presents with atrial fibrillation and is started on digoxin (but not warfarin for fear of haemorrhage from the adenomas). Six months later she is admitted with complete heart block, at which time her potassium is 2.8 mmol/L.

Comment: villous adenomas can cause profound hypokalaemia, which, in turn, increases the response to digoxin (see Ch. 4).

Idiosyncratic responses

The mechanisms underlying idiosyncratic (type B) adverse drug reactions are often poorly understood. Certain diseases seem to render patients more likely to such reactions.

Clinical sketch: increased risk of idiosyncratic adverse reactions

A man with advanced HIV disease takes co-trimoxazole as prophylaxis against *Pneumocystis carinii*. He develops a severe rash, which is attributed to the sulphonamide.

Comment: HIV disease seems to predispose towards frequent reactions to sulphonamides. The mechanism is unclear, but impaired cell detoxification of chemically reactive drug derivatives has been suggested as the cause.

Twenty

Self-assessment on Chapter 20: questions

Multiple choice questions

1. Response to the following drugs is affected adversely by the disease state:
   a. Morphine and hepatic failure
   b. Propranolol and phaeochromocytoma
   c. Gliclazide and renal failure
   d. Sulfinpyrazone and renal failure
   e. Aminophylline and cirrhosis

2. The following statements are correct:
   a. The only determinant of the effect of liver disease on response to a drug is the degree to which it is cleared by hepatic metabolism
   b. The only determinant of the effect of renal disease on response to a drug is the degree to which it is cleared, unchanged, by the kidney
   c. Heart failure has little impact on drug response
   d. Aminoglycosides should be avoided in myasthenia gravis
   e. Digoxin should be avoided in pre-excitation syndromes (such as Wolff–Parkinson–White syndrome)

Case history questions

Case history 1

A middle-aged man with chronic alcoholic liver disease is given phenytoin for generalised tonic/clonic seizures. His liver function tests are as follows (normal range in parentheses):

- albumin 37 g/L (32–42), bilirubin 14 mmol/L (2–17), gamma-glutamyltransferase 230 mg/L (<50), prothrombin time 32 seconds (control 13 seconds).

The plasma phenytoin concentration is closely watched for 3 years thereafter: the concentration remains within the therapeutic range and seizure frequency declines. He becomes lost to follow-up. The patient is admitted to hospital 5 years later with severe ataxia. His plasma phenytoin concentration is well above the therapeutic range and his liver function tests are as follows:

- albumin 17 g/L, bilirubin 50 mmol/L, gamma-glutamyltransferase 350 mg/L, prothrombin time 125 seconds (control 13 seconds).

1. Comment on the case: what are the likely mechanisms of the adverse reactions, and in what ways might they have been avoided?

Case history 2

An elderly woman develops atrial fibrillation, and is given digoxin to control her ventricular rate. Relevant blood results at the time are (normal values in parentheses):

- Na^+ 140 mmol/L (135–145), K^+ 3.9 mmol/L (3.5–5.4), urea 14 mmol/L (2.5–7.0), creatinine 140 mmol/L (50–130).

Two years later she develops peripheral oedema and nocturnal breathlessness. Her doctor diagnoses congestive heart failure, starts a thiazide diuretic and later adds an angiotensin-converting enzyme (ACE) inhibitor. Her symptoms improve. Two years later, she is admitted to hospital in complete heart block with the following blood results: Na^+ 138 mmol/L, K^+ 1.4 mmol/L, urea 45 mmol/L, creatinine 360 μmol/L.

1. Comment on the case: what are the likely mechanisms of the adverse reactions and in what ways might they have been avoided?

Extended matching items questions

Theme: Drugs for concern in disease states

Options

A. Carbamazepine

B. Diclofenac

C. Gliclazide

D. Ibuprofen

E. Metformin

F. Morphine

G. Paracetamol

H. Subcutaneous insulin

I. Tolbutamide

For each of the following clinical scenarios, select the drug from the list of options above that is most likely implicated (drug X), giving rise to most concern under the circumstances described.

1. A 50-year-old woman has chronic liver disease as a result of primary biliary cirrhosis. She is given an analgesic (drug X) for abdominal pain caused by her ascites. Several hours later her conscious level is reduced and she is taken to intensive care.

2. A 50-year-old woman has chronic renal failure as a result of diabetes. She is given an analgesic (drug X) for abdominal pain. Several hours later she is very drowsy and difficult to rouse.

3. A 60-year-old man is admitted to hospital with type 2 respiratory failure secondary to an infective exacerbation of chronic obstructive pulmonary disease. He also develops ischaemic chest pain and a nurse wants to give him analgesia (drug X). The doctor is concerned by this.

4. A 60-year-old man with type 2 diabetes is admitted to hospital with an acute anterior myocardial infarction. His usual anti-hyperglycaemic medication (drug X) is stopped and he is transferred to an insulin infusion because of concern regarding toxicity.

5. A 25-year-old woman with epilepsy (treated with an anticonvulsant, drug X) is admitted to hospital following an overdose of paracetamol. Her paracetamol levels are well below the 'normal risk' treatment line, but the specialist registrar treating here decides to give her N-acetylcysteine anyway.

Self-assessment on Chapter 20: answers

Multiple choice answers

1. a. **True.** Morphine may precipitate fatal coma.

   b. **True.** Phaeochromocytoma is a rare cause of hypertension, in which a tumour secretes catecholamines. The main effect is an increase in peripheral vascular resistance caused by noradrenaline (norepinephrine). Paradoxically, beta-blockers may worsen blood pressure control by opposing β_2-effects and by preventing the binding of noradrenaline to β_1-adenoceptors, thereby increasing its binding to α-adrenoceptors.

   c. **True.** Gliclazide is a sulphonylurea hypoglycaemic agent that is mainly excreted unchanged; it produces profound hypoglycaemia in patients with renal failure.

   d. **True.** Sulfinpyrazone is a uricosuric used in gout (Ch. 9). For the drug to work, there must be adequate renal function; furthermore, sulfinpyrazone clearance is reduced by renal failure.

   e. **True.** Aminophylline clearance is reduced in chronic liver disease.

2. a. **False.** Hepatocellular disease may cause hypoalbuminaemia: drugs extensively bound to albumin may, therefore, be more potent. Such patients have impaired clotting, increasing the effect of anticoagulants and antiplatelet drugs (such as aspirin).

   b. **False.** The accumulation of metabolic waste in patients with renal failure occupies binding sites on albumin and other plasma proteins: some protein-bound drugs may, therefore, be potentiated.

   c. **False.** Severe heart failure reduces the volume of distribution of some drugs (notably lidocaine).

   d. **True.** Aminoglycosides may cause a degree of non-depolarising blockade at the motor end-plate. This is usually of no consequence, but in myasthenia gravis, aminoglycosides may worsen weakness.

   e. **True.** Digoxin slows the rate of conduction across the atrioventricular (AV) node and may encourage aberrant conduction in WPW syndrome: this may cause ventricular tachycardia.

Case history answers

Case history 1

The lack of linearity between the dose of phenytoin and its plasma concentration (i.e. zero-order pharmacokinetics) should be covered. The extensive binding of phenytoin to plasma proteins should be mentioned and the fact that phenytoin is largely cleared by hepatic metabolism. This man had impaired liver function to start with, but during his loss from follow-up, the situation worsened: he probably continued to drink. The liver function tests give good guidance of this worsening status. Clearance of phenytoin is almost certainly lower and, given the low albumin, its free fraction is probably higher (you should discuss the importance of free drug fractions at this point). This man's problems might have been avoided had regular follow-up been undertaken, but he defaulted. You may want to discuss the problem of giving potentially toxic drugs such as phenytoin or warfarin to patients who are likely to default.

Case history 2

It should be stressed at the start that digoxin is cleared almost entirely by renal excretion and that its effects are potentiated by hypokalaemia (the mechanism of this should be presented). This patient had renal impairment to start with and probably had a low digoxin clearance. Her renal function deteriorated, however (possibly caused by the ACE inhibitor), and this, together with the thiazide-induced hypokalaemia, caused severe toxicity. She should have been followed more closely, with estimations of renal function, K^+ and plasma digoxin concentration.

Extended matching items answers

Theme: Drugs for concern in disease states

1. F. Morphine is the drug of concern here. Morphine is metabolised in the liver and may precipitate coma in patients with hepatic impairment. Although it may still be possible to use this very effective painkiller cautiously

in patients with liver disease (by using smaller doses) and many patients do tolerate it well, this patient is particularly at risk because she is already showing evidence of decompensation.

2. F. Morphine is also the drug of concern here. Morphine demonstrates altered pharmacokinetics in the presence of renal failure, resulting in the accumulation of morphine itself or an active metabolite. Morphine is metabolised to morphine-3-glucuronide and morphine-6-glucuronide, both of which are renally excreted: the half-life of these compounds is greatly increased in those patients with significant renal impairment. Patients can therefore be at risk of potentially life-threatening toxicity.

3. F. Yet another example of where morphine may cause problems, this time because of pharmacodynamic concerns rather than through any changes in metabolism or excretion. Morphine is a respiratory depressant and may cause problems in a patient who already has respiratory failure. Although no patient should have to suffer pain, use of morphine under these circumstances must be very cautious, with very small doses given in highly monitored environments.

4. E. Metformin would be stopped because of the risk of lactic acidosis in the setting of cardiac and renal failure, both potential complications of an acute myocardial infarction. Moreover, such patients are usually transferred to an insulin infusion regimen anyway, because tighter glycaemic control has been shown to improve outcome in the immediate period following a myocardial infarction.

5. A. Carbamazepine is an enzyme inducer and potentially would increase the formation of the toxic metabolite in paracetamol overdose, hence a lower threshold for treating than would normally be the case.

Chapter 21

Adverse drug reactions and drug interactions

21.1	Adverse drug reactions	283
21.2	Drug interactions	285
	Self-assessment on Chapter 21: questions	287
	Self-assessment on Chapter 21: answers	290

Overview

Adverse drug reactions are a common cause of iatrogenic morbidity and mortality. They may affect as many as 20% of patients in some form. Simple measures may prevent some of these. You should report all serious or novel adverse drug reactions to the appropriate drug licensing agency.

Drug interactions may be pharmacokinetic or pharmacodynamic. They may be useful or harmful. Certain drugs and certain patients are particularly likely to be involved in adverse interactions and we should be aware of these.

21.1 Adverse drug reactions

Learning objectives

At the end of this section you should:
- be aware of the importance of adverse drug reactions in causing morbidity and mortality
- be able to describe the simple classification of adverse drug reactions
- understand some of the mechanisms of adverse drug reactions
- understand the importance of reporting adverse drug reactions and know how to do this.

Any drug has the potential to cause an adverse drug reaction (ADR). ADRs can be defined as any unintended harmful effect of a drug. Before prescribing, the potential risks of any drug must be weighed against the possible benefits; doctors should only prescribe when the benefits outweigh the risks. ADRs are very common. It is estimated that ADRs occur in 10–20% of all patients prescribed drugs and are the cause of up to 10% of all GP consultations, 6% of all hospital admissions and about 1 in 1000 deaths. ADRs may mimic natural disease and are generally not well detected or reported by doctors. Adverse drug reactions are a significant issue for public health.

Classification

A useful classification of ADRs is as follows.

Type A: the *augmented* effects. These are dose related and are where the ADR is caused by an excessive response to the drug. This may result from pharmacokinetic or pharmacodynamic problems. These ADRs are predictable from the known effects of the drug and are dose related, e.g. hypoglycaemia in patients with diabetes treated with insulin, hypotension in patients taking antihypertensives, or excessive sedation in a patient taking carbamazepine. Such effects are very common but are often not severe. Type A ADRs can be managed often by dose modification.

Clinical sketch

An elderly patient is prescribed benzodiazepines for an inability to sleep after a recent bereavement. Two days later the patient crashes his car. Although not badly injured he has no recollection of the event leading up to the crash.

Comment: this is probably a type A reaction to benzodiazepines: increased sedation or incoordination if the patient is not used to such sedative drugs. Such adverse events are more likely to occur in the elderly, who are more sensitive to benzodiazepines. The patient should have been warned not to drive while taking the drug, or at least not drive until it was clear to what extent it would cause such sedation.

Type B: the *bizarre* effects. These are not predictable from the known effects of the drug and are not dose related. These often have an immunological basis: as such, there is often no clear relationship to the dose of drug. Such ADRs are relatively rare but are disproportionately important because the ADR is often very serious, e.g. anaphylaxis with penicillin or agranulocytosis with carbimazole. Withdrawal of the drug is necessary.

Type C: effects of *chronic* administration. These effects are caused by adaptation, change in receptor sensitivity, etc. For example, the on–off phenomenon with levodopa.

Type D: *delayed* effects. These are the long-term effects such as carcinogenesis or effects on reproduction, e.g. stilbestrol (Ch. 19).

Type E: *end of use* or *withdrawal* reactions. These occur if there have been changes such as receptor upregulation, e.g. rebound angina on withdrawal of beta-blockers. The withdrawal syndrome seen when stopping selective serotonin reuptake inhibitors (SSRIs) is another example of such a reaction.

Type F: *unexpected failure of therapy*. These are common and dose related. They are sometimes caused by drug interactions, e.g. failure of the oral contraceptive in a woman prescribed the enzyme inducer carbamazepine.

Drug testing

Premarketing testing of a new drug will involve its administration to an average of about 3000 subjects in clinical trials (this number continues to rise as drug testing becomes ever more rigorous). This will show up many common ADRs, especially type A. However, type B reactions may be relatively rare, perhaps with an incidence of only 1 in 10 000 prescriptions or less, and so are unlikely to be seen in trials. These may only become apparent after the drug is launched and the numbers of patients treated

with it rises. Likewise the late type C and D effects are only likely to be seen after the drug has been available for some years. It may be difficult to connect an adverse event with the drug, especially if the ADR resembles other disease. For example liver damage was seen in those prescribed perhexilene, an antianginal drug now withdrawn. The drug caused histological changes identical to those resulting from alcoholism and was initially not recognised as an ADR.

It is important, therefore, that when new drugs are prescribed, doctors observe closely for any possible adverse effects and report them to the proper authorities. In the UK, the Commission on Human Medicines (CHM, formerly the Committee on Safety of Medicines, or CSM) is the statutory body responsible for collecting these data and reports to CHM can be made on special yellow cards, which are widely available. Reporting can also now be undertaken via the internet. This system has been responsible for identifying many previously undescribed and serious ADRs. The CHM is particularly keen to have reports of all *serious* reactions to any drug and of *any* reaction to new drugs, identified in the advertising and the British National Formulary by a black triangle (▼).

In addition, specific postmarketing safety surveillance is often carried out on new drugs by the manufacturer, using computerised records from hospitals and primary care.

Patients particularly at risk of adverse reactions

Patients particularly at risk are:

- the elderly: little physiological reserve and altered phamacokinetics and pharmacodynamics
- the very young
- patients with renal disease
- patients with liver disease
- genetically predisposed patients: e.g. patients with glucose 6-phosphate dehydrogenase deficiency who may get haemolysis when treated with many drugs such as sulphonamides or antimalarials such as primaquine; patients with acute intermittent porphyria, who may get exacerbations if given many drugs that are metabolised by the liver and interfere with haem breakdown, such as oestrogens. There are many other genetic variations which alter both the response to drugs and the risks of adverse reactions. Research is helping us understand more about genetic variability and drug toxicity.

Ways to avoid adverse drug reactions

Prescribe drugs only when necessary, for the shortest time and in the lowest dose possible. Try to prescribe only drugs with which you are familiar – this is one of the virtues of using a limited drug formulary. Warn the patient of any common or major adverse reactions. Genetic variation is now being explored and will in the future allow us to tailor therapy to a patient more carefully.

21.2 Drug interactions

Learning objectives

At the end of this section you should:
- understand the mechanisms of drug interactions
- be aware of the drugs and patients most likely to be involved in such adverse reactions.

Drug interactions may be harmful or beneficial. Not all interactions are of clinical importance, and, like ADRs, they may not occur in every patient. Constant vigilance is, therefore, required to avoid drug interactions and to spot them when they do occur. Many lists of possible drug interactions are available. Rather than learn lists, it is better for the most part to consider which patients are at risk, which drugs are most likely to be involved and what the possible mechanisms are. Some common or dangerous interactions are mentioned but the list is not complete: check carefully if there is any doubt before prescribing. Many general practitioners now prescribe using computers and many pharmacies also use computers in their dispensing: suitable software is available to aid the detection of potential interactions.

Patients who are at risk of interactions

Patients most at risk are:

- the elderly (see Ch. 19): polypharmacy, poor homeostatic mechanisms, etc.
- severely ill patients: for similar reasons and also because a drug interaction may be difficult to distinguish from the natural history of the disease, e.g. heart failure treated with diuretics may be exacerbated by NSAIDs, which cause fluid retention
- patients who depend on prophylactic therapy for disease suppression, e.g. epileptics, patients on immunosuppressants or oral contraceptives
- patients with liver or renal disease
- patients with more than one doctor, when confusion may arise over what drugs the patient is taking
- patients who take non-prescribed drugs, e.g. those bought 'over the counter' such as theophylline, pseudoephedrine in decongestants and, of course, ethanol; always ask the patient about such drugs – many patients do not think of such drugs when asked about what medicines

they are taking. Herbal remedies are generally considered 'safe' by patients but this is not necessarily the case.

Drugs at risk

Some drugs are particularly likely to be involved in serious interactions:

- drugs with a narrow therapeutic index (Ch. 1), e.g. warfarin, digoxin, cytotoxics, lithium, aminoglycosides, theophylline
- drugs with a steep dose–response curve (Ch. 1), where a minor change in plasma concentration may make a major change in effect, e.g. oral antihyperglycaemic drugs, warfarin
- drugs with a major effect on a vital process such as clotting (warfarin)
- drugs where a loss of effect may lead to disease breakthrough, e.g. antiepileptics
- drugs that may induce or inhibit mixed function oxidase enzymes and so may decrease metabolism of other drugs, and drugs that depend on these enzymes for their metabolism (e.g. theophylline, warfarin, phenytoin, oral contraceptives, cyclosporin and many others)
- drugs that affect cardiac conduction: many drugs cause prolongation of the QT interval on the ECG, a marker of altered intracardiac conduction as a result of effects on ion channels in cardiac cells; such drugs may cause cardiac arrhythmias, especially if combined, e.g. the antihistamine terfenadine and the prokinetic agent cisapride.

Mechanisms

Drug interactions may be considered to be pharmacodynamic or pharmacokinetic.

Pharmacokinetic mechanisms

This is where the interaction causes a change in the plasma concentration of one or other drug leading to a greater or lesser effect.

Absorption. Drugs such as cholestyramine may bind to other drugs (e.g. digoxin, thiazides) in the gastrointestinal tract and prevent their absorption. Some drugs (e.g. opiates) may slow transit time and so may slow absorption, but the total amount absorbed may be unchanged. Some drugs depend on enterohepatic circulation, e.g. they are excreted in a conjugated form in bile, the conjugation is broken down by bacteria in the gastrointestinal tract and the free drug is reabsorbed, enhancing drug effect, e.g. oral contraceptive oestrogens. If this is prevented, for example by amoxicillin altering gut flora, the drug may lose its effect.

Metabolism. Enzyme inducers (e.g. phenytoin, carbamazepine, rifampicin) will decrease the effects of many drugs; since enzyme induction requires synthesis of new protein, it may take 2–3 weeks to reach its maximum effect. Enzyme inhibitors (erythromycin, ciprofloxacin, isoniazid, cimetidine, sodium valproate, metronidazole, allopurinol, ketoconazole, sulphonamides and many others), however, are effective very rapidly. Problems may arise, therefore, when a patient stable on a drug is prescribed either an enzyme inducer or an enzyme inhibitor. Problems may also arise if a patient is stabilised on a drug while receiving an enzyme inducer or inhibitor which is then withdrawn.

Distribution. Only free drug is pharmacologically active, but many drugs are heavily protein bound, e.g. warfarin to albumin. If another drug with a high affinity for protein is prescribed, the result may be a displacement of warfarin from the protein-binding sites, increasing the free drug and its effects (but this is transient, see Ch. 1). This may cause confusion if therapeutic drug monitoring is used, because this usually measures total rather than free drug.

Excretion. Drugs can interfere with excretion, for example thiazides and NSAIDs interfere with the excretion of lithium. This effect can sometimes be beneficial, e.g. reducing the clearance of penicillin by giving probenecid.

Pharmacodynamic mechanisms

Pharmacodynamic mechanisms are, in general, more common but are predictable from the known effects of the drug, e.g. two antihypertensives may be used to lower the blood pressure more than either alone. Interactions can be either synergistic or antagonistic. Alternatively, the actions of diuretics are opposed by NSAIDs, which may cause fluid retention, or the effects of oral antihyperglycaemics may be opposed by thiazides. Other pharmacodynamic interactions can arise from the effects of drugs on electrolyte or fluid balance, e.g. diuretic-induced hypokalaemia enhances digoxin toxicity.

Self-assessment on Chapter 21: questions

Multiple choice questions

1. Adverse drug reactions:
   a. Are a common source of morbidity
   b. Type A reactions are rare
   c. Type B reactions are often serious
   d. Type B reactions will generally have been identified before a drug is marketed
   e. Serious adverse reactions to all drugs should be reported to the CHM

2. Drug interactions:
   a. May result from altered metabolism
   b. May be caused by plasma protein displacement
   c. Are always harmful
   d. Are more likely in the elderly
   e. Are more likely in patients with ischaemic heart disease

3. The following drugs may interact:
   a. Glibenclamide and rifampicin
   b. Heparin and phenytoin
   c. Erythromycin and theophylline
   d. Co-proxamol and warfarin
   e. Benzodiazepines and ethanol

Case history questions

Case history 1

A 68-year-old woman with type 2 diabetes mellitus is treated with glibenclamide. She is found unconscious one evening, and taken to hospital. Her blood sugar is found to be low.

1. How would you classify this adverse reaction?

When she has been treated and has recovered, she describes how she was given fluconazole for a fungal infection the day before.

2. Is this relevant?

She is prescribed amoxicillin instead for the infection but develops bronchospasm for the first time in her life.

3. What class of adverse reaction is this?
4. Will decreasing the dose be adequate to prevent such an adverse effect?

Case history 2

A 35-year-old woman with epilepsy is prescribed ciprofloxacin for a urinary tract infection. She is currently taking carbamazepine. Five days later she has her first fit in 5 years.

1. What is the likely cause of the fit?
2. What would have been an appropriate antimicrobial choice in this patient?

Short note questions

Write short notes on:

1. The distinction between type A and type B adverse drug reactions
2. The key means to identify adverse drug reactions

Extended matching items questions

Theme: Adverse drug reactions

Options
A. Glyceryl trinitrate
B. Amoxicillin
C. Verapamil
D. Trimethoprim
E. Teratogenicity
H. Immune-mediated toxicity

I. Drug accumulation

J. Carcinogenicity

K. Phenoxymethylpenicillin

L. Exaggeration of the therapeutic effect

M. Mutagenicity

N. Atenolol

O. Placental damage

For each of the case histories below, choose the most appropriate answer from the options above. Each option may be used once, more than once, or not at all.

1. A 40-year-old cigarette smoker consults his doctor about episodic chest pain: the doctor finds the patient's feet are a little cold, and that his chest is a little wheezy, but otherwise there are no positive signs. The ECG is abnormal, suggestive of ischaemic heart disease, and the doctor diagnoses the chest pain as angina pectoris: a drug is started. Two weeks later the patient sees the GP again: he is very wheezy, indeed he can hardly talk, and for the past 2 weeks he has been unable to walk because of severe pain in his calves.

   Which drug did the GP give for the angina?

2. A young woman presents with severe dysuria. Dipstick testing of her urine reveals 'protein +++, blood +++': the doctor diagnoses a urinary tract infection. He prescribes a drug, but 2 days later the woman returns with a florid rash.
   i. Which drug was prescribed?
   ii. What is the likely mechanism?

3. A 20-year-old man has a very severe psoriasis and is under the care of a team of dermatologists. They have tried him on a number of regimens without success and eventually start him on methotrexate. This drug seems to work, and so the man doubles the dose without seeking medical advice; he also defaults from clinic for a month. When he next presents to clinic he is not well: he has a sore throat, conjunctivitis and a temperature of 40°C. His total white cell count is found to be very low at 1.0×10^9 cells/L; he is anaemic with a haemoglobin of 9.5 g% (95 g/L). The methotrexate has caused this problem, but by what mechanism?

4. A 30-year-old woman is given an antibiotic by i.v. injection for pneumonia. Five minutes later, she is found collapsed with profound hypotension, a generalised rash and is dyspnoeic with wheezing.
   i. What antibiotic is she likely to have been given?
   ii. What is the mechanism of this reaction?

Theme: Adverse effects of drugs

Options

A. Nausea

B. Dyspepsia

C. Rash

D. Bleeding

E. Agranulocytosis

F. Constipation

G. Headache

H. Dizziness

I. Ankle swelling

J. Sedation

K. Diarrhoea

L. Cold hands

M. Drug interactions

N. Peptic ulceration

For each of the drugs listed below, select from the options listed above the two or three most serious adverse effects about which you would wish to warn patients for whom you are prescribing. (Serious is taken to mean frequent or severe.) Options can be used once, more than once, or not at all.

1. Amlodipine

2. Carbimazole

3. Warfarin

4. Diclofenac

Theme: Adverse drug reactions

Options

A. Cough

B. Gastrointestinal bleeding

C. Gynaecomastia

D. Hypoglycaemia

E. Hypokalaemia

F. Lactic acidosis

G. Lowering of seizure threshold

H. Rhabdomyolysis

From the options above, select from the list below the drug most associated with each adverse reaction.

1. Simvastatin
2. Captopril
3. Ciprofloxacin
4. Metformin
5. Spironolactone

Theme: Drug interactions

Options

A. Bendroflumethiazide
B. Cefotaxime
C. Ethanol
D. Furosemide
E. Indometacin
F. Nifedipine
G. Spironolactone
H. Warfarin

From the options above, select the drug most likely to be associated with the drug interactions listed below.

1. Increased risk of life-threatening hyperkalaemia when prescribed with enalapril
2. Increased risk of CNS depression in a patient treated with chlorphenamine for hay fever
3. Increased risk of ototoxicity when given to a patient already being given gentamicin
4. Worsening of antihypertensive control when given with hydrochlorothiazide
5. Worsening of glycaemic control in a patient with type 2 diabetes mellitus treated with oral therapy

Multiple choice answers

1. a. **True.** For instance, in the elderly, adverse reactions may cause between 10 and 20% of hospital admissions (less commonly a cause in younger patients).

   b. **False.** These are related to the expected pharmacological effects of a drug and are common.

   c. **True.** Often immunological in origin and generally more serious and unpredictable than type A.

   d. **False.** Given their relatively low frequency and the small numbers of patients treated before a drug is marketed, it is less likely that type B reactions will be seen before marketing.

   e. **True.** Also all adverse reactions (serious or not) with new drugs.

2. a. **True.** For example, liver enzyme induction or inhibition.

   b. **True.** These are not usually of major importance, because the body clears free drug and a temporary increase in free drug because of protein displacement will be followed by increased clearance to restore free drug concentrations.

   c. **False.** For example, penicillin and probenecid, ACE inhibitors and diuretics.

   d. **True.** Because of polypharmacy, because of increased susceptibility to the harmful effects of drugs and because of altered pharmacokinetics and dynamics.

   e. **False.** More likely in patients with congestive cardiac failure, liver or renal disease.

3. a. **True.** The metabolism of glibenclamide and other sulphonylureas is increased because of enzyme induction by the rifampicin and the result may be hyperglycaemia.

   b. **False.** But phenytoin does interact with warfarin.

   c. **True.** Concentrations of theophylline may rise and cause serious adverse effects.

   d. **True.** Co-proxamol is a combination of paracetamol and dextropropoxyphene (a drug-metabolising enzyme inhibitor) and so may increase warfarin concentrations and cause bleeding.

   e. **True.** A pharmacodynamic interaction leading to increased drowsiness.

Case history answers

Case history 1

1. At first glance, this seems to be type A (augmented effect) adverse drug reaction. Given its severity, the doctor should report it to the CHM.

2. Now it seems more likely to be a drug interaction, caused by liver enzyme inhibition by the fluconazole.

3. This is a type B (bizarre, not predictable from the pharmacological action of a drug) adverse drug reaction.

4. No: the offending drug must be withdrawn.

Case history 2

1. Ciprofloxacin inhibits some liver enzymes but not those involved in the metabolism of carbamazepine. It is, therefore, unlikely to have had a pharmacokinetic interaction with carbamazepine. Even if it did inhibit the metabolism of carbamazepine, one would have anticipated that this would cause increased drowsiness and ataxia through raised carbamazepine concentrations rather than loss of control. Ciprofloxacin and other 5-quinolones can inhibit the inhibitory effects of GABA (gamma-aminobutyric acid). This can lead to overactivity of the CNS, e.g. vivid dreams or hallucinations, confusion in the elderly and a lowering of the seizure threshold. In this patient, the quinolone has probably lowered the seizure threshold to the extent that it is no longer adequately controlled by the carbamazepine, leading to the fit.

2. Trimethoprim would have been a more appropriate choice with no risk of either kinetic or dynamic interactions with the carbamazepine. The quinolone was contraindicated in an epileptic.

Short note answers

1. The distinct features of type A and B adverse drug reactions are:

   type A: common, usually not severe, predictable, dose related, augmented effect of the drug

   type B: rare, often severe, often immunological in origin, unpredictable from the known pharmacology of the drug.

2. This should include pre-licensing testing in drug trials, which will mainly reveal type A adverse reactions, post-licensing surveillance (either formal post-marketing surveillance or specific cohort or case control studies), case reports in medical literature, and yellow card reporting to licensing authorities. These are not unconnected; for instance, an increase in yellow card reports may prompt the undertaking of a cohort study or specific prescription event monitoring.

Extended matching items answers

Theme: Adverse drug reactions

1. i. N. These are classical adverse reactions to beta-blockers (even relatively cardioselective ones like atenolol), although rarely seen in such a severe form. This patient was clearly at risk of developing these reactions, and atenolol was a bad choice.

2. i. D. The most likely drug here is trimethoprim.

   ii. H. The mechanism is immune mediated. (The other antibiotics are not commonly used for urinary tract infections, although all might cause a rash.) This is a type B or bizarre reaction and was not predictable unless the patient had previously had a similar effect.

3. L. Methotrexate inhibits the conversion of folic to folinic acid and interferes therefore with purine and ultimately DNA formation. Hence it is used in conditions with a high cell turnover, like some malignant conditions, psoriasis and some inflammatory conditions. What has happened here is predictable from the pharmacology of the drug and is an exaggerated pharmacological effect (type A adverse drug reaction), so that the methotrexate is now affecting the blood precursors.

4. i. B. The antibiotic is probably penicillin.

   ii. H. This is classical anaphylaxis. The mechanism is immune mediated, through IgE. The patient may have had a history of previous penicillin exposure, and possibly previous adverse effects.

   iii. Supplementary question: how would you treat this patient? See Chapter 10 for the answers.

Theme: Adverse effects of drugs

1. Best answers are I, G and H. Amlodipine causes vasodilatation and as such may cause ankle swelling and headache. It sometimes causes relaxation in the smooth muscle of the gastro-oesphogeal junction and causes dyspepsia. In some patients, postural hypotension and dizziness may be a concern.

2. Best answers are E and C. Carbimazole can cause agranulocytosis, a rare but potentially fatal adverse effect. Patients must be warned to look out for any evidence of infection, such as a sore throat; if there is such evidence then a full blood count measuring white cells needs to be undertaken. If carbimaxole does cause agranulocytosis, withdrawal alone is usually adequate to restore white cell numbers. A much more common adverse effect of carbimazole, however, is rash. If this occurs it may be necessary to discontinue the carbimazole and try propylthiouracil instead.

3. Best answers are D and M. Warfarin inhibits the formation of the clotting factors II, VII, IX and X. In excess, therefore, it is prone to cause bleeding. Warfarin is probably the drug most commonly involved in serious adverse drug interactions as drugs which potentiate the warfarin (e.g. by inhibiting its metabolism), which reduce the tendency to clotting in other ways (e.g. antiplatelet effect) or which cause a risk of bleeding (e.g. by peptic ulceration) may all interact with warfarin. Patients need to be carefully warned about alerting their doctor or pharmacist before taking any prescribed or over-the-counter medicines while on warfarin. If in any doubt of the safety of a drug in combination with warfarin seek advice from the British National Formulary or your local drug information centre.

4. Best answers are N, B and C. Diclofenac like most non-steroidal anti-inflammatory drugs can cause dyspepsia (a direct effect of the acidic drug in the stomach) or peptic ulceration (inhibition of cyclo-oxygenase inhibiting maintenance of the gastric mucosa). Dyspepsia is not a reliable warning of the peptic ulceration. These drugs should clearly be avoided in patients with a previous history of peptic ulceration. Diclofenac has a range of other adverse effects, of which the most common is probably rash. However, it can also cause headache and drug interactions (for instance with diuretics its effects may be inhibited, leading to poor control of hypertension or to heart failure).

Theme: Adverse drug reactions

1. H. Muscle toxicity is rare with the statins but can be significant. Rhabdomyolysis can lead to renal failure, and this can sometimes be fatal.

2. A. A persistent cough is very typically seen with ACE inhibitors such as captopril. The patient may be able to put up with it. Alternatively another drug could be used, such as an angiotensin receptor blocker.

3. G. Ciprofloxacin can lower the seizure threshold and hence should be used only with caution in patients with epilepsy when no alternative drug exists.

4. F. The biguanide antidiabetic drugs classically have been linked to cases of lactic acidosis. This is actually quite rare, but the risk of this increases with renal, cardiac and hepatic failure.

5. C. Spironolactone can cause hyperkalaemia, particularly when used in conjunction with ACE-inhibitors. However, gynaecomastia is also listed as a typical adverse drug reaction.

Theme: Drug interactions

1. G. Spironolactone and ACE-inhibitors can each, individually, lead to hyperkalaemia. Together this can be a problem, although this need not preclude their use together. The renal function should be monitored. An example of a pharmacodynamic interaction.

2. C. Antihistamines such as chlorphenamine are centrally depressant; so is alcohol.

3. D. Furosemide and gentamicin both can cause ototoxicity.

4. E. NSAIDs such as indometacin can antagonise the antihypertensive effects of thiazide diuretics.

5. A. Bendroflumethiazide can deteriorate glycaemic control in patients with diabetes. However, this need not stop the two drugs being used together.

New drugs and clinical trials

22.1	New drugs	293
22.2	Testing new drugs	294
22.3	Prescribing new drugs	297
	Self-assessment on Chapter 22: questions	299
	Self-assessment on Chapter 22: answers	301

Overview

This chapter considers the process of developing new drugs: where they come from and how they are tested. The basic issues in designing a clinical trial are considered.

22.1 New drugs

Learning objectives

At the end of this section you should:
- be able to explain the stages of new drug development
- be aware of the likely sources for new drugs.

New drugs are developed and marketed, and the drugs learned by a doctor as a medical student will almost certainly be obsolete within his professional career. The doctor must understand where new drugs come from, how they are developed and licensed and how their value in therapy should be assessed.

How are new drugs found?

In the past, therapeutics was empirical, and drugs were natural substances or their derivatives and found by chance and experience to be valuable, e.g.

digitalis. With the development of the chemical industry, new synthetic chemicals were produced and screened for activity in various animal models or diseases, e.g. benzodiazepines. Existing drugs were purified to extract the active component and ensure more consistent quality, e.g. digoxin. These were slow and cumbersome processes and are less common today.

As our understanding of the pathophysiology of diseases grew, drugs were developed to imitate or replace naturally occurring compounds e.g. levo-dopa. Later still, the ability developed to design drugs to attach to an important receptor in the pathophysiology of the disease, e.g. β-adrenoceptor agonists or antagonists. Some drugs are enzyme inhibitors (e.g. angiotensin-converting enzyme (ACE) inhibitors, proton pump inhibitors). New targets for drugs are identified as a result of better understanding of the pathophysiology of a condition and of how the body works. In the future, these targets might be identifying and replacing a single gene to produce an altered gene product within the body, e.g. in therapy for inborn errors of metabolism.

Where do new drugs come from?

Almost all new drugs are the result of research conducted by the pharmaceutical industry, based on extensive work to understand the mechanisms behind the disease. Drug development involves a considerable commercial risk – less than 1 in 1000 molecules studied reach clinical trials and less than 1 in 100 drugs that enter trials are ever marketed. On average, it costs in the region of £500 million (approximately US$1 billion) to develop a novel drug, and it can take anything from 8 to 15 years.

22.2 Testing new drugs

Learning objectives

At the end of this section you should be able to explain:
- the advantages of the randomised controlled trial design for a new drug evaluation
- drug licensing and its significance.

Promising molecules undergo tests initially in animals (but increasingly in in vitro systems to reduce the numbers of animals involved) to detect their pharmacokinetics, pharmacodynamics and toxicity, including teratogenicity and carcinogenicity. However, animal studies, although essential, do not always predict effects in humans. Drugs that show a likelihood of therapeutic benefit and acceptable toxicity will be subsequently tested in humans. Testing in humans is generally divided into four phases, but the exact duration and size of these studies will be determined by the nature of the drug and its proposed indication for use. For instance, an antihypertensive that will be taken for many years needs to be more carefully evaluated in humans and to be less toxic than a cancer chemotherapy drug, which will be used for short periods in patients with a poor prognosis.

Clinical trials are usually considered in four phases:

Phase I. Small studies of the basic clinical pharmacology of a drug involving 50–100 healthy volunteers. These trials will examine pharmacokinetics and pharmacodynamics and will involve the use of various doses. Typically a single low dose, many orders of magnitude lower than a comparable nontoxic dose in animals, is administered first in controlled circumstances. The dose is then increased to give information on tolerability. Multiple doses are then studied, as are other factors such as the effect of food on absorption. Although no estimation of drug effect can properly be made in this group, pharmaceutical companies are increasingly keen to show evidence of potential effect, using *biomarkers*, or *surrogates* for efficacy (e.g. showing an analgesic drug does actually reduce pain by using a model of pain).

Phase II. The early clinical investigations to determine if the drug has the intended therapeutic effect in patients. A group of 50–300 patients will be studied, looking at efficacy and also at pharmacokinetics, pharmacodynamics and adverse effects using various doses. This may be the first indication that the drug is efficacious (or not) in its intended indication.

Phase III. If the early trials show promise, advanced clinical investigations will follow. These will involve 300–5000 patients with the relevant condition and will look at efficacy and adverse effects. They may compare the new drug with existing treatments. Study of special patient groups, e.g. elderly, patients with renal disease, etc., will also be undertaken.

Licence application. If all of these studies show that the drug is effective and relatively safe compared with existing therapies, the company may apply for a licence to market the drug. The evidence will be considered by the licensing authority and if considered satisfactory, a licence, or marketing authorization, will be granted. The drug may then be marketed for specific indications, but testing does not end here.

Phase IV. The average number of humans studied before a new drug is marketed is approximately 3000; it is clear that common adverse effects will, therefore, have been identified at this stage, but rarer effects, for instance with an incidence of 1 in 10 000, may not. After marketing, the number of patients who use the drug will rise rapidly, and previously undetected adverse effects may appear. These may be very significant and lead to the withdrawal of the drug from the market. It is imperative, therefore, that trials continue after marketing: these test the drug as it is used in the real world but focus more on adverse effects (*post-marketing surveillance*) and less on efficacy. They may involve 2000–10 000 or more patients. Other trials exploring other uses of the drug (license extensions) will also continue.

Design of clinical trials

The design of clinical trials is complex but of great importance, since poorly designed trials delay progress and waste resources. There are many possible designs depending on the drug and the nature of the condition to be treated. Some features are essential.

A clear question to be answered should be established in advance. A trial should be designed to answer a specific hypothesis. For example, the question 'What happens if we give drug X to hypertensives?' is too vague, with no clear focus of what is being sought – how will you know when you find it? The question 'Drug X will not lower blood pressure by 5 mmHg in hypertensive patients' is clear-cut. A hypothesis is usually stated as a negative ('the null hypothesis') and then the trial is designed to disprove the hypothesis. This double negative may seem perverse but it makes the trial much more rigorous than a positive hypothesis. Most trials can really only answer the one question for which they were designed ('hypothesis testing'): too often, trials are badly designed with multiple ill-defined endpoints and end up with no useful information or, even worse, misleading information. Sometimes people try to extract answers other than to the original question from trials. This is unreliable, since a trial will rarely provide a definitive answer to any other question; however, it may raise questions that can be answered in further trials ('hypothesis generation').

Comparison with other treatments. Where there is an effective treatment already in existence for the condition in question, it is inadequate simply to compare the new drug with placebo: rather it should be compared with the best current treatment.

The subjects of the trial. These should be appropriate. For example, if the drug for heart failure is to be used mainly in elderly patients, then it should be tested in such patients and not in younger patients. The trial should also include enough subjects to allow the question posed to be answered.

The duration of the trial. The trial should be of an appropriate duration. For example, for antibiotics a few days may be appropriate, but for an antihypertensive, trials should be measured in months or years.

The trial should be analysed statistically. The statistical analysis of the trial is of vital importance and should be clearly established *before* the trial is performed. This needs to address questions such as the size of the trial (is it large enough?). How will the results be analysed? In any treatment with any drug, some patients will do well and some will do badly. If you conduct a trial, you could get an unfavourable result by chance. Think about tossing a coin: imagine that heads is a good outcome and tails a bad outcome. You would expect to get an equal number of heads and tails (unless the coin is biased). Now toss a coin 10 times – how many heads and how many tails? By chance you may have hit a streak of heads or of tails. Similarly, in a trial, an unfavourable or favourable result might have arisen by chance. How do you know whether your result is correct or not? One way is to increase the size of your trial (the more times you toss the coin, the closer the ratio of heads to tails becomes). In clinical trials this is expensive and may expose more patients to adverse events. So we test the probability of a trial to give us accurate results, and report the results as statistically significant or not. Statistically significant by convention means that the result we got was only likely to occur by chance 1 time in 20 (also known as the 5% significance level). You may have hit on the 1 in 20 chance of course, but we have to draw a line somewhere. The results of a trial analysed in this way are therefore *probably* accurate – there is little absolute certainty in medicine. Finally, we need to distinguish statistical significance from clinical significance: a statistically significant result could be so small that it may mean nothing in terms of benefit to patients.

The ethics of the trial should be considered. Trials should be designed so as to minimise any possible harm to the patients (or healthy volunteers) who participate. The patients should be made fully aware that they are participating in a trial and consent to this. To protect both patients and themselves, investigators should have the protocol considered by an expert ethical review committee. However, trials that are poorly designed are also unethical even if they are unlikely to harm patients – poor science is a waste of time and resources, and of patients' goodwill. In any trial there are risks (of adverse effects) and benefits (that a potential treatment will be found effective, or ineffective and so we do not need to waste any more time or money on it). A poorly designed study that cannot provide the benefits of answering these key questions exposes the patients to the hazards of a new treatment for no good reason: the balance of risks and benefits is firmly against the study.

Twenty-two

Clinical sketch

A doctor is asked by a pharmaceutical company to enter the next five depressed patients he sees into a clinical trial in which they will be given a newly licensed drug. There is a payment for each patient he enters. The doctor agrees.

Comment: this sounds like a 'seeding' study, an attempt to get the doctor used to prescribing the new drug so that he will continue it later. The payment per patient could be interpreted as an out and out bribe. A non-comparative study of this kind sounds scientifically useless. The doctor needs to be clear on the aims and design of the study and its ethical approval. He also needs to inform patients they are taking part in a clinical trial and obtain their consent.

Clinical sketch

A pharmaceutical company wants to develop a new drug for the treatment of depression. They have designed the first ever study in humans administering a single low dose of the drug to healthy volunteers. The volunteers are going to be paid £600 for taking part, but the research ethics committee thinks the amount of money proposed is too much and ask for the payment to be reduced to £450.

Comment: it is unethical for potential study subjects to be offered payments that may be coercive, i.e. offering an amount that is difficult to refuse. Typically healthy volunteers are offered payment for their participation in a study that reflects the amount of time and inconvenience involved. In no way is risk accounted for in this payment. Patients with a disease may (or may not) derive some therapeutic benefit from the participation and hence are usually not paid, other than having their expenses refunded. Furthermore, patients in clinical trials often have closer medical monitoring and supervision than they would otherwise enjoy.

Placebo

Investigators must consider the placebo effect whereby patients may seem to improve when given any treatment, effective or not. Trials are often placebo controlled, i.e. patients are divided at random into two groups, of whom half are given a placebo and half the active drug; the difference in response between the two groups gives a measure of the effectiveness of the drug. If there is an effective treatment already available for a disease, then a placebo-controlled trial may be unethical: the comparison should be the standard treatment. Alternatively, if the new treatment is an add-on to existing treatment rather than a replacement for it, the patients in both arms could receive the standard treatment and then, in addition, half new drug, half placebo.

Blinding

Often trials are conducted in a double-blind fashion whereby neither the patients nor the investigator seeing the patients and measuring the effects of the drug know which patients are taking which drug or placebo; this reduces the possibility of bias on the part of either the patient or the investigator. Blinding is not always possible, depending on the circumstances, but if not included in the trial protocol, the reasons why not should be carefully justified.

Randomisation

One problem in trials is ensuring that the patients receiving the trial drug and the comparator are similar, so that any difference between the treatments can be confidently attributed to the treatments and not to the selection of patients. For example, if all the smokers or all the women went into the placebo arm of a trial of a new drug for airways obstruction, would that bias the results? Quite probably, but there are other areas where the bias might not be so apparent or even where we just do not know what other factors might influence the outcomes. To get around this we randomly select patients into the different arms of the trial. In this way, we hope that any unknown factors that might bias the results will appear in equal numbers in both arms of the trial and will cancel each other out, leaving us able to attribute any difference in outcome to the treatments studied.

Size of trial

A common design fault is to include too few subjects in a trial. This may cause an indeterminate result when the trial is analysed statistically – a waste of effort. Conversely, a trial should not include so many subjects that it is impossible to complete nor should it expose an excessive number of patients to unknown risks. A statistician should be consulted to calculate the optimum size for a trial likely to give a definite result in favour of or against new therapy.

Drug licensing

Drugs are licensed for sale according to the evidence presented to the licensing authority. In the UK, the licensing authority is the Secretary of State for Health, guided by the Medicines and Healthcare Products Regulatory Agency (MHRA, formerly the Medicines Control Agency and Medical Devices Agency) and one of its committees, the Commission on Human Medicines (CHM). The MHRA also has a role in regulating clinical trials in the United Kingdom, issuing clinical trials authorisations that must be obtained (alongside ethical approval) before any trial with an investigational medicinal product (IMP) commences. Increasingly, drug licensing takes place at a European level where the agencies are the European Medicines Evaluation Agency (EMEA). The Food and Drug Administration (FDA) has a similar role in the USA. Factors considered in the licensing process are the quality of the drug (is it well and safely manufactured?), its efficacy (does it work in the condition for which the licence is sought?) and its relative safety (is it as safe as the existing therapy or, if not, does its greater efficacy justify its greater toxicity?). Note that the efficacy of the drug relative to existing drugs is not generally considered, only its relative toxicity.

The CHM is also responsible for monitoring reports of adverse drug reactions and reviewing new knowledge that may allow an extension or a reduction in the terms of the licence of a drug, or even its withdrawal.

Drug licensing is mainly concerned with drug safety: many countries now have separate agencies that advise not only whether a drug may be prescribed but also whether it should be prescribed from the point of view of its effectiveness or value for money. In the UK this agency is the National Institute for Health and Clinical Excellence (NICE).

22.3 Prescribing new drugs

Learning objectives

At the end of this section you should be able to:
- explain the principles of being a good prescriber
- list sources of information for updating knowledge in therapeutics.

The true role of any new drug in therapeutics and its adverse effects is often unclear at first and may only become apparent with time. Comparative data with existing drugs are often inadequate. Very few new drugs are true innovative advances, and the majority are minor variations on existing drugs ('me too' drugs). In general, doctors should prescribe new drugs only when they are sure that the new drug is an improvement on existing therapy, in terms of efficacy, safety or cost, and never simply because they are new. New drugs should be prescribed with particular caution (see Ch. 21) and any adverse effect reported to the CHM.

Where do doctors get their information about new drugs?

Many of the most commonly used drugs today were not available at the time that many doctors were medical students. Doctors must, therefore, keep up to date with pharmacology and therapeutics, since existing knowledge may rapidly become obsolete. The most common source of information about new drugs for doctors may be the pharmaceutical companies and their representatives; however, doctors must be aware that companies aim to sell their products and that the information they supply may, therefore, be biased. Doctors should be capable of critically reviewing the evidence presented and should use independent evaluations of new drugs, such as those in the *Drugs and Therapeutics Bulletin* or in peer-reviewed journals. There are several other sources of information about drugs in general and not just new drugs.

The British National Formulary **(BNF)** is updated every 6 months and distributed free to doctors in the UK. It lists drugs by their therapeutic uses and provides information on indications for the drugs, formulations and doses, and adverse effects. It also has useful sections on prescribing in general, prescription writing, drugs in the elderly and in children, and in renal and liver disease, as well as drug interactions. It is a most valuable resource and prescribing doctors should always carry one and refer to it regularly.

Drug information services are pharmacist operated and sited in regional health authorities. They are available for consultation by letter or telephone (telephone numbers are in the BNF). Many produce local drug information bulletins.

A 'summary of product characteristics' or drug data sheet is produced by the pharmaceutical company and approved by the regulatory authorities. Other material may be more promotional than informational.

Clinical sketch

A drug company representative comes to see a GP and tells him of the highly effective new antidepressant produced by his company. This drug is claimed to be effective in 95% of patients and to have no significant adverse effects. This is supported by a large amount of literature, which the drug representative gives the doctor. The doctor is impressed and prescribes the drug to the next depressed patient who consults.

Comment: doctors should not depend on drug company promotional activities as their only source of information about new drugs but should seek out independent sources as well. These will often take a rather more jaundiced view of the company's product. Experience with other antidepressants tells us that no drug is effective in such a high percentage of patients: it would take very strong evidence to convince doctors that the new drug will be substantially different in this area. Such a high percentage response rate may be a consequence of careful patient selection before entry to the trial or a placebo effect, and it is unlikely to be reflected in clinical practice. Similarly, adverse drug reactions are often not well identified in clinical trials and new drug monographs often report few adverse drug reactions in comparison to those for older drugs. With experience, more adverse effects will appear! Doctors should, therefore, be extremely cautious in prescribing new drugs and report all adverse drug reactions. Do not think that such promotional activities of companies will not affect you!

Twenty-two

Marketing

Drug companies survive by selling their product and must make a profit both to fund further research on new products and to remain in business. Companies, therefore, spend large amounts – hundreds of millions of pounds a year in the UK – promoting their products to doctors, but the enthusiasm of a company for its products sometimes exceeds the critical opinion of an independent reviewer. Doctors should, therefore, exercise particular care in considering promotional material and always seek independent evidence.

Prescribing

Prescribing may be defined as the practical everyday use of drugs. It is, therefore, based on the clinical pharmacology of a drug but also includes factors such as the diagnosis, the patient's previous medical history, as well as other sociological and medical factors. Doctors often prescribe for reasons other than the pharmacological effects of the drug, although this might be deplored. Other reasons include the placebo effect, meeting patient demand, maintaining the vital relationship with the patient or even terminating the consultation. Prescribing for these reasons may be wasteful and harmful to the patient.

Good prescribing is therefore:

- appropriate (is a drug needed at all?)
- effective and safe (given the diagnosis and consideration of patient factors, which drug is best and in what dosage?)
- cost-effective (takes due account of the costs of drugs: where efficacy and safety are equal then the least expensive drug is the most appropriate; however, more expensive drugs may be justified for a better effect or because they are safer); doctors should bear in mind that money spent unnecessarily on inappropriate or unnecessary drugs is wasted and deprives other patients of essential care.

Doctors must consider all prescribing as an experiment, in which the outcome may be beneficial or harmful to the patient. In each case, the risks and benefits must be weighed and a drug administered only if the expected benefits outweigh the risks. This constitutes the risk–benefit analysis undertaken before every single prescription. Sometimes this is clear-cut; frequently it is less so.

How to be a good prescriber

- Stay up to date with information from independent sources.
- No one can know all about the 5000 preparations in the BNF. Use a limited range of drugs with which you are familiar. Most doctors do 70–80% of their prescribing from a personal formulary of about 50 drugs. Drugs should be added to or subtracted from this only after careful consideration and review of evidence. Most hospitals have written formularies for their staff to use, and increasingly GPs are developing their own formularies as a useful way to rationalise drug therapy.
- Prescriptions should be written with the generic name of the drug and not its proprietary name where possible.
- Prescribing for individual patients should be reviewed regularly, and unnecessary drugs stopped; communication between doctors in hospitals and in general practice is particularly important.
- If in any doubt about dose or any other details of a drug, look it up in the BNF or other appropriate resource; be especially careful when prescribing new or unfamiliar drugs.
- Individualise prescriptions, do not prescribe in a routine manner: consider the patient, the disease, the choice of drug and formulation, the dose, other possible interacting diseases or drugs (including drugs that a patient might buy themselves over the counter without prescription). Consider also patient convenience, and keep drug therapy as simple as possible to minimise interactions and adverse effects.
- Educate the patient. Drugs may not be the most appropriate way of managing a problem. The patient should know what they have been prescribed and why, how they are to use the medication, and for how long, and what the possible adverse effects are.

In long-term treatment, patients on average take only about 60–70% of prescribed drugs: this is particularly so when patients are unsure of points mentioned above, or when the drug regimen is complex. Both of these may represent failure on the part of the doctor. We must help our patients to make best use of their medicines in any way we can.

Self-assessment on Chapter 22: questions

Multiple choice questions

1. The following statements are correct:
   a. Phase I trials involve large numbers of patients
   b. Phase IV trials are completed before a drug is marketed
   c. Drug licensing considers efficacy, safety and cost
   d. New drugs are superior to older drugs and so should be widely prescribed
   e. New drugs may be designed for effect at specific receptors

2. Clinical trials:
   a. That are double blind means that neither the doctor nor the patient know what drug the patient is taking at a particular time
   b. That are placebo controlled are appropriate to show that a new drug is more effective than existing therapy
   c. Should be reviewed by an ethics committee before being undertaken
   d. Results that come from several small but similar trials are inevitably more reliable than the results of a single large trial
   e. That are analysed statistically can prove that a new drug is effective

3. The following statements are correct:
   a. The BNF contains up-to-date information about drugs, doses and formulations
   b. 'Me too' drugs generally have little major advantage over existing drugs
   c. Comparative data on efficacy between new and existing drugs are essential before a new drug gets a licence
   d. All prescribing is an experiment
   e. Drugs should be prescribed by brand name

4. A good prescriber:
   a. Stays up to date
   b. Usually prescribes new drugs
   c. Uses a wide range of drugs to treat all conditions
   d. Never looks anything up
   e. Communicates well with colleagues and patients

Case history questions

A drug manufacturer wishes to study a new antihypertensive drug and compare its efficacy with an existing drug. It decides to conduct the study in primary care and seeks to recruit GPs to help.

1. What will the GP need to know about the drug before agreeing to take part?
2. What will the GP need to know about the kind of patient required?
3. What reassurances would a GP need that the study was scientifically sound?

Short note question

Compare and contrast the criteria for drug licensing with those for good prescribing.

Extended matching items questions

Theme: Clinical trials and licensing

Options
A. Phase 1
B. Phase 2
C. Phase 3
D. Phase 4
E. Medicines and Healthcare Products Regulatory Agency (MHRA)
F. European Medicines Evaluation Agency (EMEA)
G. Food and Drug Administration (FDA)
H. National Institute for Health and Clinical Excellence (NICE)
I. Commission on Human Medicines (CHM)

For each of the questions below, select the most appropriate options from the list above. Each option may be used once, more than once, or not at all.

Questions

1. The regulatory authority with responsibility for licensing and monitoring of drugs in the USA.

2. The UK agency that examines the safety of new therapies.

3. The UK agency that examines the cost-effectiveness of new therapies.

4. Clinical trials using healthy volunteers designed to study pharmacokinetics and tolerability.

5. Pre-marketing clinical trials designed to study efficacy in large number of patients.

Self-assessment on Chapter 22: answers

Multiple choice answers

1. a. **False.** Usually involve healthy volunteers or small numbers of patients if the drug is considered too toxic to give to healthy volunteers, e.g. anticancer agents.

   b. **False.** These are post-marketing surveillance studies.

   c. **False.** Cost may not be considered by law. Cost may need to be considered by other agencies such as NICE but is not part of the licensing process.

   d. **False.** Despite what drug company advertising might have you believe.

   e. **True.** For example, sumatriptan as a serotonin analogue.

2. a. **True.** Though it should be possible to break a code to find out what the patient is taking in case of emergency. This is code-breaking and is quite rarely necessary.

   b. **False.** The comparison should be against the best existing therapy (although this is often not the case in advertising).

   c. **True.** To protect both the patient and the investigator. Additionally, clinical trials must be approved and authorised by the regulatory authority – in the UK, the MHRA.

   d. **False.** Many trials are too small to show a genuine significant clinical effect: a single trial of adequate size is generally superior.

   e. **False.** Statistics can only give a probability, never certainty, especially at commonly used levels of significance such as $P < 0.05$. Statistical significance is also not the same as clinical significance.

3. a. **True.** The best available source and should be carried by all prescribing doctors.

   b. **True.** Again, a drug company may not like to admit this and will go to great lengths to demonstrate a minor or supposed advantage as a selling point.

   c. **False.**

   d. **True.** An important attitude for safe prescribing.

   e. **False.** There are, however, exceptions such as some fixed drug combinations or slow-release preparations.

4. a. **True.** Using reliable independent sources.

   b. **False.** A good prescriber will use new drugs where appropriate, i.e. where there is evidence of a clear therapeutic or other advantage.

   c. **False.** In general, good prescribers will work from a formulary of drugs (written or not) with which they are familiar.

   d. **False.** This attitude is arrogant. Doctors should always make suitable checks to ensure they are correct in what they do.

   e. **True.** An essential component.

Case history answers

1. The GP would need to know the likely adverse effects of the drug, their likely frequency compared with existing therapies and what evidence there was, to date, in small studies of the drug.

2. The GP would need to know exactly what the entry criteria are, since it may be that the practice will, in fact, have few patients who meet the entry criteria, or who fall out because the exclusion criteria are so strict. In general, there always seem to be lots of suitable patients – until you go to look for them!

3. The GP would need to be reassured that the study has been approved by an ethics committee which takes account not only of the likelihood of patient harm, and this harm is outweighed by the likelihood of patient benefit, but also that the study is scientifically sound and will add useful information to medical knowledge. The key factors the ethics committee will have to consider are the design of the study, randomisation, duration, entry and exclusion criteria, suitability of comparator, size and analysis of the trial. These factors are complex and probably beyond the ability of the average doctor to interpret. It is important, therefore, that the doctor ensure that such matters have been

considered by an ethical review board, such as an ethics committee.

Short note answer

Drugs are licensed on the basis of their efficacy, their safety and their quality of manufacturer. Good prescribing must be effective: this is not quite the same as efficacy, which may be based on a surrogate marker, e.g. lowering blood pressure rather than preventing strokes. Effectiveness is also a measure of what the drug will actually do in the real world rather than in the idealised circumstances of the clinical trial. The trial regimen may be such that it is impossible to apply in practice.

Safety. The doctor must select the patients carefully. It is unlikely he or she would be able to select in exactly the same way as using the clinical trial and, therefore, the risks and benefits of the drug may vary. Also for a new drug the doctor may prefer to wait until there is more experience available.

Appropriate. A key question for a doctor is, is the drug better than the one already being used? If not, the doctor should carry on with the current prescrip-

tion and reserve a new drug for very occasional use or not use it at all. Prescribing should be cost-effective. If a drug is no better than existing therapy and if it is more expensive than existing therapy then it should not be used.

Extended matching items answers

1. G. The USA is one of the most important markets for drug companies and their products.
2. I (or E). The Commission on Human Medicines used to be the Committee on Safety of Medicines (CSM) and reports to the MHRA on matters of drug safety.
3. H. NICE will look at all the evidence and advise doctors on what to prescribe.
4. A. Usually only relatively small numbers of subjects.
5. C. Thousands of subjects, probably comparing the new drug with placebo, or more likely, standard therapy.

Index

A

Abdominal sepsis 195
Absence seizures (petit mal) 87
    treatment 90
Absorption 3
    disease-related changes 273
    drug interactions 286
    in elderly people 267
    factors affecting rate/degree 4
        blood flow 4, 273
    pregnancy-related changes 264
    through skin 233
Acamprosate 253
Acenocoumarol 74
Acetaminophen *see* Paracetamol
Acetazolamide 57
Acetylator status 200
    genetic polymorphisms 6
Acetylcholine 149
    Alzheimer's disease
        pathophysiology 97
    antagonists (non-depolarising
        muscle relaxants) 119–120
    neuromuscular transmission 119
    neurotransmission 22
    termination of action 22
Acetylcholine receptors
    muscarinic 11, 23, 154
    nicotinic 23, 119
Acetylcholinesterase 22, 119
Acetylcholinesterase inhibitors 97
    organophosphates 245
N-Acetylcysteine 244
Acetylsalicylic acid *see* Aspirin
Aciclovir 213, 214, 233
Acidic drugs
    albumin binding 5
    pharmacokinetics in pregnancy
        264
Acne 235
Acquired immune deficiency
    syndrome *see* Human

immunodeficiency syndrome
    (HIV)/AIDS
Acromegaly 179
Activated charcoal 243, 245
Activated partial thromboplastin
    time (APTT) 73
Addiction 251
    see also Substance abuse/
        dependency
Addisonian crisis 171, 174
Addison's disease 172
Adenosine 60
Adrenal medulla 21
Adrenaline (epinephrine)
    adrenal medulla secretion 21
    intravenous actions 26
    lidocaine formulations 26, 116
    therapeutic uses 26
        anaphylaxis/angioedema 142
Adrenergic receptors 23
    agonists (sympathomimetics)
        25–26
    see also α-adrenoceptors;
        β-adrenoceptors
Adrenocortical insufficiency 172
Adrenocorticotrophic hormone
    (ACTH; corticotropin) 97, 171
Adsorbents (antidiarrhoeal agents)
    156
Adult respiratory distress syndrome
    140
Adverse drug reactions 13, 283–285
    aciclovir 214
    adenosine 60
    alkylating agents 224
    allopurinol 130
    aminoglycosides 197
    aminophylline 138
    aminosalicylates 156
    amiodarone 60
    amoxicillin 195, 196, 235
    amphotericin 213
    ampicillin 195, 196, 235

angiotensin converting enzyme
    (ACE) inhibitors 38–39
antibiotics 155
anticholinergics 24, 154
anticholinesterases 120
antihypertensive agents 283
antimalarials 235, 285
antiplatelet agents 74, 75
aspirin 74, 266
autoimmune (type II) reactions
    142
azathioprine 129
bendroflumethiazide 36
benzodiazepines 86
β$_2$-adrenoceptor agonists 137
beta blockers 38
bismuth, chelated 153
bisphosphonates 180
bleomycin 226
blood dyscrasias 142
calcium channel blockers 39
carbamazepine 88, 236, 283
carbenoxolone 153
carbimazole 170, 284
cephalosporins 196
    in children 266, 285
ciclosporin 129
cimetidine 152, 267
classification 283–284
clindamycin 197
co-cyprindiol 235
colchicine 129
Commission on Human
    Medicines (CHM) monitoring
    297
contact dermatitis 142
corticosteroids 172–174
    glucocorticoids 173–174, 234,
        266
    mineralocorticoids 174
cyclo-oxygenase COX-2 inhibitors
    126
cyclophosphamide 224

cytotoxic drugs 76
danazol 176
dapsone 201
definition 283
delayed (type IV) hypersensitivity reactions 142
desmopressin 179
didanosine 215
digoxin 58, 267
disopyramide 24, 59
dopaminergic drugs 95, 96
doxorubicin 226
in elderly people 267–268, 285
epoietin 77
ergocalciferol 179
ethambutol 201
ethosuximide 90
ferrous sulphate 76
flecainide 60
fluconazole 236
flucytosine 213
foscarnet 216
fusidic acid 199
gabapentin 90
ganciclovir 216
general anaesthetic agents
    inhaled 119
    injected 117
glitazones 169
gold (sodium aurothiomalate) 128, 235
griseofulvin 212
heparin 73
high risk patient groups 285
hormone replacement therapy 177
hydralazine 142
identification 284
imidazoles 213
immediate (type I) hypersensitivity reactions 141
immune-complex (type III) hypersensitivity reactions 142
indometacin 127
insulin 167–168, 283
interferons 214
isoniazid 142, 201
isotretinoin 235
lamivudine 215
lamotrigine 89
levetiracetam 90
levodopa 95, 284
levothyroxine 171
lidocaine 59
lithium 92
local anaesthetic agents 117

loop diuretics 56–57
macrolides 197
mefloquine 217
metformin 168
methotrexate 128, 225
methyldopa 76, 142
methysergide 97
metoclopramide 154
metronidazole 199
minoxidil 41
misoprostol 153
muscle relaxants 120
neuroleptics 24, 93, 95
    atypical 94
nevirapine 216
new drugs 297
    clinical trials 294
nitrates 54
nitrofurantoin 199
non-steroidal anti-inflammatory drugs (NSAIDs) 76, 110, 127, 151
oestrogens 285
ondansetron 154
opiates 109, 155, 228
oral contraceptives, oestrogen-progesterone combinations 175
penicillamine 128
penicillin 76, 142, 195, 235, 284
pentamidine 217
phenothiazines 154
phenytoin 90
potassium-sparing diuretics 37, 57
prevention 285
progestogens 176
protease inhibitors 216
proton pump inhibitors 153
pyrazinamide 201
quinidine 24
quinolones 198
ranitidine 152
reporting 284, 297
ribavirin 215
rifampicin 201
selective serotonin reuptake inhibitors 91, 284
serum sickness 142
skin manifestations 235–236
sodium valproate 89
statins 42–43
sulfasalazine 128
sulphonamides 142, 198, 285
sulphonylureas 168
sumatriptan 97

suxamethonium (succinylcholine) 120
systemic-lupus-erythematosus-like reactions 142
tamoxifen 177, 226
teicoplanin 200
teratogenesis see Teratogenesis
tetracyclines 199
    in fetus 264
theophylline 266
thrombolytic drugs 75
topimarate 90
trastuzumab 227
tricyclic antidepressants 24, 92, 155
trimethoprim 198
type A (augmented effects) 283
type B (idiosyncratic reactions) 277, 284
type C 284
type D 284
type E (withdrawal reactions) 284
type F (unexpected failure) 284
uricosuric agents 130
vancomycin 200
vigabatrin 90
vincristine 225
warfarin 73
zalcitabine 215
zidovudine 215
Agonists 12
    endogenous 14
    full 12
    individual variation in response 14
    partial 12
Agranulocytosis, drug-induced 142
    carbimazole 170, 284
Airway protection, poisoning 241–242, 243
Akathisia 93
Albumin
    acidic drug binding 5
    age-related changes 267
    disease-related changes 274
    pregnancy-related changes 264
Alcohol
    abuse 251, 252–253
        osteoporosis risk 180
        treatment 253
    clinical pharmacokinetics 252
    drug interactions 86, 92, 109, 252, 285
    physical effects 252
    psychological effects 252

teratogenesis 264
tolerance 251
withdrawal 253
Aldosterone 37, 54, 57, 171, 172
Alemtuzumab 227
Alendronate 180
Alkaline diuresis 243
Alkylating agents 224
Allergic reactions
cephalosporins 196
penicillins 195–196
Allopurinol 11, 129–130
α_1-acid glycoprotein
basic drug binding 5
disease-related changes 274
pregnancy-related changes 264
α-adrenoceptors 23
1α-hydroxycholecalciferol 179
Alpha blockers 39, 40
hypertension 40
Alteplase 75
Aluminium hydroxide 152
Alzheimer's disease 97
Amantadine 213, 214
antiparkinsonian activity 96
Amfetamines 254
Amikacin 196
Amiloride 37, 57
Amine hypothesis 91
Aminoglycosides 192, 193, 196–197
adverse effects 197
bacterial resistance 196
clinical pharmacokinetics 196
contraindication in pregnancy
264
drug interactions 120, 128, 286
excretion 7, 275
monitoring 197
topical use 197
Aminophylline 138
overdose/poisoning 243
Aminosalicylates 156
5-Aminosalicylic acid (5-ASA) 128,
156
Amiodarone 58, 60, 61
Amitriptyline 91, 92, 227
Amlodipine 39
Amoebiasis 216
Amoxicillin 151, 194
adverse effects 195, 196, 235
clavulanic acid combination (co-
amoxiclav) 194
drug interactions 286
Amphotericin 193, 213
Ampicillin 194, 195, 196, 235, 264
Anaemia 76–77

Anaesthesia 115–120
general 117–119
local 115–117
pain prevention 115
Analgesics 107–110
compound 110
inhaled anaesthetic agents 118
migraine 96–97
non-steroidal anti-inflammatory
drugs (NSAIDs) 110
opiate 108–110
palliative care 227
paracetamol (acetaminophen)
110
Anandamide 254
Anaphylaxis 26, 141–142, 284
management 142
Anastrozole 177–178
Androgens 178–179
Angina pectoris 37, 38, 51–52, 74
hypertensive patients 41
unstable 52, 53
Angioedema 141–142
Angiotensin converting enzyme
(ACE) inhibitors 11, 38–39, 293
adverse effects 38–39
combined treatments 40
contraindications 39
drug interactions 37, 39, 57
teratogenesis 264
therapeutic uses 38
cardiac failure 55, 56, 57
hypertension 40, 41
myocardial infarction 53
Angiotensin II 11, 38, 54
Angiotensin II receptor blockers 39,
57
combined treatments 40
Anorexia, palliative care 228
Antacids 12, 152
Antagonists 12–13
individual variation in response
14
Antiandrogens 178–179
Antianginal drugs 53–54
Antiarrhythmic agents
class I 59–60
class II 60
class III 60
class IV 60
Vaughan Williams classification
59
Antibiotics 191–201
actions 191
adverse effects 155
antimicrobial resistance 193–194

bactericidal/bacteriostatic 191
in breastfeeding mothers 265
combinations 192
contraindications 264
cytotoxic 226
drug interactions 174
empirical therapy 192
first line therapy 195
Helicobacter pylori eradication 150,
151
microbial sensitivity testing
192
monitoring 192
mycobacterial infections 200–
201
in pregnant patients 264
prescribing principles 192–193
prophylactic 192–193
sites of action 193
topical 233
Anticholinergic drugs 24
adverse effects 24, 154
antiemetics 154
antimuscarinic 24–25, 120, 228
antinicotinic 24
antispasmodic actions 156
asthma 137–138
chronic obstructive pulmonary
disease 137–138
parkinsonism 96
Anticholinesterases 24, 120
Anticoagulant therapy 71–74
contraindications 72
indications 71
with liver disease 276
oral 73–74
Anticonvulsants 87–88
in breastfeeding mothers 265
drug interactions 74, 197, 201,
285, 286
neuropathic pain relief 227
teratogenicity 264
Antidepressants 91–92
Antidiuretic hormone (vasopressin)
179
Antidiuretic hormone analogues
179
Antidotes 243
Antiemetics 154
palliative care 228
Antifibrinolytic drugs 75–76
Antifungal drugs 211–213
topical 233
Antihistamines 234
anaphylaxis/angioedema
management 142

antiemetic actions 154, 155
cough suppression 140
drug interactions 86
seasonal rhinitis 141
Antihyperlipidaemic agents 42–43,
53
Antihypertensive agents 35–40
adverse effects 283
in breastfeeding mothers 265
drug combinations (ABCD rule)
40
in elderly people 268
in pregnancy 265
selection 40–41
treatment monitoring 41
Anti-inflammatory drugs
asthma 136–137
inflammatory bowel disease
156
see also Glucocorticoids; Non-
steroidal anti-inflammatory
drugs (NSAIDs)
Antimalarials
adverse effects 235, 285
rheumatoid arthritis 128
Antimetabolites 224–225
toxicity 224
Antimotility drugs 156
Antimuscarinic drugs 24–25,
120
palliative care 228
Antiplatelet agents 74–75
with liver disease 276
therapeutic uses 74
non-ST segment elevation
myocardial infarction 53
unstable angina 53
Antiprotozoal drugs 216–217
Antipyretic agents 126
Antispasmodics 156
Antithyroid drugs
in breastfeeding mothers 265
fetal effects 264
Antiviral drugs 213–216
modes of action 213
topical 233
Anxiety 85–86
Apparent volume of distribution
9–10
Aprepitant 154
Aqueous cream 233
Arachidonic acid metabolism 126,
171
Area under the curve (AUC) 8
Arginine vasopressin 179
Arrhythmias *see* Cardiac arrhythmias

Arthritis 125–130
causes 125
Aspergillosis 212
Aspirin (acetylsalicylic acid) 9, 74,
126
adverse effects 74
in children 266
antiplatelet activity 74
in breastfeeding mothers 265
drug interactions 74, 127
overdose/poisoning 7, 244
therapeutic uses 126
analgesia 110
angina pectoris prophylaxis
52
myocardial infarction 53
Asthma 26, 135, 136–139, 140, 141
acute severe attack 137, 138
management 138
anti-inflammatory drugs 136–137
bronchodilators 137
clinical features 136
in hypertensive patients 40
leukotriene pathway inhibitors
137
life-threatening attack 138
non-steroidal anti-inflammatory
drug-induced 127
pathophysiology 136
respiratory failure 139, 140
Atenolol 7, 38
contraindications 265
Athlete's foot (tinea pedis) 211
Atopy 141, 234
Atorvastatin 42–43
Atovaquone 216
Atracurium 120
Atrial arrhythmias 59, 60
Atrial fibrillation 58, 60, 61, 71
Atrial flutter 60
Atropine 24–25, 120, 245, 256
antiarrhythmic actions 60
Atypical mycobacteria 201
Atypical neuroleptic drugs 94
Autoimmune (Hashimoto's)
thyroiditis 170–171
Autoimmune (type II) reactions
142
Autonomic nervous system 21–27
function 22–23
neurotransmitters 22
receptors 22–23
structure 21–22
Azathioprine 129, 130, 156
rheumatoid disease 129
Azithromycin 197

B

Bacterial antibiotic resistance
193–194
Barbiturates
abuse 254
tolerance 251
withdrawal symptoms 254
Basic drugs
α1-acid glycoprotein binding 5
pharmacokinetics in pregnancy
264
Beclomethasone 136
Bendroflumethiazide 36
Benefits versus risks approach
clinical trial design 295
prescribing 283, 298
Benserazide 95
Benzodiazepine receptors 86
Benzodiazepines 14, 86, 253, 293
abuse/dependence 253–254
adverse effects 86
contraindications 86
in breastfeeding mothers 265
drug interactions 86
in elderly people 268
overdose/poisoning 86, 244
therapeutic uses 86
epilepsy 87
withdrawal syndrome 254
Benzoyl peroxide 235
Benzylpenicillin (penicillin G) 4, 194
bacterial resistance 193
β2-adrenoceptor agonists 13, 293
adverse effects 137
in breastfeeding mothers 265
therapeutic uses 26, 137
asthma 137, 138
β-adrenoceptors 11, 23
antagonists *see* Beta blockers
upregulation following prolonged
beta blocker use 37
β-lactamase 193, 194
Beta blockers 12, 37–38, 276, 293
adverse effects 38
rebound hypertension 14
withdrawal reactions 284
cardiac actions 37
combined treatments 40
contraindications 37, 38
drug interactions 39
therapeutic uses 38, 60, 61
angina pectoris prophylaxis
51, 52
arrhythmias 60, 61
cardiac failure 56, 57

hypertension 40, 41
hyperthyroidism 170
migraine prophylaxis 97
myocardial infarction 53
Betamethasone 234
Bethanecol 24
Bezafibrate 43
Biguanides 168
Bile acids 157
Biliary excretion 7
Bioavailability 4
Biomarkers 294
Biotransformation 6
concentration-dependent 6–7
genetic factors 6
see also Metabolism
Bipolar affective disorder 92
Bisacodyl 155
Bismuth, chelated 153
Helicobacter pylori eradication 150, 151, 153
Bisoprolol 57
Bisphosphonates 180
Bladder cancer 252
Bladder smooth muscle tone 24
Bladder toxicity, cyclophosphamide 224
Bleeding, drug-induced 76
Bleomycin 226
Blinding, clinical trial design 296
Blood
coagulation 71–76
formation 76–77
Blood dyscrasias, drug-induced 142
Blood flow
absorption relationship 4, 273
tissue distribution effects 5
Blood pressure 35
monitoring, hypertension management 41
Blood vessels, sympathetic innervation 21
Bone marrow toxicity
bleomycin 226
cyclophosphamide 224
doxorubicin 226
flucytosine 213
methotrexate 225
pyrimethamine 217
zalcitabine 215
zidovudine 215
Bone metastases, analgesia 110
Bowel disorders 155–156
Brainstem 21
vomiting centre 154

Bran 155
Breast cancer 177, 178, 224, 226, 227
Breastfeeding 8, 265–266
drugs inhibiting lactation 265
British National Formulary (BNF) 297, 298
Bromocriptine 95, 179, 265
Bronchi, sympathetic innervation 21
Bronchitis, chronic 136, 252
Bronchodilators 137
Budesonide 136
Bulking agents 155
Bumetanide 37, 56
Bupivacaine 117
Buprenorphine 109, 255
overdose/poisoning 244
Bupropion (amfebutamone) 252
Buserelin 178
Busulfan 224
Butyrylcholinesterase (pseudocholinesterase) 120

C

Cabergoline 95, 179
Calciferol 179
Calcipotriol 234
Calcitonin 180
Calcium channel blockers 39
adverse effects 39
drug interactions 39
therapeutic uses 39
angina pectoris prophylaxis 51
arrhythmias 60
hypertension 40, 41
Calcium edetate 245
Calcium metabolism 179
Cancer treatment 223
chemotherapy see Chemotherapy
opiate analgesia 109
palliative care 227–228
Candidiasis 211, 212
systemic infection 212
Cannabinoid receptors 254
Cannabis 254
Capreomycin 201
Captopril 38
Carbamazepine 6, 87, 88, 264
adverse effects 88, 236, 283
contraindications 88
drug interactions 88, 89, 90, 174, 284, 286
overdose/poisoning 243
teratogenesis 264
therapeutic uses 88, 110

Carbenoxolone 153
Carbidopa 95
Carbimazole 170
adverse effects 170, 284
in fetus 265
Carbonic acid anhydrase inhibitors 57
Carboplatin 226
Cardiac action potential 59
Cardiac arrest 26
Cardiac arrhythmias 52, 59–61
drug interactions 286
drug treatment 59–61
overdose/poisoning 242, 245
Cardiac failure 40, 54–59
causes 54
drug treatment 55, 56–59
New York Heart Association classification 55
pathophysiology 55
Cardiac toxicity
cyclophosphamide 224
doxorubicin 226
overdose/poisoning 242
trastuzumab 227
Cardiogenic shock 26, 57
Cardiopulmonary resuscitation 26
Cardiovascular disease 51–61
prevention 33–43
risk prediction 34
Cardiovascular risk factors 33–34, 42, 252
diabetes mellitus management 166
Carotid sinus massage 59
Carvedilol 57
Castor oil 155
Catchol-O-methyltransferase 22, 96
Cefalexin 196
Cefotaxime 196
Cefradine 196
Cefuroxime 196
Celecoxib 126
Cellulitis 233
Central nervous system disease 85–97
Cephalosporins 193, 196
adverse effects 196
allergic (immediate hypersensitivity) reactions 141, 196
in breastfeeding mothers 265
drug interactions 128
Cerebrovascular accident 71, 74, 75
oral contraceptives association 176

Cetrizine 141
Chelators 245
Chemoreceptor trigger zone 154
Chemotherapy 223–228
    antiemetics 154
    contraindication in breastfeeding
        mothers 265
    courses of treatment 223
    drugs 172, 224–227
        combinations 223
        interactions 286
        resistance 223
    supportive care 227
Chenodeoxycholic acid 157
Children 266–267
    adverse drug reactions 266, 285
    dosage 266
    drug licensing 266–267
    pharmacodynamics 266
    pharmacokinetics 266
Chlorambucil 224
Chloramphenicol 193, 233
    contraindication in breastfeeding
        mothers 265
Chlordiazepoxide 253
Chloride channels 86
Chloroquine 128, 217
Chlorphenamine 141
Chlorpromazine 93, 228, 264
    in breastfeeding mothers 265
Chlorpropamide 168
Cholesterol 41, 42
    target levels 42
Cholestyramine 286
Cholinergic drugs 23–25
    agonists 24
    antagonists see Anticholinergic
        drugs
Cholinergic receptors see
    Acetylcholine receptors
Chronic pain 91
Ciclosporin 156
    adverse effects 129
    drug interactions 197, 286
    rheumatoid disease 129
Cimetidine 6, 152
    adverse effects 152, 267
    drug interactions 73, 86, 152, 286
Ciprofloxacin 6, 193, 198
    contraindications
        in breastfeeding mothers 265
        in pregnancy 264
    drug interactions 73, 198, 286
Cisapride 286
Cisplatin 226
Citalopram 91

Clarithromycin 151, 197
Clavulanic acid/amoxicillin
    combination (co-amoxiclav) 194
Clearance 8–9
Clindamycin 197
Clinical trials 294–296
    blinding 296
    design 294–295
    duration 295
    ethical issues 295
    optimum size 296
    phase I 294
    phase II 294
    phase III 294
    phase IV 294
    placebo-controlled 296
    randomisation 296
    regulation 296
    statistical analysis 295
Clobetasol 234
Clodronate 180
Clomethiazole 253
Clomifene 178
Clonazepam 86
Clopidogrel 53, 74, 75
Clotrimazole 212, 233
Clozapine 94
Coagulation 71–76
    effects of liver disease 276
Coal tar preparations 234
Co-amoxiclav 194, 196
Cocaine 116, 254–255
Co-codamol 110
Co-cyprindiol 235
Codeine 109, 140, 156, 227
    abuse/dependence 255
Colchicine 11, 129
Colorectal cancer 227
Coma, overdose/poisoning 241–242
Commission on Human Medicines
    (CHM) 284, 296, 297
Conazepam 87
Conjugated equine oestrogens 177
Conjunctival antibiotics 233
Conn's syndrome (primary
    hyperaldosteronism) 37, 57
Consent, clinical trial participants
    295
Constipation 155
    palliative care 228
Contact dermatitis 142
Contraceptive steroids see Oral
    contraceptives
Coronary artery spasm 51, 53
Coronary syndromes, acute 52–53,
    71, 72, 74, 75

Corrosives ingestion 243
Corticosteroids 171–174
    adverse effects 172–174, 234
        osteoporosis 180
    in breastfeeding mothers 265
    in children 266
    physiological role 171–172
    therapeutic uses 172
        anaphylaxis/angioedema 142
        asthma 136, 138
        chronic obstructive pulmonary
            disease 136
        inflammatory bowel disease
            156
        multiple sclerosis 97
        palliative care 228
        rheumatoid disease 125,
            128–129
        seasonal rhinitis 141
    withdrawal of treatment after
        long-term use 174
    see also Glucocorticoids;
        Mineralocorticoids
Corticotropin see
    Adrenocorticotrophic hormone
Co-trimoxazole 72, 198, 217
Cough suppressants 140
    opiates 109
Crohn's disease 156
Cryptococciasis 212
Cushing's syndrome 173
Cyclizine 228
Cyclo-oxygenase COX-1 126
Cyclo-oxygenase COX-2 126
Cyclo-oxygenase COX-2 inhibitors
    126, 127
Cyclophosphamide 224
Cycloserine 201
Cyproterone acetate 179, 235
Cytarabine 213, 225
Cytochrome P450s 6
    genetic polymorphisms 6
    macrolides inhibition 197
    warfarin metabolism 73, 74
Cytomegalovirus infection 216
Cytotoxic drugs 76, 224–227
    antibiotics 226

D

Dalteparin 72
Danazol 176
Dapsone 201
Daunorubicin 226
Decontamination, poisoning
    treatment 242–243

Deep vein thrombosis 71, 175
Delayed (type IV) hypersensitivity reactions 142
Depression 90–92
  amine hypothesis 91
  drug treatment 91–92
Dermatomycoses 211, 212
Descending reticular system 21
Desferrioxamine 245
Desmopressin 179
Desogestrel 174, 175
Dexamethasone 154, 173, 228
Diabetes insipidus 179
Diabetes mellitus 165–169
  acute ketoacidosis 168
  cardiovascular risk 33, 34
  complications 165
  glucocorticoid-induced 173
  hypercholesterolaemia treatment 42
  hypertension treatment 35, 41
  insulin therapy 167–168
  management in pregnancy 265
  oral antihyperglycaemic drugs 168
  type 1 166, 275–276
  type 2 165–166, 276
Diamorphine (heroin) 109
  abuse/dependence 255
Diarrhoea 155–156
  drug absorption influence 273
  opiate treatment 109
Diazepam 5, 7, 86
Diclofenac 129
Didanosine 215
Dietary modification
  constipation 155
  diabetes mellitus 166
  hyperlipidaemia 42
  see also Lifestyle changes
Diethylstilbestrol 264, 284
Digitalis glycosides 57–59
Digitoxin 58
Digoxin 10, 12, 13, 57–59, 264, 293
  adverse effects 58, 267
  contraindications 58
  drug interactions 58, 152, 286
  excretion 7
    reduction with renal impairment 275
  monitoring 58
  in neonates 266
  plasma protein binding 5
  therapeutic uses 58, 60, 61
  toxicity management 58–59

Dihydrofolate reductase inhibitors 11, 198, 224
Dihydropyridines 39
Diltiazem 39, 60
Dimercaprol 245
Dinoprostone 178
Diphenoxylate 156
Dipyridamole 74, 75
Disease-modifying antirheumatic drugs 128–129
Disopyramide 24, 59, 60, 61
Dissociative anaesthesia 117
Distribution 3, 5
  in children 266
  disease-related changes 274
  drug interactions 286
  in elderly people 267
  pregnancy-related changes 264
Disulfiram 253
Dithranol 234
Diuretic-induced hypokalaemia 37, 56, 57
Diuretics 35–36
  cardiac failure management 55, 56
  combined treatments 40
  drug interactions 37, 58, 92, 127–128, 285, 286
  types 35
DNA polymerase inhibitors 213
Dobutamine 26, 57
Domperidone 152, 154
Donepezil 97
Dopamine 22
Dopamine receptors 23, 93, 94, 154
Dopaminergic drugs 95–96
Dosage in children/neonates 266
Dose–response curve 12–13
Doxazosin 40
Doxorubicin 226
Doxycycline 199
Drug data sheets 297
Drug information services 297
Dry-powder inhalers 137
Duodenal ulcers 150
  healing 152
Dysfunctional uterine bleeding 175, 176
Dyskinesia 95
Dysmenorrhoea 175, 176
Dyspepsia 152
  non-steroidal anti-inflammatory drug-induced 127
Dyspnoea, palliative care 228
Dystonia 93

E

EC_{50} 12
Ecstasy (methylenedioxymetamfetamine) 245, 254
Eczema 234
Edrophonium 120
EDTA 245
Efficacy 12
  clinical trials 294
  drug licensing 296
Elderly people 267–268
  adverse drug reactions 267–268, 285
  compliance 268
  diazepam elimination 86
  drug interactions risk 285
  osteoporosis risk 180
  pharmacodynamic alterations 267–268
  pharmacokinetic alterations 267
  polypharmacy 267
  recommendations for prescribing 268
E_{max} 12
Embolus 71
Emergency hormonal contraception 176
Emollients 233, 234
Emphysema 136, 252
Emulsifying ointment 233
Enalapril 6, 38
Endocrine disorders 165–180
Endogenous ligands 276
Endorphins 107
Enflurane 118–119
Enoxaparin 72
Entacapone 96
Enterohepatic circulation 7, 174, 226, 286
Enzyme inhibitors 11
Enzymes 11–12
  transmembrane 11
Ephedrine 26, 27
Epidural anaesthesia 117
Epilepsy 87–90
  definitions 87
  drug treatment 87–88
  management 87
    in pregnancy 264
  seizure types 87
Epinephrine see Adrenaline
Eplerenone 57
Epoietin 77
Eptifibatide 53

Ergocalciferol 179
Ergometrine 178
Ergot derivatives 95
Ergotamine, contraindication in breastfeeding mothers 265
Erysipelas 233
Erythromycin 6, 193, 197, 235
　adverse effects 197
　bacterial resistance 194
　drug interactions 73, 197, 286
Erythropoietin 77
Esomeprazole 152–153
Estradiol 177, 233
Ethambutol 200, 201
Ethical issues 295
Ethinylestradiol 174, 235
Ethosuximide 87, 90
Etidronate 180
Etomidate 118
European Medicines Evaluation Agency (EMEA) 296
Excretion 3, 7–8
　in children 266
　disease-related changes 275
　drug interactions 286
　in elderly people 267
　pregnancy-related changes 264
Exercise-induced angina 51, 52
Exfoliative dermatitis 235
Expectorants 140
Ezetimibe 43

F

Faecal softeners 155, 228
Famciclovir 214
Fast acetylators 6, 200
Febrile convulsions 110, 126
Fenofibrate 43
Fentanyl 109
Ferrous sulphate 76
Fetal development 263–264
　see also Teratogenesis
Fibrates 43
Fight or flight response 21
Filgrastim 77
First pass metabolism 4, 267, 274
Fixed drug eruption 235
Flecainide 60, 61
Flucloxacillin 193, 194
　adverse effects 196
　fusidic acid combination 199
Fluconazole 73, 213, 236
Flucytosine 213
Fludrocortisone 172
Fluid retention, cardiac failure 54

Flumazenil 86, 244
Fluoroquinolones 198
Fluorouracil 224, 225
Fluoxetine 91
Flupentixol 93
Flutamide 178–179
Folic acid deficiency 76–77
Follicle-stimulating hormone 174, 176, 178
Fondaparinux 73
Food and Drug Administration (FDA) 296
Formoterol 137
Foscarnet 216
Fungal infections 211
　superficial 211–212
　systemic 212–213
Furosemide 37, 56, 128
Fusidic acid 199

G

G-protein-linked transmembrane receptors 11
Gabapentin 90, 110, 227
Gallstones 156–157
　bile acid treatment 157
Gamma-aminobutyric acid (GABA) 86, 90, 117
Gamma-hydroxybutyrate 255
Ganciclovir 213, 216
Gastric acid secretion 149–153
　drug actions 150, 152–153
　pathological conditions 150–152
　regulation 149–150
Gastric clearance 152
Gastric lavage 243
Gastric ulcers 150
　healing 152
Gastrin 149
Gastrointestinal system 149–157
　sympathetic innervation 21
Gastro-oesophageal reflux 151–152
Gemeprost 178
Gemfibrozil 43
General anaesthesia 115, 117–119
General anaesthetic agents
　dissociative anaesthesia 117
　induction 117, 118
　inhaled 118–119
　injected 117–118
Generalised seizures 87
　treatment 88, 90
Genetic factors
　adverse drug reaction risk 285
　hypercholesterolaemia 42

polymorphisms 6
　acetylator status 6, 200
　thiopurine S-methyltransferase 129
receptor sensitivity 14
Gentamicin 196, 197, 233
　penicillin combined therapy 192
　plasma protein binding 5
　tissue distribution 5
Gestational diabetes 265
Gestodene 174, 175
Giardia lamblia 216
Glasgow Coma Scale 241
Glaucoma 24, 57
Glibenclamide 168
Gliclazide 7, 168
Glimepiride 168
Glitazones 166, 168–169
Glomerular filtration rate 7
　in elderly people 267
　in neonates 266
Glucagon 168
Glucocorticoid receptors 11
Glucocorticoids 171–172
　adverse effects 173–174, 234
　　in children 266
　in breastfeeding mothers 265
　therapeutic uses 172
　　topical 234, 235
　withdrawal of treatment after long-term use 174
Gluconeogenesis 172
Glucose-6-phosphate dehydrogenase deficiency 285
Glutamate 89, 90
Glyceryl trinitrate 4, 51, 54, 233
Glycoprotein IIb/IIIa receptor inhibitors 53, 74
Glycopyrolate 120
Gold (sodium aurothiomalate) 125, 128, 235
Gonadorelin (gonadotrophin-releasing hormone) 178
Gonadotrophin-releasing hormone analogues 178
Goserelin 178
Gout 125, 126, 129
Grand mal (tonic/clonic seizures) 87
　drug treatment 88, 89, 90
Granulocyte colony stimulating factors 77
Graves' disease 169, 170
Griseofulvin 212
Growth hormone disorders 179

H

Haematological malignancy 227
Haemodialysis, poisoning management 243
Haemoperfusion, poisoning management 243
Haemophilia 127
Half-life 8
Hallucinogens 256
Haloperidol 93, 228
Halothane 118, 119, 120
Haptens 141, 142
Harm reduction approach 109
Hashimoto's (autoimmune) thyroiditis 170–171
Heart
  β₁-adrenoceptors 23
  sympathetic innervation 21
Heavy metal poisoning 245
Helicobacter pylori infection
  eradication regimens 150–151
  peptic ulcers 150
Henderson–Hasselbach equation 4
Heparin 72
  adverse effects 73
  in breastfeeding mothers 265
  monitoring 73
  reversal of effects 73
  therapeutic uses 72–73
Heparinoids 73
Hepatitis A 213
Hepatitis B 213, 214, 251
  chronic hepatitis 214
Hepatitis C 213, 214, 215, 251
  chronic hepatitis 214
Herbal remedies 286
Herpes simplex 214, 233
Herpes zoster 214
Highly active antiretroviral therapy (HAART) 215, 216
Hirudins 73
Histamine 149
  H₁ receptors 154
  H₂ receptors 11, 149
Histamine H₁ receptor antagonists 141, 142, 154
Histamine H₂ receptor antagonists 152
Hodgkin's lymphoma 172, 224
Hormonal anticancer agents 226
Hormone modulating therapy 177–178
  infertility treatment 178
  pregnancy/pregnancy termination 178

Hormone replacement therapy 176–177, 180
Human immunodeficiency syndrome (HIV)/AIDS 213, 215–216, 251
  drug absorption with chronic diarrhoea 273
  highly active antiretroviral therapy (HAART) 215, 216
  management 215
  systemic fungal infections 212
  viral infections 213
Hydralazine 6, 39, 142, 265
  autoimmune (type II) reactions 142
  in breastfeeding mothers 265
Hydrocortisone 171, 234
  adverse effects 173
  therapeutic uses
    acute asthma/chronic obstructive pulmonary disease 136
    inflammatory bowel disease 156
3-Hydroxy-3-methylglutaryl-CoA reductase inhibitors *see* Statins
Hydroxychloroquine 128
Hydroxycobalamin 76
5-Hydroxytryptamine
  amine hypothesis of depression 91
  migraine pathophysiology 96
  organ-specific effects 96
5-Hydroxytryptamine agonists, migraine 97
5-Hydroxytryptamine 5-HT₃ antagonists 154
5-Hydroxytryptamine receptors 11
Hyoscine 154, 155, 228
Hyperaldosteronism, primary (Conn's syndrome) 37, 57
Hypercalcaemia of malignancy 180
Hyperlipidaemia 41–43
  cardiovascular risk 33
  genetic factors 42
  target cholesterol levels 42
  treatment 42–43
Hypersensitivity 140–142
  type I (immediate) 141
  type II (autoimmune) 142
  type III (immune-complex) 142
  type IV (delayed) 142
Hypertension 34–41
  cardiovascular risk 33, 34
  causes 35
  diagnosis 35
  monitoring 41

  oral contraceptives association 176
  in pregnancy 265
  rebound 14
  resistant 41
  treatment 35
    blood pressure targets 35
    coexistent disease 40–41
    drug combinations (ABCD rule) 40
    drugs 35–41
    emergencies 41
    non-pharmacological 35
    tailored care approach 40–41
  type 2 diabetes association 166
Hyperthyroidism 169–170
  in pregnancy 265
Hypertriglyceridaemia 42
Hypnotics 86
  abuse 253–254
Hypoglycaemia 167–168
Hypokalaemia, diuretic-induced 37, 56, 57
Hypomania 90–92
Hypothalamic-pituitary-adrenal axis 171, 174
Hypothalamus 21
Hypothesis generation 295
Hypothesis testing 295
Hypothyroidism 170–171

I

Ibuprofen 110, 126
Idiosyncratic (type B) adverse reactions 277, 284
Idoxuridine 213
Imantinib 226
Imidazoles 212, 213
Immediate (type I) hypersensitivity reactions 141
Immune-complex (type III) hypersensitivity reactions 142
Immunomodulating anticancer drugs 227
Immunosuppressed patients
  protozoal infections 216
  systemic fungal infections 212
Immunosuppressive agents
  drug interactions 285
  glucocorticoids 173
  psoriasis 235
  rheumatoid arthritis 125, 128
Impetigo 233
Indinavir 213, 216
Indometacin 126, 127, 129

Infants 266
Infective endocarditis 192, 193
Infertility 178
Inflammatory bowel disease 156
Inflammatory response 126
Infliximab 129, 156
Influenza virus 213, 214
Information sources 297, 298
Inhaled anaesthesia 118–119
    clinical stages 118
    mode of action 118
Inotropic agents, cardiac failure 55, 56, 57
Insomnia 85–86
Insulin 166
    actions 166
    formulations 167
    regimens 167
    therapy 167–168
        adverse effects 167–168, 283
        in pregnancy 265
        type 1 diabetes mellitus 166
        type 2 diabetes mellitus 166
Insulin aspart 167
Insulin glargine 167
Insulin lispro 167
Insulin receptor 11
Insulin resistance 166, 276
Insulin zinc suspensions 167
Interactions 285–286
    aciclovir 214
    alcohol 86, 92, 109, 252, 285
    allopurinol 130, 286
    aminoglycosides 120, 128, 286
    aminophylline 138
    amiodarone 58
    amitriptyline 92
    amoxicillin 286
    ampicillin 196
    angiotensin converting enzyme (ACE) inhibitors 37, 39, 57
    antacids 152
    antibiotics 174
    anticonvulsants 74, 197, 201, 285, 286
    antihistamines 86
    aspirin (acetylsalicylic acid) 74, 127
    azathioprine 130
    benzodiazepines 86
    beta blockers 39
    calcium channel blockers 39
    carbamazepine 88, 89, 90, 174, 284, 286
    cephalosporins 128
    cholestyramine 286

ciclosporin 197, 286
cimetidine 73, 86, 152, 286
ciprofloxacin 73, 198, 286
cisapride 286
co-trimoxazole 73
cytarabine 225
cytotoxic drugs 286
detection 285
digoxin 58, 152, 286
diuretics 37, 58, 92, 127–128, 285, 286
drugs at risk 286
in elderly people 285
erythromycin 73, 197, 286
fluconazole 73
fluorouracil 225
furosemide 128
immunosuppressive agents 285
isoniazid 201, 286
ketoconazole 286
levodopa 96
levofloxacin 198
lithium 37, 91, 92, 128, 286
with liver disease 285
loop diuretics 37, 57
6-mercaptopurine 130, 225
methotrexate 225
metronidazole 73, 199, 286
monoamine oxidase inhibitors 27, 92, 96
muscle relaxants 120
neuroleptic drugs 94
non-steroidal anti-inflammatory drugs (NSAIDs) 37, 92, 127–128, 285, 286
oestrogens 286
omeprazole 153
opiates 109, 286
oral antihyperglycaemic drugs 286
oral contraceptives 88, 90, 174, 196, 201, 284, 285, 286
patients at risk 285–286
penicillin 128, 196, 286
pharmacodynamic mechanisms 286
pharmacokinetic mechanisms 286
phenytoin 90, 201, 286
potassium-sparing diuretics 37, 57
probenicid 127, 214, 286
pseudoephedrine 285
quinidine 58
quinolones 198
with renal impairment 285

rifampicin 74, 174, 201, 286
sedatives 86
selective serotonin reuptake inhibitors 91
sodium valproate 88, 89, 286
sulfinpyrazone 127
sulphonamides 286
sulphonylureas 168
sympathomimetics (adrenergic agonists) 27
terfenadine 286
tetracycline 152
theophylline 90, 198, 285, 286
thiazide diuretics 37, 286
6-thioguanine 225
tricyclic antidepressants 92
verapamil 58
warfarin 73–74, 88, 90, 127, 130, 197, 199, 201, 212, 286
Interferon-alfa 214
Interferon-beta 97
Interferons 213, 214
Intermittent porphyria, acute 285
International normalised ratio (INR) 73
Intravenous general anaesthetic agents 117–118
Iodine 170
    contraindication in breastfeeding mothers 265
Ion channels 11
Ion pump inhibitors 12
Ionisation 4
Ipecacuanha 243
Ipratropium 24, 138
Irinotecan 227
Iron deficiency anaemia 76
Iron dextran 76
Iron poisoning 245
Irritable bowel syndrome 156
Ischaemic heart disease 51–54
    cardiovascular event risk 34
    rebound angina following prolonged beta blockers 37
Isoflurane 118–119
Isoniazid 6, 200–201
    adverse effects 142, 201
        autoimmune (type II) reactions 142
    contraindication in pregnancy 264
    drug interactions 201, 286
    genetic polymorphism in metabolism 6, 200
Isoprenaline 26
Isosorbide dinitrate 54, 57

Isosorbide mononitrate 54
Isotretinoin 235
Ispaghula 155
Itraconazole 233

K

Kaolin 156
Keratolytics, topical 234
Ketamine 117
Ketoconazole 213, 286
Kidney, diuretics mode of action
    loop 37
    potassium-sparing 37
    thiazide 35–36

L

Labetalol 265
Labour 178
Lactation
    drugs inhibiting 265
    see also Breastfeeding
Lactulose 155
Lamivudine 214, 215
Lamotrigine 87, 89
Lansoprazole 152
Laxatives 155, 228
Lead poisoning 245
Leprosy 201
Leukaemia 172, 224
Leukotriene receptor antagonists
    137
Levetiracetam 90
Levodopa 95, 293
    adverse effects 95, 284
    contraindications 95
    drug interactions 96
Levofloxacin 198
Levomepromazine 228
Levonorgestrel 174
    emergency contraception 176
Levonorgestrel-releasing interuterine
    device 176
Levothyroxine 171
Licensing
    new drugs 294, 296–297
    prescribing for children 266–267
Lichen-planus-like skin reaction
    235
Lidocaine 116
    adrenaline (epinephrine)-
        containing formulation 26,
        116
    adverse effects 59
    antiarrhythmic actions 59, 61

Lifestyle changes
    hypertension treatment 35
    see also Dietary modification
Lincosamides 197
Linezolid 200
Lipid solubility 4
Lipid-lowering agents see
    Antihyperlipidaemic agents
Lipocortin 171
Lipodystrophy 168
Liquid paraffin 155
Lisuride 95
Lithium 13, 92
    adverse effects 92
    contraindications 92
        in breastfeeding mothers 265
    drug interactions 37, 91, 92, 128,
        286
    monitoring 92
    overdose/poisoning 243
Liver
    cholesterol metabolism 41–42
    pregnancy-related metabolic
        changes 264
Liver disease
    adverse drug reaction risk 285
    anticoagulant/antiplatelet agent
        effects 276
    drug interactions 285
    drug metabolism alterations 7,
        274–275
    fluoxetine accumulation 91
Liver toxicity
    antituberculous drugs 200, 201
    imidazoles 213
    methotrexate 225
    paracetamol overdose 244
Local anaesthetic agents 115–117
    adverse effects 117
    clinical pharmacokinetics
        116–117
    mode of action 116
Loop diuretics 37
    adverse effects 56–57
    drug interactions 37, 57
    mode of action 56
    therapeutic uses 56
Loperamide 156
Loratidine 141
Lorazepam 86, 87, 154
Lormetazepam 86
Losartan 39
Low-molecular-weight heparins 53,
    72, 73
Lower oesophageal sphincter
    pressure 152

LSD (lysergic acid diethylamide)
    256
Lung cancer 224, 227, 252
Luteinising hormone 174, 176, 178
Lymphoblastic leukaemia, acute 227
Lymphoma 227
Lysergic acid diethylamide (LSD)
    256

M

Macrolides 197
Magnesium enemas 155
Magnesium sulphate 138
Magnesium trisilicate 152
Malaria 216, 217
Malignant hyperthermia 119, 120
Mannitol 10, 12, 57
Mantoux test 142
Marketing 298
Mebeverine 156
Medicines and Healthcare Products
    Regulatory Agency (MHRA) 296
Medroxyprogesterone 176
Mefloquine 217
Meningitis 195
Menopause 176, 180
    clinical symptoms 177
6-Mercaptopurine 224
    drug interactions 130, 225
Mercury poisoning 245
Mesalazine 156
Mescaline 256
Mesna, cyclophosphamide
    combination 224
Metabolism 3, 5–6
    in children 266
    disease-related alterations 7,
        274–275
    drug interactions 286
    first pass effect 4
Metered dose inhalers 137
Metformin 166, 168
Methadone 109, 255
    overdose/poisoning 244
Methicillin 193
Methimazole 170
Methionine 244
Methotrexate 11, 128, 224–225, 235
    adverse effects 128, 225
    drug interactions 225
Methyldopa 39, 265
    adverse effects 76
        autoimmune (type II) reactions
        142
    in breastfeeding mothers 265

Methylenedioxymetamfetamine (ecstasy) 245, 254
Methysergide 97
Metoclopramide 152, 154, 228
Metolazone 56
Metoprolol 38, 57
Metronidazole 151, 199, 216
    adverse effects 199
    drug interactions 73, 199, 286
    teratogenicity 264
    therapeutic uses 199
Mexiletine 59
Miconazole 212
Midazolam 86
Mifepristone 178
Migraine 96–97
    drug treatment
        acute attack 96–97
        prophylaxis 97
    5-hydroxytryptamine in pathophysiology 96
Milrinone 57
Mineralocorticoids 171, 172
    adverse effects 174
Minoxidil 41
Miosis (pupillary constriction) 24
Mirtazepine 92
Misoprostol 151, 153
Moclobemide 92
Molecular mechanisms of action 10–13
Monoamine oxidase 22
Monoamine oxidase inhibitors 11, 200
    drug interactions 27, 92, 96
Montelukast 137
Morbilliform skin reaction 235
Morphine 6, 109, 156, 227, 228
    abuse/dependence 255
Motion sickness 154, 155
Motor end-plate 119
Multiple sclerosis 97
Mupirocin 233
Muscarine 256
Muscarinic acetylcholine receptors 11, 23, 154
Muscle relaxants 24, 115, 119–120
    depolarising 120
    non-depolarising (acetylcholine antagonists) 119–120
Myasthenia gravis 120
Mycobacterial infections 200–201
Mydriasis (pupillary dilatation) 24
Myeloid leukaemia, chronic 226

Myocardial infarction 52–53, 71, 74, 75, 176
    management 53, 109

N

Nabilone 154, 254
Nalidixic acid 198
Naloxone 110, 244
Naltrexone 255
Naproxen 126
Naratriptan 97
Nasal decongestants 27
Nateglinide 168
National Institute for Health and Clinical Excellence (NICE) 297
National Poisons Information Service (NPIS) 241
Nausea 153–155
    palliative care 227–228
Nebulised drug solutions 137
Nedocromil 137
Neomycin 233
Neonates 266
Neostigmine 119, 120
Neuralgia 90, 91, 107, 110
Neurokinin receptor antagonists 154
Neuroleptic drugs 93–94
    adverse effects 24, 93
        parkinsonism 95, 96
    atypical 94
    in breastfeeding mothers 265
    contraindications 94
    drug interactions 94
    therapeutic uses 93
Neuroleptic malignant syndrome 93
Neuropathic/neurogenic pain 90, 107, 110, 227
Neurotoxicity
    methotrexate 225
    vincristine 225
Neurotransmitters 22
Nevirapine 215, 216
New drugs 293–294
    clinical trials 294–296
    development process 293
    information sources 297
    licensing 294, 296–297
    post-marketing surveillance 284, 294
    premarketing testing 284
    prescribing 297–298
Nicorandil 51, 54
Nicotine 233, 252
    replacement therapy 252

Nicotinic acetylcholine receptors 23
    motor end-plate 119
Nicotinic acid 43
Nifedipine 39
Nitrates 53–54
    adverse effects 54
    therapeutic uses
        angina pectoris prophylaxis 51
        cardiac failure 56, 57
    tolerance 54
Nitrofurantoin 199
Nitrous oxide 118
Non-nucleoside reverse transcriptase inhibitors (NNRTIs) 215
Non-rapid eye movement (NREM) sleep 86
Non-ST segment elevation myocardial infarction 52, 53
Non-steroidal anti-inflammatory drugs (NSAIDs) 110, 126–128, 227
    adverse effects 76, 110, 127
        peptic ulcers 151
        prophylactic acid secretion reduction 153
    contraindications 127
    drug interactions 37, 92, 127–128, 285, 286
    in elderly people 268
    therapeutic uses 110, 126
        gout 129
        osteoarthritis 125
        rheumatoid arthritis 125
Noradrenaline (norepinephrine)
    amine hypothesis of depression 91
    cardiac failure pathophysiology 54
    intravenous actions 25–26
    sympathetic neurotransmission 22, 23
    termination of action 22
Norepinephrine see Noradrenaline
Norethisterone 174, 176
Normal distribution curve 13
Nortriptyline 91
Nucleoside reverse transcriptase inhibitors (NRTIs) 215
Null hypothesis 295
Nystatin 212

O

Obesity, type 2 diabetes association 166

Obstetric analgesia 118
Obstructive pulmonary disease, chronic 135, 136–139
    anti-inflammatory drugs 136–137
    bronchodilators 137
    clinical features 136
    hypertensive patients 40
    leukotriene pathway inhibitors 137
    respiratory failure 139, 140
Octreotide 179
Oesophageal varices 179
Oestrogens 174, 265
    adverse effects 285
    drug interactions 286
    hormone replacement therapy 177
Off-label prescribing for children 266–267
Ofloxacin 198
Olanzapine 94
Olsalazine 156
Omeprazole 12, 151, 152
    drug interactions 153
Ondansetron 154
Onychia 211, 212
Opiates 107, 108–110, 227
    abuse/dependence 109, 255
    administration routes 227
    adverse effects 109, 155, 228
        antiemetics use 155
    antagonists 110
    clinical pharmacokinetics 109
    contraindications 109
    cough suppression 140
    drug interactions 109, 286
    metabolism with liver disease 7
    mode of action 108–109
    overdose/poisoning 244
    therapeutic uses 109
    tolerance 109, 251
    withdrawal symptoms 255
Opioid receptors 107
Oral anticoagulants 73–74
Oral antihyperglycaemic drugs 166, 168
    contraindications 265
    drug interactions 286
Oral contraceptives 174–176
    drug interactions 88, 90, 174, 196, 201, 284, 285, 286
    emergency contraception 176
    enterohepatic circulation 7
    metabolism 6
    oestrogen-progesterone combinations 174–175, 176

    adverse effects 175
    contraindications 176
    progestogen-only pill 176
Organophosphate poisoning 245
Oseltamivir 214
Osmotic diuretics 57
Osmotic laxatives 155
Osteoarthritis 125, 126
Osteomalacia 179
Osteomyelitis 195
Osteoporosis 178, 179–180
    glucocorticoid-induced 173
    high-risk patients 180
    menopause-related 177, 180
    prevention 180
    treatment 180
Otitis externa 233
Ototoxicity
    aminoglycosides 197
    furosemide 56
    vancomycin 200
Ovarian failure 176
Over the counter medicines 285
Overdose see Poisoning
Ovulation 174, 178
Oxcarbazepine 88
Oxycodone 227
Oxygen therapy 139–140
    overdose/poisoning 241
Oxytetracycline 199
Oxytocin 178

P

Paclitaxel 226–227
Paget's disease of bone 180
Pain 107
    palliative care 227
    prevention (anaesthesia) 115
    relief see Analgesics
Palliative care 227–228
Pamidronate 180
Pancuronium 119
Pancytopenia, drug-induced 142
Para-aminosalicylate 201
Paracetamol (acetaminophen) 110, 227
    clinical pharmacokinetics 110
    mode of action 110
    overdose/poisoning 6, 243–244
    therapeutic uses 110, 126
        migraine 96
Parasympathetic nervous system 21
    function 22–23

    neurotransmitters 22
    receptors 22–23
    structure 21–22
Parkinsonism 94–96
    anticholinergic drug treatment 96
    dopaminergic drug treatment 95–96
Parkinson's disease 95
Paroxetine 91
Partial agonists 12
Partial seizures 87
    drug treatment 88, 89, 90
Penicillamine 125, 128, 245
Penicillin 13, 193, 195–196
    adverse effects 76, 142, 195–196, 235, 284
        immediate (type I) hypersensitivity 141
        immune-complex (type III) hypersensitivity 142
    allergic reactions 195–196
        anaphylaxis 142, 284
    bacterial resistance 193, 195
    in breastfeeding mothers 265
    drug interactions 128, 196, 286
    gentamicin combined therapy 192
    in neonates 266
    pharmacokinetics 195
    probenicid combination 286
    renal handling 7
Pentamidine 217
Pentazocine 255
Peptic ulcers 150–151
    drug treatment
        gastric acid secretion reduction 152–153
        protective elements enhancement 153
        healing 152, 153
        Helicobacter pylori infection-related 150–151
        non-steroidal anti-inflammatory drug-related 127, 151
        prophylaxis 153
Pergolide 95
Pernicious anaemia 76
Pethidine 109
Petit mal see Absence seizures
pH
    absorption effects 4
    urinary manipulation, overdose/poisoning management 243
Phaeochromocytoma 276

Pharmacodynamics 10–14
   in children 266
   clinical trials 294
   disease-related alterations 275–277
   drug interactions 286
   in elderly people 267–268
   interindividual variation 14
   target macromolecules 10, 11–12
Pharmacokinetics 3–8
   in children 266
   clinical trials 294
   disease-related changes 273–275
   drug interactions 286
   in elderly people 267
   inhaled anaesthetics 118
   parameters 8–10
   pregnancy-related changes 264
Phase I reactions 6
Phase I studies 294
Phase II reactions 6
Phase II studies 294
Phase III studies 294
Phase IV studies 294
Phenindione 74
Phenobarbital 6, 90
   overdose/poisoning 243
Phenothiazines 154
   antiemetic actions 154, 155
Phenoxymethylpenicillin (penicillin V) 194
Phenytoin 6, 7, 13, 89–90, 264
   adverse effects 90
   in children 266
   drug interactions 90, 201, 286
   monitoring 89
      in pregnancy 264
   teratogenesis 264
   therapeutic uses 89
Phosphate enemas 155
Physicochemical drug effects 12
Physostigmine 120
Pilocarpine 24
Pioglitazone 168
Piperacillin 195
   tazobactam combination 195
Pirenzipine 24
Pituitary hormones 179
Pizotifen 97
Placebo 296
Plant alkaloids 225–226
Plasma protein binding 5
   disease-related changes 274
   pregnancy-related changes 264
Plasmin 75
Plasminogen 75

Platelets 74
Pneumocystis carinii pneumonia 216, 217
Pneumonia, respiratory failure 139, 140
Poisoning 241–245
   airway protection 241–242, 243
   antidotes 243
   cardiovascular toxicity 242
   coma 241–242
   decontamination 242–243
   elimination enhancement 243
   initial management 241
   renal failure 242
   seizures 242
   specific drugs 243–245
   supportive care 241–242
Polyethylene glycols 155
Polypharmacy 267
Postganglionic neurones
   cholinergic receptors 23
   neurotransmitters 22
   parasympathetic nervous system 22
   sympathetic nervous system 21
Postmarketing surveillance 284, 294
Postoperative antiemetics 154
Postpartum haemorrhage 178
Potassium iodide 170
Potassium permanganate 234
Potassium supplements 37, 57
Potassium-sparing diuretics 37, 57
Potency 12
Pralidoxime 245
Prazosin 40
Prednisolone 156, 227, 228
Pre-eclampsia (toxaemia of pregnancy) 265
Pregabalin 110, 227
Preganglionic neurones
   neurotransmitters 22
   parasympathetic nervous system 22
   sympathetic nervous system 21
Pregnancy 263–265
   antiemetics 154
   diabetes mellitus 265
   epilepsy 264
   hypertension 265
   hyperthyroidism 265
   infections 264
   labour 178
   pharmacokinetic changes 264
Pregnancy termination 178
Premarketing testing 284
Prescribing 283, 298

Prevention, primary/secondary 34
Primaquine 285
Probenicid 130, 195
   drug interactions 127, 214, 286
   penicillin combination 286
Procainamide 6
Prochlorperazine 154, 267
Procyclidine 96
Prodrugs 6
Progesterone 174, 233
Progestogen-only pill 176
Progestogens 265
   adverse effects 176
   hormone replacement therapy 177
Prokinetic agents 152
Promethazine 154
Propantheline 156
Propofol 117, 120
Propranolol 10, 38, 170, 264, 267
Propylthiouracil 170
Prostaglandin synthetase 126
Prostaglandins
   acid secretion reduction 153
   uterine actions 178
Prostate cancer 178–179, 224, 226
Prostatic hypertrophy 24
Prosthetic heart valves 71
Protamine 73
Protease inhibitors 213, 215, 216
Prothrombin time 73
Proton pump inhibitors 152–153, 293
   adverse effects 153
   gastro-oesophageal reflux 152
   Helicobacter pylori eradication 150, 151
Protozoal infections 216–217
Pseudoephedrine 285
Pseudomembranous colitis 199, 200
Psilocybin 256
Psoralen 235
Psoriasis 234–235
Pulmonary embolism 71, 75, 175
   respiratory failure 139, 140
Pulmonary fibrosis 139
Pulmonary oedema 56
   respiratory failure 139
   treatment 54, 109
Pupillary constriction 24
Pupillary dilatation 24
Pupillary muscles, sympathetic innervation 21
Purine analogues 213
Pyrazinamide 200, 201
Pyridostigmine 120

Pyrimethamine 217
Pyrimidine analogues 213

Q

Quetiapine 94
Quinidine 24, 58
Quinine 217
Quinolones 198
    contraindication in pregnancy
        264

R

Radioactive iodine therapy 170
Raloxifene 178, 180
Ramipril 11, 38
Randomisation, clinical trial design
    296
Ranitidine 152
Rapid eye movement (REM) sleep
    86
Receptors 11
    agonists 12
    antagonists 12–13
    autonomic nervous system
        22–23
    drug-induced downregulation/
        upregulation 14
    interindividual variation 14
Referred pain 107
Reflux oesophagitis 152
Renal artery stenosis 38, 39
Renal function 7
    neonates 266
Renal impairment
    adverse drug reaction risk 285
    anaemia (erythropoietin
        deficiency) 77
    drug excretion reduction 275
        fluoxetine 91
    drug interactions 285
Renal toxicity
    aminoglycosides 197
    disease-modifying antirheumatic
        drugs 128
    lithium 92
    non-steroidal anti-inflammatory
        drugs 127
    overdose/poisoning 242
    sulphonamides 198
    vancomycin 200
Renin 54
Renin-angiotensin-aldosterone
    system 38, 171
    activation in cardiac failure 55

Repaglinide 168
Reproductive steroid hormones
    174–179
Reserpine 91
Resins 12
Restlessness, palliative care 228
Respiratory disorders 135–140
Respiratory failure 139–140
    benzodiazepine overdose/
        poisoning 244
    opiate overdose/poisoning 244
    type I 140
    type II 140
Respiratory stimulants 139–140
Respiratory syncytial virus 215
Respiratory tract infection 195
Respiratory tract secretions, palliative
    care 228
Retinoids 235
Reverse transcriptase inhibitors 213
Reversible inhibitors of monoamine
    oxidase A (RIMA) 92
Reye's syndrome 266
Rheumatoid arthritis 125, 126, 268
    disease-modifying antirheumatic
        drugs 128–129
Ribavirin 213, 214, 215
Rickets 179
Rifampicin 6, 193, 200, 201
    adverse effects 201
    contraindication in pregnancy
        264
    drug interactions 74, 174, 201,
        286
Ringworm (tinea) 211, 212
Risperidone 94
Ritonavir 216
Rituximab 227
Rocuronium 120
Rofecoxib 126
Ropinirole 95
Rosiglitazone 168

S

St John's wort 92
Salbutamol 26, 137
Salicylic acid 10, 126, 234
    overdose/poisoning 243, 244
Salivary excretion 8
Salmeterol 137
Schizophrenia 93
    neuroleptic drug treatment
        93–94
Seasonal rhinitis 141
Second messengers 11, 23

Sedatives 86
    abuse 253–254
    drug interactions 86
Seizures
    management 87
    overdose/poisoning 242, 244,
        245
    types 87
Selective oestrogen receptor
    modulators (SERMs) 177–178
Selective serotonin reuptake
    inhibitors 91
    withdrawal reactions 284
Selegiline 11, 96
Senna 155
Septicaemia 195
Serotonin see 5-Hydroxytryptamine
Sertraline 91
Serum sickness 142
Short stature 179
Simvastatin 42
    adverse effects 42–43
Skin
    adverse drug reaction 235–236
    disorders 233–235
        primary 234–235
    drug absorption 233
Skin infection 195
    fungal 211–212
Slow acetylators 6, 200
Smoking 252
    cardiovascular risk 33
Sodium bicarbonate 152, 243, 245
Sodium channels 11, 88, 90
    depolarising muscle relaxant
        actions 120
    local anaesthetic agent effects
        116
Sodium cromoglycate 137
    seasonal rhinitis 141
Sodium retention, cardiac failure 54
Sodium valproate 87, 88–89, 264
    adverse effects 89
    contraindications 89
    drug interactions 88, 89, 286
    teratogenesis 264
    therapeutic uses 89
Solvents abuse 256
Somatic pain 107, 115
    opiate analgesia 109
Somatostatin 179
Somatropin 179
Sotalol 60
Spironolactone 37, 57
ST elevation myocardial infarction
    52

Statins 42–43, 53
Statistical analysis 295
Status epilepticus 87
    management 89
Steroid card 174
Steroid responsive elements 171
Stevens–Johnson syndrome 198, 236
Stimulant laxatives 155
Stimulants, overdose/poisoning
    245
Streptokinase 75, 76
Streptomycin 196, 201
Stress response 172
Stroke *see* Cerebrovascular accident
Structural protein drug targets
    11–12
Substance abuse/dependency
    251–256
    associated risks 251
    definitions 251–252
Succinylcholine *see* Suxamethonium
Sucralfate 153
Sulfamethoxazole 198
Sulfapyridine 128, 156
Sulfasalazine 128, 156
Sulfinpyrazone 127, 130
Sulphonamides 193, 197, 198, 217
    adverse effects 142, 198, 285
        immune-complex (type III)
        hypersensitivity 142
    contraindication in breastfeeding
        mothers 265
    drug interactions 286
Sulphonylureas 166, 168, 276
    contraindication in breastfeeding
        mothers 265
    excretion reduction with renal
        impairment 275
Sumatriptan 97
Supportive care
    chemotherapy 227
    poisoning 241–242
Supraventricular tachycardia 59,
    60
Surface area, absorption effects 4
Surrogate markers 294
Suxamethonium (succinylcholine) 6,
    120
Sympathetic nervous system 21
    cardiac failure pathophysiology
        54
    drug actions 25–27
    function 22–23
    neurotransmitters 22
    receptors 22–23
    structure 21

Sympathetic trunk 21
Sympathomimetics (adrenergic
    agonists) 25–26
    drug interactions 27
    therapeutic uses 26–27
Systemic-lupus-erythematosus-like
    reactions 142, 201

T

Tamoxifen 177, 226
Tardive dyskinesia 93
Taxanes 226–227
Tazobactam, piperacillin combination
    195
Teicoplanin 200
Temazepam 253
Tenecteplase 75
Teratogenesis 263, 264
    alcohol 264
    angiotensin converting enzyme
        (ACE) inhibitors 264
    anticonvulsants 264
    carbamazepine 88, 264
    diethylstilbestrol 264
    isotretinoin 235
    metronidazole 199, 264
    phenytoin 264
    sodium valproate 89, 264
    trimethoprim 264
    warfarin 263
Terbinafine 211, 212, 233
Terbutaline 137
Terfenadine 286
Terminal care
    analgesia 109, 110
    cough suppression 140
    palliative care 227–228
Testosterone 174, 178
Tetracycline 151, 193, 199, 235
    adverse effects 199
        in fetus 264
    bacterial resistance 193
    contraindications
        in breastfeeding mothers
        265
        in pregnancy 264
    drug interactions 152
Thalidomide 263
Theophylline 13
    in breastfeeding mothers 265
    in children 266
        adverse effects 266
    drug interactions 90, 198, 285,
        286
Therapeutic drug monitoring 13

Therapeutic window/therapeutic
    index 13
Thiazide diuretics 13, 35–36, 265
    cardiac failure 56
    combined treatments 40
    drug interactions 37, 286
    hypertension 36, 40
Thiazolidinediones 166, 168
6-Thioguanine 225
Thiopental 5, 117
Thiopurine S-methyltransferase,
    genetic polymorphism 129
Thiouracils 170
Thrombolytic drugs 75
Thrombosis 71–76
Thromboxane A_2 74
Thyroid crisis 170
Thyroid disease 169–171
Thyroid hormone receptors 11
Thyroid-stimulating hormone 169,
    171
Thyroxine 169, 170, 171
Tinea (ringworm) 211, 212
Tinidazole 151
Tiotropium 138
Tirofiban 53, 74, 75
Tissue distribution 5
    disease-related alterations 274
Tissues
    drug apparent volume of
        distribution 9–10
    drug mechanisms of action
        10–13
Tobacco 252
Tobramycin 196
Tolerance 14, 251
    nitrates 54
Tonic/clonic seizures (grand mal)
    87
    drug treatment 88, 89, 90
Topimarate 90
Toxaemia of pregnancy (pre-
    eclampsia) 265
Toxoplasmosis 216, 217
Tramadol 109
Tranexamic acid 75, 176
Transient ischaemic attack 74
Transit time
    absorption effects 4
    disease-related alterations 273
Transmembrane enzymes 11
Transmembrane receptors 11
Transport mechanisms 12
Trastuzumab 227
Tretinoin 235
Triamterene 37, 57

Tricyclic antidepressants 9, 10, 91–92
adverse effects 24, 92, 155
in breastfeeding mothers 265
contraindications 92
drug interactions 92
overdose/poisoning 244–245
therapeutic uses 91
migraine prophylaxis 97
neuropathic pain relief 110, 227
Triglycerides 41, 42
Trihexyphenidyl 24, 96
Trimethoprim 193, 197, 198, 224
adverse effects 198
bacterial resistance 194
teratogenicity 264
Troglitazone 169
Tropicamide 24
Tuberculosis 200–201, 215
drug regimens 200
drug-resistance 200
reserve drugs 201
Tubocurarine 119

U

Ulcerative colitis 156
Unstable angina 52, 53
Unwanted (toxic) effects 13
see also Adverse drug reactions
Uric acid excretion 130
Uricosuric agents 129, 130
Urinary pH manipulation, overdose/poisoning management 243
Urinary retention 24
Urinary tract infection 195
management in pregnancy 264
Ursodeoxycholic acid 157

V

Vagus nerve 22, 149, 154
digoxin actions 58
Valaciclovir 214
Valdecoxib 126
Valsaratan 39
Vancomycin 200
Variation in drug response 14
Vasopressin (antidiuretic hormone) 179
Vaughan Williams classification of antiarrhythmic agents 59
Vecuronium 120
Venlafaxine 92
Venous thromboembolic disease 71
oral contraceptives association 175
risk factors 71–72
Ventricular arrhythmias 59, 60
Ventricular tachycardia 59, 61
Verapamil 39, 60, 267
adverse effects 39
drug interactions 58
Vestibular disease 154
Vidarabine 213
Vigabatrin 90
Vinblastine 225
Vincristine 225
Viral hepatitis 213, 214
Viral infections 213
Visceral pain 107, 115
opiate analgesia 109
Vitamin B_{12} deficiency anaemia 76
Vitamin D_2 179
Vitamin K-dependent clotting factors 73
Voltage-dependent calcium channels 39

Vomiting 153–155
induction in overdose/poisoning management 243
palliative care 227–228

W

Warfarin 10, 73–74
adverse effects 73
in breastfeeding mothers 265
drug interactions 73–74, 88, 90, 127, 130, 197, 199, 201, 212, 286
monitoring 73
plasma protein binding 5
reversal of effects 74
teratogenesis 263
therapeutic uses 73
Withdrawal reactions 251, 284
Wolff–Parkinson–White syndrome 60

X

Xanthine oxidase 129, 130
Xanthine oxidase inhibitors 11

Z

Zafirlukast 137
Zalcitabine 215
Zaleplon 86
Zanamivir 214
Zero order processes 7, 89, 252
Zidovudine (AZT) 213, 215
Zollinger–Ellison syndrome 152
Zolpidem 86
Zopiclone 86